FUNDAMENTALS OF VETERINARY SCIENCE

Fundamentals of Veterinary Science

Editor:

Stephen Rego, Ph.D.

Delve Publishing
www.delvepublishing.com

Fundamentals of Veterinary Science
Editor: **Stephen Rego, Ph.D.**

708 3rd Avenue, 6th Floor

New York, NY 10017

United States of America

www.delvepublishing.com

ISBN: 978-1-68095-858-4

Library of Congress Control Number: 2016951611

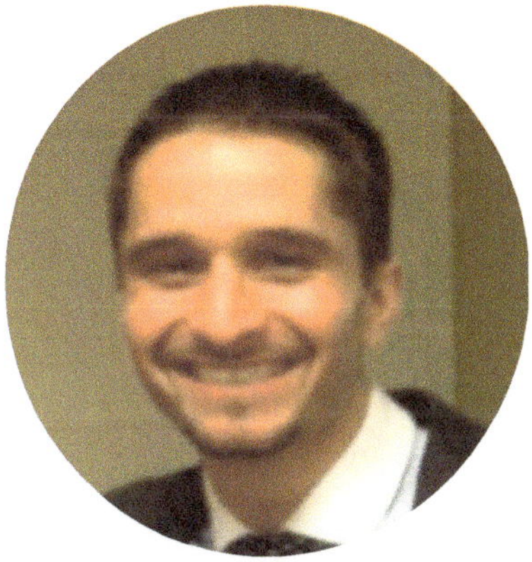

About the Editor

Stephen Rego, Ph.D.

Stephen obtained his PhD from the University of North Carolina at Charlotte in 2013 where his graduate research focused on cancer immunology and the tumor microenvironment. He received postdoctoral training in regenerative and translational medicine, specifically gastrointestinal tissue engineering, at the Wake Forest Institute of Regenerative Medicine. Currently, Stephen is an instructor for anatomy and physiology and biology at Forsyth Technical Community College.

Contents

List of Contributors

Lowell Ackerman
Westborough, Boston, Massachusetts, USA

DVM DACVD MBA MPA
Westborough, Boston, Massachusetts, USA

Miyu Mercier
VCA Aurora Animal Hospital, 2600 West Galena Blvd, Aurora, Illinois, 60506, USA

Heidi L. Barnes Heller
VCA Aurora Animal Hospital, 2600 West Galena Blvd, Aurora, Illinois, 60506, USA

Mickael Weber
Royal Canin Research Center, Aimargues, France

Laura Sams
Royal Canin Research Center, Aimargues, France

Alexandre Feugier
Royal Canin Research Center, Aimargues, France

Sandrine Michel
Royal Canin Research Center, Aimargues, France

Vincent Biourge
Royal Canin Research Center, Aimargues, France

Carina Helmer
Clinic for Swine and Small Ruminants, University of Veterinary Medicine Hannover, Foundation, Hannover, Germany

Regina Eibach
Clinic for Swine and Small Ruminants, University of Veterinary Medicine Hannover, Foundation, Hannover, Germany

Esther Humann-Ziehank
Clinic for Swine and Small Ruminants, University of Veterinary Medicine Hannover, Foundation, Hannover, Germany

Philip C. Tegtmeyer
Clinic for Swine and Small Ruminants, University of Veterinary Medicine Hannover, Foundation, Hannover, Germany

Daniela Bürstel
Tierseuchenkasse (Animal Diseases Fund) Baden-Wuerttemberg, Fellbach, Germany

Kathrin Mayer
Small Ruminant Health Service, Sächsische Tierseuchenkasse (Animal Diseases Fund), Dresden, Germany

Udo Moog
Animal Health Service Thuringia e.V., Thüringer Tierseuchenkasse (Animal Diseases Fund), Jena, Germany

Sieglinde Stauch
Schafpraxis (sheep veterinary practice) Stoffenried, Stoffenried, Germany

Heinz Strobel
Schafpraxis (sheep veterinary practice) Stoffenried, Stoffenried, Germany

Katja Voigt
Clinic for Ruminants, Ludwig Maximilians University (LMU) Munich, Oberschleißheim, Germany

Philipp Sieber
Clinic for Ruminants, Ludwig Maximilians University (LMU) Munich, Oberschleißheim, Germany

Matthias Greiner
Federal Institute for Risk Assessment (BfR), Berlin, Germany
University of Veterinary Medicine Hannover, Foundation, Hannover, Germany

Martin Ganter
Clinic for Swine and Small Ruminants, University of Veterinary Medicine Hannover, Foundation, Hannover, Germany

Paa Kobina Turkson
Department of Animal Science, School of Agriculture, University of Cape Coast, Cape Coast, Ghana

Iheanacho Okike
International Livestock Research Institute, Nigeria, Ibadan, Nigeria

Kristin Kirkby Shaw
Animal Surgical Clinic of Seattle, Seattle, Washington, USA

Lesley C. Rausch-Derra
Aratana Therapeutics, Inc., Kansas City, Kansas, USA

Linda Rhodes
Aratana Therapeutics, Inc., Kansas City, Kansas, USA

Adriana Tomoko Nishiya
Department of Pathology, School of Veterinary Medicine and Animal Science, University of São Paulo, Av. Prof. Dr. Orlando Marques de Paiva, 87, CEP 05508-270, São Paulo, Brazil

Cristina Oliveira Massoco
Department of Pathology, School of Veterinary Medicine and Animal Science, University of São Paulo, Av. Prof. Dr. Orlando Marques de Paiva, 87, CEP 05508-270, São Paulo, Brazil

Claudia Ronca Felizzola
Department of Pathology, School of Veterinary Medicine and Animal Science, University of São Paulo, Av. Prof. Dr. Orlando Marques de Paiva, 87, CEP 05508-270, São Paulo, Brazil
Surgical Oncology Rua Antônio Alves Magan, 124, CEP 01251-150, São Paulo, Brazil

Eduardo Perlmann
Department of Surgery, School of Veterinary Medicine and Animal Science, University of São Paulo, CEP 05508-270, São Paulo, Brazil

Karen Batschinski
Department of Pathology, School of Veterinary Medicine and Animal Science, University of São Paulo, Av. Prof. Dr. Orlando Marques de Paiva, 87, CEP 05508-270, São Paulo, Brazil

Marcello Vannucci Tedardi
Department of Pathology, School of Veterinary Medicine and Animal Science, University of São Paulo, Av. Prof. Dr. Orlando Marques de Paiva, 87, CEP 05508-270, São Paulo, Brazil

Jéssica Soares Garcia
Department of Pathology, School of Veterinary Medicine and Animal Science, University of São Paulo, Av. Prof. Dr. Orlando Marques de Paiva, 87, CEP 05508-270, São Paulo, Brazil

Priscila Pedra Mendonça
Department of Surgery, School of Veterinary Medicine and Animal Science, University of São Paulo, CEP 05508-270, São Paulo, Brazil

Tarso Felipe Teixeira
Pathology Veterinary Medicine, FEPI Itajubá University Center, Dr. Antonio Braga Filho Street, 687, Itajubá, 37.501-002 Minas Gerais, Brazil

Maria Lucia Zaidan Dagli
Department of Pathology, School of Veterinary Medicine and Animal Science, University of São Paulo, Av. Prof. Dr. Orlando Marques de Paiva, 87, CEP 05508-270, São Paulo, Brazil

Nikolaos Dervisis
Virginia Maryland College of Veterinary Medicine, 245 Duck Pond Dr., Blacksburg, VA 24061, USA

Shawna Klahn
Virginia Maryland College of Veterinary Medicine, 245 Duck Pond Dr., Blacksburg, VA 24061, USA

Jyotika Varshney
Department of Surgery, University of Minnesota Medical School, Moos Tower, 11-212420 Delaware Street, S.E.; MMC 195, Minneapolis, MN 55455, USA
Masonic Cancer Center, University of Minnesota, Minneapolis, MN 55455, USA

Milcah C. Scott
Masonic Cancer Center, University of Minnesota, Minneapolis, MN 55455, USA
Animal Cancer Care and Research Program, University of Minnesota, St. Paul, MN 55455, USA
[4]Department of Veterinary Clinical Sciences, College of Veterinary Medicine, University of Minnesota, St. Paul, MN 55108, USA

David A. Largaespada
Department of Pediatrics, University of Minnesota, Minneapolis, MN 55455, USA
[1]Masonic Cancer Center, University of Minnesota, Minneapolis, MN 55455, USA

Subbaya Subramanian
Department of Surgery, University of Minnesota Medical School, Moos Tower, 11-212420 Delaware Street, S.E.; MMC 195, Minneapolis, MN 55455, USA
Masonic Cancer Center, University of Minnesota, Minneapolis, MN 55455, USA

Claire M. Cannon
University of Tennessee College of Veterinary Medicine, 2407 River Drive, Knoxville, TN 37996, USA

Rachael Thomas
Department of Molecular Biomedical Sciences, College of Veterinary Medicine & Center for Comparative Medicine and Translational Research, North Carolina State University, Raleigh NC 27607, USA;

Domenico Santoro
Department of Small Animal Clinical Sciences, College of Veterinary Medicine, University of Florida, Gainesville, FL 32610, USA

Rosanna Marsella
Department of Small Animal Clinical Sciences, College of Veterinary Medicine, University of Florida, Gainesville, FL 32610, USA

Basil Alexander
Department of Farm Animal Production and Health, Faculty of Veterinary Medicine and Animal Science, University of Peradeniya, Sri Lanka
Department of Biomedical Sciences, Ontario Veterinary College (OVC), University of Guelph, Ontario, Canada

Gabriela Mastromonaco
Reproductive Physiology, Toronto Zoo, 361A Old Finch Avenue, Scarborough, ON, M1B 5K7
Department of Biomedical Sciences, Ontario Veterinary College (OVC), University of Guelph, Ontario, Canada

W. Allan King
Department of Biomedical Sciences, Ontario Veterinary College (OVC), University of Guelph, Ontario, Canada

Micaela Cipolla
Department of Veterinary Science and Public Health (DIVET), Università degli Studi di Milano, via Celoria 10, 20133 Milano, Italy

Luigi Bonizzi
Department of Veterinary Science and Public Health (DIVET), Università degli Studi di Milano, via Celoria 10, 20133 Milano, Italy

Alfonso Zecconi
Department of Veterinary Science and Public Health (DIVET), Università degli Studi di Milano, via Celoria 10, 20133 Milano, Italy

Jelalu Kemal
College of Veterinary Medicine, Haramaya University, Ethiopia

Preface

With the increasing domestication of animals worldwide, especially in developed countries, the importance of veterinary science is becoming more evident. Numerous studies have linked both domestic and commercial animal health to human health and it make sense that decreasing the occurrence and spread of disease in domestic animals would also decrease transmission of those diseases into humans. The field of veterinary science is broad and may focus on domestic or commercial animals, various breeds and species and specific diseases. This book introduces a broad range of topics in veterinary science including dermatology, inflammation, diet, influenza, pain and various forms of cancer. The animal species discussed in this book include felines, canines, sheep, goats, rabbits along with other animal species. To conclude, the Fundamentals of Veterinary Science mentions how animal health is closely linked to human health to highlight the importance of this field.

Editor

Stephen Rego, Ph.D.

1

CHAPTER

SEVEN COMMON MISTAKES TO AVOID IN ACHIEVING LONG-TERM SUCCESS WITH DERMATOLOGY PATIENTS

Lowell Ackerman

Westborough, Boston, Massachusetts, USA

ABSTRACT

Managing a pet's chronic dermatologic conditions can be frustrating for both clients and clinicians, but there are steps to making the process easier for everyone. Avoid the following seven mistakes sometimes made in managing dermatology cases and you will find the process considerably easier in the future.

NOT APPRECIATING APPROPRIATE CLINICAL TIMELINES

While most veterinarians focus on the needs of the client and pet at the time of a specific office visit, it is important to realize that for many dermatologic conditions opportunities exist on a time continuum for intervention and client education. In some instances, the first discussions with the owner may take place long before there is even a skin problem to treat. So, for the owner of a breed at risk for atopic dermatitis, discussions should actually start during puppyhood, long before there might be any clinical evidence of allergies (Ackerman 2011). This is the best time to instruct owners to be vigilant looking for early signs of disease, such as licking and chewing at the feet, ear infections, or rashes in the axillary and inguinal areas. Perhaps more importantly, this provides an opportunity to discuss that if atopic dermatitis is eventually diagnosed in the pet that this is a lifelong condition without a cure, but early detection provides the most options for successful long-term management. This might also prompt a discussion of

Citation: Lowell Ackerman, Seven common mistakes to avoid in achieving long-term success with dermatology patients, DOI: 10.1002/vms3.1

the likely costs associated with long-term management, so the owners might consider their options for risk management strategies, including pet insurance.

Appreciating appropriate timelines also helps in treatment selection. When a two-year-old atopic patient presents with pruritus, the first tendency might be to treat with glucocorticoids (corticosteroids) to achieve short-term relief. However, when you reflect on how that same patient might look at 8 or 10 years of age with such treatment, there is often a different perspective on what the long-term liabilities are for such short-term gains, and alternative more targeted treatments might be selected, given the need for sensible long-term solutions.

It is also important to schedule effectively. No one can solve a complicated dermatology case in a single visit, regardless of the appointment's duration, or the clinician's expertise. You can address the client's primary concerns, but be clear with the client that the pet's problems will likely not be solved with that single visit. The key to successful dermatology management is scheduling frequent re-evaluation appointments. The success of this strategy is predicated on sharing the action plan with pet owners, so they can understand and appreciate what is expected to be accomplished, and according to what timeline.

For a young dog with localized juvenile demodectic mange, the owner should expect regular re-evaluations over a several-month period. They also need to realize that the underlying problem could be some form of immune dysfunction, which might be transitory or long-lasting. Regardless, the condition is characterized by the overpopulation of mites normally resident in the skin (these are not external invaders), which in turn typically causes bacterial infections in the hair follicles, and the sequel to that is inflammatory changes and hair loss. The initial goal might be to control the associated bacterial folliculitis, provide supportive care in terms of frequent shampooing with a follicular-flushing agent, ensure there is no evidence of other internal or external parasites, assess immune function, and put the pet on an improved plane of nutrition. Actually killing the mites might not even be necessary as a first treatment attempt. If the owner realizes that a cure without miticidal therapy is possible because many young animals 'self-cure' with appropriate supportive therapy, they are more likely to understand why you are approaching the problem in stages, rather than just reaching for the strongest mite-killing therapy on the shelf. Miticidal therapy can always be used if this otherwise healthy young animal fails to self-cure in a reasonable amount of time. The pathway to resolution might include supportive care, decreasing mite numbers, resolution of the secondary bacterial folliculitis and, finally hair regrowth. It is also important for owners to realize that clinical cure often precedes microscopic cure, so it is important to continue to monitor with recheck examinations and skin scrapings before stopping therapy prematurely; otherwise, recurrence is more likely. When owners understand the plan, they can also appreciate the timeline to achieve it.

There are many dynamics at work in the development and resolution of skin problems and they can either work for or against the clinician depending on how they are relayed to pet owners.

The skin is not a sterile surface and is home to a large population of resident organisms. There are also lots of occasions for the skin to be colonized by the opportunistic overgrowth of organisms typically present in small numbers, the most common of which are bacteria (such as*Staphylococcus pseudintermedius*) and yeasts (such as *Malassezia pachydermatis*). As it is neither possible nor desirable to try to sterilize the skin, the goal needs to be to address the underlying reason for the microbial overgrowth (allergies, hypothyroidism, immune dysfunction, skin folds, etc.), manage it effectively (possibly long term) and use sensible systemic and topical therapies to help curb the microbial populations. The population dynamics also dictates reasonable treatment intervals. If staphylococcal populations can double in number within minutes to hours on the skin surface, can an every-other-week bathing schedule ever have much of an impact? Probably not. If owners want to help control surface bacterial numbers with topical therapies, they need to realize that more frequent treatments are likely needed, at least initially.

Similarly, when it comes to epidermal turnover rates in keratinization disorders (e.g. seborrhea), we are at the mercy of those skin cell dynamics. Even if you could wave a magic wand and immediately correct the problem, it would still take weeks for the 'normal' skin to grow through the epidermal layers and replace the abnormal skin cells on the skin surface. Without a magic wand it takes many more weeks and even months for progress to be noted. When clients realize this, it helps them be more realistic with their expectations.

NOT APPROPRIATELY FRAMING CLIENT EXPECTATIONS

Many pet skin problems cannot be cured, regardless of the medication selected, so set realistic expectations with clients early in the process. Fortunately, control of the condition and a better quality of life for the pet can be attained with appropriate management. For the pet with atopic dermatitis, you might explain to clients that this is no different than addressing other incurable but manageable medical conditions such as diabetes mellitus or degenerative joint disease (osteoarthritis). We can often achieve excellent long-term control with ongoing treatment and close monitoring, but it is unlikely that we will be able to 'fix' the underlying problem. Usually once owners appreciate that the goal is control rather than cure, their expectations tend to be more reasonable and realistic.

Similarly, it is important to manage expectations around the metrics of treatment success and the timeframe in which such judgment can be anticipated. For example, in a dog with demodicosis and associated hair loss, the pet owner may judge success as hair regrowth, while the clinician will likely be more focused on controlling mite numbers initially. So, how long after treatment initiation should the client expect to see hair regrowth if the treatment is working? If the owners are told to expect the likely onset of hair regrowth eight weeks or so after the mite population has been satisfactorily reduced, they will not be expecting that hair growth shortly after starting treatment; hopefully they will appreciate that mite population control must happen first, before hair regrowth can start. They should also then be attentive at recheck visits and use progress on mite control reported by the clinician as a signpost for the path to eventual resolution (and hair regrowth).

For the dog with sarcoptic mange, it is important to notify the owner that the pruritus is likely to persist for another week or two even after successful treatment has been initiated. This occurs because mite faecal pellets that remain in the epidermal burrows still trigger hypersensitivity reactions, and because dead and decaying mite fragments in the skin tend to be irritating. Aggressive topical therapy and some pruritus-relieving medications will definitely help, but complete resolution requires the elimination of all mite-related remnants from the skin. With absolute adherence to veterinary recommendations regarding treatment of the pet and in-contact animals, the itching should start to substantially abate after two weeks, with complete resolution to be anticipated within 6–8 weeks if the pet is not reinfested from its environment.

Setting realistic expectations with clients is critical because ultimate success and client satisfaction will be measured by the owner's perception. Similarly, if you perform a flawless surgery but discharge the animal soiled with faecal matter, the client's perception of the procedure's success may differ significantly from your own. As it is the client who is paying for the service and the one (by definition) who ultimately determines customer satisfaction, the client's interpretation takes precedence. Accordingly, take the time to understand those expectations so you can plan to meet and even exceed them, or be prepared to discuss more realistic expectations with the owner before starting treatment.

NOT VIEWING THE SITUATION IN TERMS OF QUALITY OF LIFE

Veterinarians might sometimes view dermatologic problems as minor medical issues because often the pet's life is not at risk, but pet owners may not share that same perspective. Pet owners may not know what a diseased liver looks like, but they are certainly aware when their pet keeps them awake at night while scratching, has bald patches in its fur, or harbours offensive odours, rashes, parasites, or skin colour changes associated with a variety of skin diseases. There might also be a certain amount of guilt associated with friends and relatives asking why they have not done a better job of treating their pet's skin ailments, even when the pet owner has done everything they have been instructed to do. Veterinarians and hospital staff would do well to consider what pet owners find stressful, in addition to what might be causing the pet discomfort.

Pet owners are often concerned with the responsibility of successfully managing their pet's problems at home. In many instances, it is stressful for clients to have to regularly administer medications, bathe their pets, apply parasite-control products on schedule, and other tasks often assigned by hospital staff. Even something as basic as applying ear drops can be a trying experience if the pet demonstrates discomfort, cries, or retreats from the owner, adversely affecting the human–animal bond. People own pets for the positive connection that develops between them and anything that interferes with that is likely to be stressful for both. Veterinary staff should do everything in their power to set clients up for success at home. This includes honestly assessing the recommendations being made and the likelihood that they can be successfully accomplished at home.

When medically prudent to do so, the use of injectable medications is often preferred because it frees the owner up from having to administer medication to their pet. Rather than asking the pet owner to do something at home that might cause their pet discomfort, such as applying ear drops to a painful inflamed ear, the pet might be admitted into the hospital, sedated and appropriately treated and administered anti-inflammatory therapy or pain management so that the owner is not required to contend with an objectionable experience at home. This might not be possible in all instances, but hospital staff should always strive to make the pet owner's tasks easier at home and to reinforce the human–animal bond at every opportunity by offering such services.

NOT FOLLOWING EVIDENCE-BASED STANDARDS OF CARE

Most pet owners do not want their pets to serve as learning tools, so they appreciate knowing that veterinarians know what they are treating, the chances of success, what problems might be encountered, and the alternatives available should the need arise. Pet owners also appreciate that such knowledge is evidence-based and reflects established expertise, even if not direct experience. They find comfort in consistent messaging from hospital staff, specialists, and even Internet resources.

Having an evidence-based action plan assures owners that their pet is not the first to experience this problem, and that there is collective wisdom and experience in how it is best managed (Ackerman 2014).

Standards of care should be created by hospitals to provide this assurance, and to guarantee the best care to all patients and all pet owners, regardless of the individual experience and expertise of the clinician currently treating that pet. Protocols are often used for standardized approaches to basic preventive and acute care (e.g. parasite control, treatment of sarcoptic mange) while care pathways represent a model for approaching problems that might require long-term or even lifelong care (e.g. atopic dermatitis, demodicosis, pemphigus foliaceus, etc.) (Ackerman *et al.* 2013).

One of the benefits of standards of care is that owners realize that even with a well-conceived plan, outcomes cannot be guaranteed, and contingency plans may be needed. For example, when treating a dog with bacterial pyoderma, you might select an antibiotic empirically based on the likelihood that the organism is *Staphylococcus pseudintermedius* and that there is a predictive rate of susceptibility and resistance to specific antibiotics. If the pet owner realizes that your plan is based on the likelihood that the organism will be sensitive to the antibiotic selected, but cannot be guaranteed, they can likely also appreciate the need to re-evaluate the pet at some point and for a bacterial culture and susceptibility test to be performed if there is no evidence of substantial improvement by that time. In fact, following a plan of action allows the owner to feel more engaged in the decision-making process. They might even participate more fully in the discussion, asking if it might be worthwhile to consider the culture even before starting empirical therapy. This is much more desirable than dispensing treatment, and if it does not seem to be working the owner just decides to get the opinion of another primary-care veterinarian. Sharing your action plan and thought processes with pet owners can make all the difference in client engagement, consent, and satisfaction.

As the majority of dermatologic cases have underlying disorders, it makes sense to perform tests to try to identify them, so they may be addressed, if possible. Utilizing the basic diagnostic tests, such as skin scrapings, cytology, and fungal cultures, is good medicine and good business. And, if you do have something such as sarcoptic mange on your list of differential diagnoses, it is reasonable to do a parasite-control trial – even if you do not find parasites on skin scrapings. A properly conducted dietary trial also yields a lot of useful information in the workup of a pruritic animal. However, it is important to have a clear diagnostic plan and to proceed logically. For example, the results from biopsies are more likely to be useful if a thorough history, clinical description and differential diagnoses are provided to the pathologist (images are a nice touch as well). Also, it is worth deciding how and if the test results will potentially change your treatment plan. If they will not alter your decisions, what is the purpose of running the tests?

Because most dermatologic presentations have underlying disorders, you should anticipate recurrence if that underlying problem cannot be permanently corrected. Reaching for a stronger medication just temporarily masks the underlying problem, and clients are quick to recognize this. The answer is to start looking more intently for the primary causes. So, tell clients that you will consider attempting symptomatic therapy at first with an appropriate product, but also tell them that if the problem recurs when the medication is discontinued, more investigation may be warranted before stronger medications are considered. In fact, it is possible that methicillin-resistant staphylococci might potentially arise in some cases from the unnecessary escalation of antibiotic therapy, among many other theoretical causes (Weese *et al.* 2012).

Dermatologists will tell you that many clients come to referral appointments with a plastic bag full of products that have been ineffective. Clients are often looking for the magic bullet, the one special drug that the dermatologist has access to, but the primary-care veterinarian does not. The reality is that dermatologists do not have any magic bullets, and rarely rely on one product to address all the needs of their patients. Dermatology patients often have multiple issues to contend with, and treating only one may not be enough to resolve the clinical problem.

For example, many pets with dermatologic issues also have secondary microbial overgrowth (bacterial and/or yeast dermatitis) that needs to be addressed. If those secondary infections are not properly managed, it may be difficult – or impossible – to assess the response to other treatments.

We must also be aware that even well-accepted theories of cause and effect can and do change over time, and our standards of care must be prepared to change with them. For example, we once thought of atopic dermatitis as a classic Type I hypersensitivity reaction primarily driven by mast-cell dynamics in response to inhaled allergens. We now know that the major allergen presentation occurs across the skin surface via Langerhans cells and that inflammatory mediators such as interleukin-31 (IL-31) and other pruritogenic cytokines are most responsible for the scratching that we see in our allergic patients (Marsella *et al.* 2012). This helps explain why antihistamines are often of limited benefit, and points the way to more targeted therapies that can and should be considered.

When creating standards of care for your hospital, remember to build into the model specific points at which referral to a specialist should take place. The best referral happens as part of a well-conceived plan, not as an afterthought. It helps to prepare clients early on that the first course of treatment may not resolve the problem, and if so, that you may try other options or recommend the assistance of a specialist. Clients will appreciate your efforts to inform them now, rather than when they are frustrated, upset, and depleted of funds.

For example, dogs with recurrent pyoderma may be controlled adequately with a combination of medications and topical therapies, but including a dermatologist in the decision-making process early in the course of the condition has many benefits, including helping to determine the underlying causes, and exploring long-term solutions before chronic changes have occurred in the skin, which might limit the benefits of some treatment options. This can also decrease reliance on medications over the long term, and perhaps stave off the development of antibiotic resistance, so has the potential of saving the owner money, health risks, and effort over time. It is much better for all concerned to have specialists involved early in the course of the disease, when they can play an invaluable role as part of the pet's health care team.

In addition to Standards of Care, Consistency of Care is important in multi-doctor hospitals. Consistent messaging to clients only occurs when the process of creating standards helps clinicians achieve consensus in their approaches to common clinical entities, so there can be alignment of hospital team members around an established evidence-based approach, whenever possible.

Underestimating the role of compliance

When it comes to managing many skin conditions, client compliance is an issue that must be considered.

Before dispensing any medications to owners, be realistic in your expectations for what can be reasonably accomplished at home. Better yet, have that exact conversation with owners, including asking open-ended questions of their previous experiences, so you can plan your treatment accordingly. Owners are more likely to be compliant treating clinical signs they can judge (e.g. control of scratching or pain), and can be less compliant with things that are not as obvious, such as administering antibiotics orally at specific intervals or remembering to give parasite-control products on schedule when no parasites are seen.

Because compliance is such an important issue in the resolution of most dermatologic problems, clinicians must recognize this and create treatment plans accordingly. If it is medically prudent to do so, injectable medications should be first-line therapy, if available, because they offer convenience to the owner and guaranteed compliance. The next preferred medications are ones that can be administered once daily, followed by those that can be administered every 12 h. It is unlikely that oral medications needing to be administered more often than twice daily will be given on schedule other than by the most dedicated of pet owners (Adams, *et al*, 2005). It is also important to remember that administering a medication twice daily is not the same as administering it every 12 h, so even clients that remember to give a medication twice in any given day might not give it at the appropriate interval consistent with the drug's pharmacokinetics. If so, the pet is not receiving the true intended benefit of that medication.

Finally, cost might be one consideration in medication selection, but if the goal is for the pet to actually receive all the benefit of any selected medication, compliance should be the main selection attribute. The most costly medication (in terms of time and medical outcomes) is actually the medication that fails to deliver the anticipated benefits because it was not administered appropriately.

LACKING REALISTIC PRODUCT AND PRICING MODELS

Veterinary hospitals benefit from carrying appropriate products in inventory, pricing them competitively, and tracking compliance to ensure that pets and owners are actually receiving the full benefit of products dispensed and administered.

While clients might want to browse retail store shelves for the best bargains, when it comes to treating their pets with medical issues, they typically want a firm recommendation made by the veterinarian, not a list of possible treatments that the owner can consider. Be prepared to make clear product recommendations, and be prepared to explain why this is the best option for a particular pet. Some clients will always want the least costly option, but veterinarians owe it to their clients to make firm recommendations, based on evidence-based criteria of what is in the pet's best interest.

Dermatology patients tend to be managed long-term, so consider which products and pricing models work best for you and your clients to keep that revenue in your practice. It pays to stock products that are priced appropriately for the value delivered, and that have been researched, safety tested, and labelled for use in the species to which they are being administered. However, inventory should be kept lean and there is little need to keep multiple products on the shelf that do essentially the same thing.

CONSIDERING DERMATOLOGY CLIENTS A NUISANCE

You are in business to serve the needs of your clients. Owing to the nature of dermatologic diseases, you will see most of your dermatologic patients and their owners many times during the year, for many years to come. That gives you a great opportunity to bond with these pet owners and help shape a positive and mutually beneficial veterinarian–client–patient relationship. These are exactly the clients that you should crave for your practice. The next time the pollen count rises and your telephone starts ringing frequently from clients with itchy pets – do not curse – give thanks! If properly counselled, these are probably the most dedicated clients you will have in your practice.

REFERENCES

1. Ackerman L. (2011) The Genetic Connection, 2nd edn: A Guide to Health Problems in Purebred Dogs & Cats. 329pp. AAHA Press: Lakewood, CO.

2. Ackerman L. (2014) Standards of care & care pathways. In: Five-Minute Veterinary Practice Management Consult (ed L.J. Ackerman), 2nd edn, pp 384–387. John Wiley & Sons, Inc.: Ames, Iowa.

3. Ackerman L., Ball E., Brunt J., Chmiel D., Felsted K., Glickman L. et al. (2013) The Zoetis Lifelong Care Initiative: Putting the Promise into Practice. Clinician's Update, pp 1–8. This is a stand-alone supplement to Clinician's Brief, published by the North American Veterinary Community.

4. Adams V.J., Campbell J.R., Waldner C.L., Dowling P.M. & Shmon C.L. (2005) Evaluation of client compliance with short-term administration of antimicrobials to dogs. J Am Vet Med Assoc 226(4), 567–574.

5. Marsella R., Sousa C.A., Gonzales A.J. & Fadok V.A. (2012) Current understanding of the pathophysiologic mechanisms of canine atopic dermatitis. Journal of the American Veterinary Medical Association 241, 194–207.

6. Weese J.S., Faires M.C., Frank L.A. et al. (2012) Factors associated with methicillin-resistant versus methicillinsusceptible Staphylococcus pseudintermedius infection in dogs. Journal of the American Veterinary Medical Association 240, 1450–1455.

2
CHAPTER

EFFICACY OF GLUCOCORTICOID MONOTHERAPY FOR TREATMENT OF CANINE MENINGOENCEPHALOMYELITIS OF UNKNOWN ETIOLOGY: A PROSPECTIVE STUDY IN 16 DOGS

Miyu Mercier and Heidi L. Barnes Heller

VCA Aurora Animal Hospital, 2600 West Galena Blvd, Aurora, Illinois, 60506, USA

ABSTRACT

Canine non-infectious, inflammatory meningoencephalomyelitis is termed meningoencephalomyelitis of unknown etiology (MUE) and may affect dogs of any age, breed or gender. Treatment with immunosuppressive medication has been widely reported, however no prospective clinical trials with a standard glucocorticoid monotherapy are available. The objectives were to compare the cerebrospinal fluid (CSF) analysis at diagnosis and after treatment with a standard glucocorticoid (GC) dose and to determine the survival time in dogs with MUE. We hypothesized that abnormal CSF findings would normalize in dogs with MUE, and survival time would be longer than previously reported for glucocortocoid therapy alone. Inclusion criteria were: (1) normal minimum database, (2) no GC use within 5 days, (3) magnetic resonance imaging performed, (4) negative infectious disease titres, and (5) abnormal CSF analysis. All dogs received GC therapy at 1 mg/kg *per os* q 12 h. Responders had normal CSF analysis at 1 month. Sixteen dogs met the inclusion criteria. Median total nucleated cell count (TNCC) and protein concentration at time of diagnosis were 39 cells/μL (0–1400 cells/μL), and 49 mg/dL (25–293 mg/dL), respectively. Median TNCC and protein concentration at 1 month were 1 cell/μL (0–120 cells/μL), and 24 mg/dL (13–175 mg/dL), respectively. Seven of 16 dogs (44%) were responders. There was no significant difference in survival

Citation: Miyu Mercier and Heidi L. Barnes Heller, Efficacy of glucocorticoid monotherapy for treatment of canine meningoencephalomyelitis of unknown etiology: a prospective study in 16 dogs, DOI: 10.1002/vms3.4

between the CSF responders and CSF non-responders ($P = 0.85$). Overall median survival was 602 days (45–654 days). This study supports using GC therapy in dogs with MUE.

INTRODUCTION

Canine meningoencephalomyelitis is a heterogeneous collection of inflammatory and infectious diseases of the central nervous system (CNS). In the majority of dogs, meningoencephalomyelitis has an inflammatory non-infectious etiology. There are several non-infectious inflammatory forms of meningoencephalomyelitis, including granulomatous meningoencephalitis (GME), necrotizing meningoencephalitis (NME), necrotizing leukoencephalitis (NLE) and eosinophilic meningoencephalitis (EME). Due to the distinctive high eosinophil presence in CSF and on histopathology, EME can be readily distinguished from GME, NME, and NLE. Dogs with GME, NME, and NLE may be any age, breed, or sex. Many dogs diagnosed with GME, NME, or NLE are small-breed dogs, but the presence of the disease is not restricted to this population. (Granger *et al.* 2010) Diagnostic imaging for GME, NME, or NLE often involves magnetic resonance imaging (MRI) and may be normal or show focal or multifocal changes. Mononuclear pleocytosis is often present but this varies widely, and cerebrospinal (CSF) analysis may be normal in 12–22% of cases. (Granger *et al.* 2010) In the absence of histopathologic examination, GME, NME, and NLE are indistinguishable on the basis of clinical presentation, breed, sex, age, advanced imaging, and CSF analysis. When histopathologic examination is not available for a given dog, the term meningoencephalomyelitis of unknown etiology (MUE) is used to describe suspected GME, NME, or NLE. (Zarfoss *et al.* 2006; Granger *et al.* 2010; Talarico & Schatzberg 2010)

Following a diagnosis of MUE, initial therapy consists of glucocorticoid (GC) drugs, with or without the addition of other immunosuppressant medications. (Adamo *et al.* 2007; Coates *et al.* 2007; Menaut *et al.* 2008; Pakozdy *et al.* 2009; Talarico & Schatzberg 2010; Wong *et al.* 2010; Flegel *et al.* 2011; Lowrie *et al.* 2013) Glucocorticoid monotherapy has been considered the standard therapy (Zarfoss *et al.* 2006; Adamo *et al.*2007; Jung *et al.* 2007; Pakozdy *et al.* 2009; Talarico & Schatzberg 2010; Wong *et al.* 2010; Flegel *et al.* 2011); however, its efficacy without adjunct immunosuppression in the treatment of MUE has been evaluated in only a limited number of studies. (Munana & Luttgen 1998; Jung*et al.* 2007; Pakozdy *et al.* 2009; Flegel *et al.* 2011) Use of GC drugs, with variable dosing within each study, has been reported in 59 dogs. The doses have ranged from 5–30 mg/kg per day (Pakozdy *et al.* 2009), 0.17–2.5 mg/kg per day (Flegel *et al.* 2011), 1 mg/kg per day (Jung*et al.* 2007), and 0.5–4 mg/kg per day. (Munana & Luttgen 1998) Therefore, the aims of the current study were compare the CSF analysis at diagnosis and after treatment with a standard GC dose in dogs with MUE. The second aim was to determine the survival time in dogs with MUE treated with GC monotherapy. We hypothesized that abnormal CSF findings would normalize in dogs with MUE, and survival time would be longer than in previous studies utilizing variable GC protocols.

MATERIALS AND METHODS

Study population and inclusion criteria

In this prospective study, client-owned dogs were accrued continuously between September 2006 and May 2009. All clients signed informed consent forms prior to enrollment. Complete physical and neurologic examinations were performed by 1 of the authors. Dogs were included in the study if the following inclusion criteria were met: (1) normal minimum database; (2) GC was not administered within 5 days prior to presentation; (3) MRI consistent with meningoencephalitis/myelitis; (4) negative infectious disease titres, including, tick-borne agents (*Borrelia bergdorferi*, *Rickettsia rickettsii*, and *Ehrlichia canis*), protozoa (*Neospora caninum*), fungi (*Histoplasma, Blastomyces, Aspergillus, Coccidioidomyces*, and *Cryptococcus*) and paired serum and CSF distemper virus titers; and (5) abnormal CSF findings without evidence of neoplastic or infectious etiology. A minimum database was defined as a complete blood count, serum biochemical panel, urinalysis, and three-view thoracic radiographs. Large breed dogs with cervical hyperpathia only were excluded from the study.

Diagnostic testing

Magnetic resonance imaging (GE Horizon 1.0 Tesla magnet, Pittsburg, PA, USA) was performed under general anesthesia in all dogs based on lesion localization from the neurologic examination. Dogs were pre-medicated with hydromorphone (Baxter Pharmaceutical, Deerfield, IL, USA) at 0.1 mg/kg IV and diazepam (Valium; Hospira, Lake Forest, IL, USA) at 0.25 mg/kg IV and induced with propofol (PropoFlo; Abbott Animal Health, Abbott Park, IL, USA) at 4 mg/kg IV to effect. Anesthesia was maintained with isoflurane (IsoFlo®; Abbott Animal Health). The standard MRI protocol for this study included T1- and T2- weighted images in sagittal and transverse planes, fluid attenuated inversion recovery images in the transverse planes, and T1-weighted images after administration of Gadolinium (MultiHance; Bracco Diagnostics, Monroe Township, NJ, USA) in transverse and sagittal planes. Magnetic resonance imaging findings were classified as normal, focal or multifocal for this study.

Cerebrospinal fluid (CSF) was collected from the cerebellomedullary or lumbar cisterns during the same anesthetic episode as neuroimaging. Normal CSF analysis was defined as nucleated cell count (TNCC) <5 cells/μL and protein concentration <25 mg/dL for cerebellomedullary cistern puncture and <40 mg/dL for lumbar puncture. (Platt & Olby 2004) After collection, the CSF sample was divided into two aliquots for transportation; in 1 sample, a 1:10 dilution of CSF to autologous serum was made to improve cell stabilization for transportation, and the other sample was CSF only. (Cellio 2001) All samples were transported in additive-free sterile glass tubes. Analysis was performed by an affiliated laboratory (Antech Diagnostic Laboratory, Oakbrook, IL, USA) within 12 h of collection and analysed according to standard procedure. Correction factors were not applied to the data, and all reported values were uncorrected. (Summers *et al.* 1995) Approximately 1 month after initial CSF analysis, a second CSF sample was collected from the same cistern, using the same anesthetic protocol, and analysed as detailed above.

Treatment protocol

Immediately upon recovery from anesthesia all dogs received intravenous methylprednisolone (Solu-Medrol; Pfizer, New York, NY, USA) at 30 mg/kg IV followed by 15 mg/kg IV 3 h after the initial dose and 10 mg/kg IV 3 h after the second dose was administered. Following treatment with methylprednisone, prednisone (West-Ward Pharmaceutical, Eatontown, NJ, USA) or prednisolone (Lloyd, Inc., Shenandoah, IA, USA) at 1 mg/kg PO q12 h, sulfadimathoxine/ormetoprim (Primor® tablets; Pfizer) at 15 mg/kg PO q12 h, doxycycline (Doxycycline tablets; West Ward Pharmaceutical) at 5–10 mg/kg PO q24 h, and famotidine (Famotidine tablets; Wockhardt, Ltd, Morton Grove, IL, USA) at 1 mg/kg PO q24 h were initiated. After obtaining negative results for infectious disease testing, sulfadimathoxine/ormetoprim and doxycycline were discontinued.

If the second CSF results were within reference intervals, the dog was classified as a CSF responder and a gradually decreasing dose of prednisone or prednisolone was administered as follows: 1 mg/kg *per os* q24 h × 30 days, then 1 mg/kg *per os* q48 h × 30 days and then discontinued. If the second CSF results were abnormal, the dog was classified as a CSF non-responder and the same dose of prednisone or prednisolone was continued for an additional 30 days. If dogs did not improve at 60 days or greater following the above treatment, or worsened during treatment, additional immunosuppressive agents were recommended.

Referring veterinarians were contacted by telephone within 48 months after diagnosis of MUE and questioned about the survival of each dog. If the dog had died, the reason for the death was noted. Referring veterinarians were asked if clinical signs had recurred for CSF responders. Relapse was defined as a reoccurrence of clinical signs in CSF responders, after discontinuing GC therapy.

Statistical analysis

Descriptive statistics including medians, minimums and maximums were recorded for continuous data. A Kaplan–Meier survival curve was created for survival data. Overall survival time and survival time of CSF responders and CSF non-responders was evaluated with the Mantel-Cox Log-Rank test comparison.

RESULTS

Sixteen dogs met the inclusion criteria. Breeds included Lhasa apso ($n = 2$), Dachshund ($n = 2$), and 1 each of the following breeds: Golden Retriever, Retriever mix, Pug, Welsh Springer Spaniel, Boston Terrier, Pug-Beagle mix, Beagle, Jack Russell Terrier, Rottweiler, Collie, Maltese terrier and mixed breed. The median age was 4.5 years (2–11 years) and the median weight was 12.0 kg (5.2–38.4 kg). Neuroanatomical lesion localization, based on the neurologic examination, was prosencephalon (5/16 dogs), brainstem (3/16 dogs), T3-L3 myelopathy (2/16 dogs), L6-S2 radiculopathy (1/16 dogs) and peripheral neuropathy (1/16 dogs) involving the vestibulocochlear nerves. Four of 16 dogs were diagnosed with multifocal lesion localization. Magnetic resonance imaging findings were normal in 2 dogs, focal in 3 dogs and multifocal in 11 dogs. Abnormalities on MRI corresponded with the neuroanatomic lesion localization in all dogs. The median prednisone or prednisolone dose was 1 mg/kg (0.8–1.2 mg/kg) PO q12 h. Sulfadimethoxine/ormetoprim and doxycycline were discontinued by day 7 of treatment in all dogs.

Initial CSF analysis

Initial CSF samples were collected from the cerebellomedullary cistern in 13 dogs and the lumbar cistern in 3 dogs. See Table 1 for median CSF TNCC and protein concentration. Results indicated mixed mononuclear or lymphocytic pleocytosis (n = 15) and neutrophilic pleocytosis (n = 1); in 3 dogs the TNCC was within the reference interval, but the protein concentration was increased.

Table 1: Median CSF TNCC and protein concentration for dogs diagnosed with MUE

	Median CSF TNCC (cell/μL)		Median CSF protein (mg/dL)	
	Initial	1 month	Initial	1 month
Responder	8.5 (0–1160)	0 (0–1)	40.5 (25–251)	19 (13–24)
Non-responder	59 (0–1400)	15 (0–120)	68.5 (28–293)	38 (17–175)
Combined	39 (0–1400)	49 (25–293)	1 (0–120)	24 (13–175)

CSF, cerebrospinal fluid; TNCC, total nucleated cell count; MUE, meningoencephalomyelitis of unknown etiology. Responders achieved normal CSF results at 1 month; non-responders did not achieve normal CSF results at 1 month. Combined values refer to CSF responders and CSF non-responders together.

Second evaluation and CSF analysis

In seven of 16 dogs (44%), CSF analytes were within reference intervals and they were therefore considered CSF responders. One dog did not have sufficient sample to perform CSF protein concentration therefore this dog was considered a CSF responder based on the TNCC. Median TNCC and protein concentration for CSF responders and CSF non-responders are listed in Table 1.

The neurologic examination was normal in 10 of 16 dogs (63%) and abnormal in 6 dogs (38%). In 5 of 10 dogs (50%) with normal neurologic examinations, CSF analysis was also normal. In 2 of 6 dogs (33%) with abnormal neurologic examinations, CSF analysis was normal. All abnormalities on neurologic examination indicated persistent changes; no new abnormalities were detected. Three CSF non-responders started adjunct immunosuppression at a median of 68 days (62–75 days) from diagnosis due to a failure to improve on GC treatment. All 3 dogs received cytosine arabinoside (Generic; Hospira Inc, Lake Forrest, IL, USA) at 50 mg/m² *subcutaneous* q 12 h. for 48 h, repeated every 3 weeks as needed.

Survival time

Follow-up information was obtained within 48 months (45–1100 days) of initial diagnosis in all dogs. One of seven CSF responders (14%) was reported to have clinical signs consistent with relapse and was euthanized without additional diagnostic testing or treatment. Two CSF non-responders were euthanized because of progressive disease; two CSF non-responders and one CSF responder were euthanized due to unrelated causes; and two CSF responders and one CSF non-responder were euthanized or died acutely of unknown causes. The remaining three CSF responders and four CSF non-responders dogs were alive at the time of writing (Median 485 days). Median survival for all dogs based on Kaplan–Meier survival analysis was 602 days (45–654 days). Median survival for CSF responders was 602 days and the median was not reached in the CSF non-responders. (Fig. 1) There was no significant difference in survival between the CSF responders and CSF non-responders ($P = 0.85$). Due to the small number of dogs that died due to disease, reporting of survival time between CSF responders and CSF non-responders was not accurate. Additional statistical analysis was not performed due to small sample size.

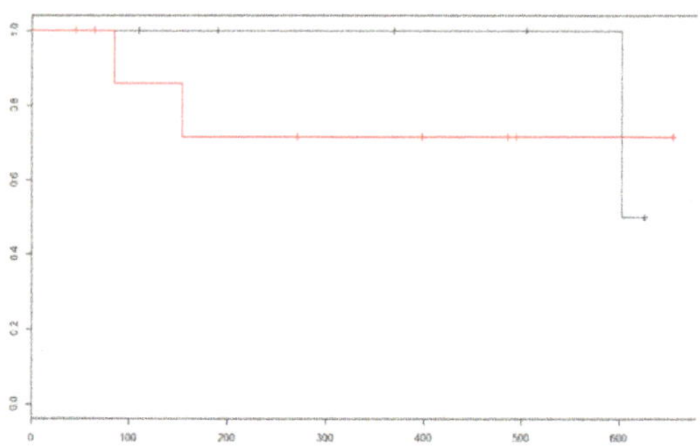

Figure 1: Kaplan-Meier survival curves for 7 responder dogs (black line) and 8 non-responder dogs (red line) with meningoencephalomyelitis of unknown etiology (MUE). Tick marks represent dogs censured for events other than progression of disease.

DISCUSSION

Treatment of dogs with MUE using standardized GC monotherapy resulted in normalization of the CSF analytes in 44% of dogs. None of the previous studies evaluating solo GC therapy has evaluated repeated CSF analysis as a marker for immunosuppression in canine MUE. However, repeated CSF analysis has been evaluated for other immunosuppressant protocols used in treating MUE (Lowrie *et al.* 2013), as well as other inflammatory CNS diseases. (Cizinauskas *et al.* 2000) One study suggested that serial monitoring of CSF TNCC and protein concentrations is a sensitive indicator of successful treatment of inflammatory disease; however, clinical relapse was not evaluated statistically. (Cizinauskas *et al.* 2000) Another study failed to find an association between normal CSF analysis and improved outcome, but did find an association between abnormal CSF analysis and relapse or poor outcome. (Lowrie *et al.* 2013) In the current study, only one CSF responder was reported to have relapsed, suggesting that CSF analysis may be a valid tool for monitoring success or failure of treatment in dogs diagnosed with MUE and treated with GC monotherapy. Larger studies are needed to evaluate this association more fully.

Survival times for dogs in the current study were longer than those in all previous studies of dogs treated with GC monotherapy. Median survival times were reported to be 28 (Pakozdy *et al.* 2009), 91 (Lowrie *et al.* 2013), and 323 (Lowrie *et al.* 2013) days, compared with 602 days in this study. The difference in survival times among studies may reflect different immunosuppression protocols or the prospective nature of the current study. In the current study, we evaluated an immunosuppressive dose of GC that was standardized for all 16 dogs. Methylprednisolone was administered intravenous following the initial diagnosis in all dogs to try to achieve rapid immunosuppression. In studies of treatment protocols using GC in combination with other immunosuppressant agents, median survival times ranged from 26 to 1834 days (Adamo *et al.* 2007; Coates *et al.* 2007; Menaut *et al.* 2008; Pakozdy *et al.* 2009; Talarico & Schatzberg 2010; Wong *et al.* 2010; Flegel *et al.* 2011; Lowrie *et al.* 2013), with a combined median survival time of 375 days. Some of these studies attributed the survival times exclusively to the alternative immunosuppressant. Based on the current study, GC immunosuppression may be a contributing factor to survival times reported for studies, using combination treatments. Furthermore, the long median survival time in this study supports the use of GC monotherapy for dogs diagnosed with MUE.

Lack of a histopathologic diagnosis was a limitation of this study. Although antemortem diagnostic criteria have been established for MUE, inclusion of patients with acute phase infectious disease or neoplasia is an inherent risk in the diagnosis of MUE. (Granger *et al.* 2010) To partially address this possibility, extensive serologic testing was performed at the time of diagnosis for the most common infectious disease in the geographic area as well as paired CSF and serum titres for distemper virus. Serologic testing evaluates immune response to a specific pathogen, therefore it is possible that a dog with acute infectious disease may not yet have mounted an immune response and therefore had negative serology when initially tested. Death or euthanasia due to worsening signs would be expected for dogs with infectious diseases receiving immunosuppressive treatment without concurrent long-term antimicrobial treatment. All dogs included in the study survived for the first 30 days of treatment; therefore it is unlikely that dogs with infectious meningoencephalomyelitis were included. Although neoplastic cells were not identified in CSF, histopathologic examination of the CNS would be expected to be more sensitive than CSF analysis for detection of neoplasia. Brain biopsy was not performed in the dogs in this study due to the risk of complications. Additionally, necropsy was not required and was not obtained in any of the deceased dogs. Requiring diagnosis by either CNS biopsy or necropsy may have resulted in bias towards shorter survival. Therefore, although considered unlikely, occurrence of neoplastic diseases mistakenly diagnosed as meningoencephalomyelitis cannot be excluded. Other limitations of this study included the small size of the study population and limited follow-up time. Larger studies may be able to detect prognostic variables, such normalization differences in CSF protein or TNCC for dogs with MUE that were not evaluated in the current study.

CONCLUSIONS

In dogs with MUE, 44% had normal CSF analysis after 1 month of GC immunosuppression; further studies are needed to determine if a relationship exists between prognosis and results of CSF analysis. Dogs with normal CSF findings at 1 month had longer survival times than dogs with abnormal CSF findings at 1 month. Glucocorticoid therapy in this study, resulted in median survival time longer than previously reported times in studies evaluating combination immunosuppressant protocols; therefore a positive GC effect on survival time in those studies should be considered. Dogs may benefit from the administration of combination immunosuppression protocols if the side effects of GC warrant limited use of GC. In conclusion, this study supports the use of immunosuppression with GC monotherapy in dogs diagnosed with MUE.

REFERENCES

1. Adamo P.F., Rylander H. & Adams W.M. (2007) Ciclosporin use in multi-drug therapy for meningoencephalomyelitis of unknown aetiology in dogs. The Journal of Small Animal Practice 48, 486–496.
2. Cellio B.C. (2001) Collecting, processing, and preparing cerebrospinal fluid in dogs and cats. Compendium Continuing Education for Veterinarians 23, 786–792.
3. Cizinauskas S., Jaggy A. & Tipold A. (2000) Long-term treatment of dogs with steroid-responsive meningitisarteritis: clinical, laboratory and therapeutic results. The Journal of Small Animal Practice 41, 295–301.
4. Coates J.R., Barone G., Dewey C.W., Vitale C.L., Holloway-Azene N.M., Sessions J.K. (2007) Procarbazine as adjunctive therapy for treatment of dogs with presumptive antemortem diagnosis of granulomatous meningoencephalomyelitis: 21 cases (1998–2004). Journal of Veterinary Internal Medicine 2, 100–106.
5. Flegel T., Boettcher I.C., Matiasek K., Oevermann A., Doherr M.G., Oechtering G., Henke D. (2011) Comparison of oral administration of lomustine and prednisolone or prednisolone alone as treatment for granulomatous meningoencephalomyelitis or necrotizing encephalitis in dogs. Journal of the American Veterinary Medical Association 238, 337–345.
6. Granger N., Smith P.M. & Jeffery N.D. (2010) Clinical findings and treatment of non-infectious meningoencephalomyelitis in dogs: a systematic review of 457 pub-lished cases from 1962 to 2008. Veterinary Journal 184, 290–297.
7. Jung D.I., Kang B.T., Park C., Yoo J.H., Gu S.H., Jeon H.W., Kim J.W., Heo R.Y., et al. (2007) A comparison of combination therapy (cyclosporine plus prednisolone) with sole prednisolone therapy in 7 dogs with necrotizing meningoencephalitis. Journal of Veterinary Medical Science 69, 1303–1306.
8. Lowrie M., Smith P.M. & Garosi L. (2013) Meningoencephalitis of unknown origin: investigation of prognostic factors and outcome using a standard treatment protocol. The Veterinary Record 172, 527–533.

9. Menaut P., Landart J., Behr S., Lanore D., Trumel C. (2008) Treatment of 11 dogs with meningoencephalomyelitis of unknown origin with a combination of prednisolone and cytosine arabinoside. The Veterinary Record 162, 241–245.

10. Munana K.R. & Luttgen P.J. (1998) Prognostic factors for dogs with granulomatous meningoencephalomyelitis: 42 cases. Journal of the American Veterinary Medical Association 212, 1902–1906.

11. Pakozdy A., Leschnik M., Kneissl S., Gumpenberger M., Gruber A., Tichy A., Thalhammer J.G. (2009) Improved survival time in dogs with suspected GME treated with cyclosporin. The Veterinary Record 164, 89–91.

12. Platt S.R. & Olby N.J. (2004) In BSAVA Manual of Canine and Feline Neurology, 35–53. British Small Animal Veterinary Association: Gloucester.

13. Summers B.A., Cummings J.F., deLahunta A. (1995) Inflammatory diseases of the central nervous system. In: Veterinary Neuropathology, (This is the only edition of this book), pp. 95–162. Mosby: St. Louis

14. Talarico L.R. & Schatzberg S.J. (2010) Idiopathic granulomatous and necrotizing inflammatory disorders of the canine central nervous system: a review and future perspectives. The Journal of Small Animal Practice 51, 138–149.

15. Wong M.A., Hopkins A.L., Meeks J.C., Clarke J.D. (2010) Evaluation of treatment with a combination of azathioprine and prednisone in dogs with meningoencephalomyelitis of undetermined etiology: 40 cases (2000–2007). Journal of the American Veterinary Medical Association 237, 929–935

16. Zarfoss M., Schatzberg S., Venator K., Cutter-Schatzberg K., Cuddon P., Pintar J., et al. (2006) Combined cytosine arabinoside and prednisone therapy for meningoencephalitis of unknown aetiology in 10 dogs. The Journal of Small Animal Practice 47, 588–595.

3

CHAPTER

INFLUENCE OF THE DIETARY FIBRE LEVELS ON FAECAL HAIR EXCRETION AFTER 14 DAYS IN SHORT AND LONG-HAIRED DOMESTIC CATS

Mickael Weber, Laura Sams, Alexandre Feugier, Sandrine Michel, and Vincent Biourge

Royal Canin Research Center, Aimargues, France

ABSTRACT

Hairballs are a common problem in cats and may result in intestinal obstruction. Dietary fibre has been recommended to stimulate hair faecal excretion. The objective of this study was to assess the influence of psyllium and different levels of total dietary fibre (6% vs. 11% vs. 15% TdF) on hair faecal excretion in short and long-haired (LH) domestic cats. Twenty-one adult cats were divided into three panels: shedding panel, short-haired (SH) panel and LH panel. Shedding panel was used to assess shedding throughout the study with a normalized brushing. In parallel, SH panel and LH panel were used to evaluate the impact of the diets on faecal hair excretion. They were fed a low-fibre diet during phase 1 (diet 6, 6.0% TdF). In phase 2, panels were fed either diet 11 (11% TdF) or diet 15 (15% TdF). In phase 3, cats returned to diet 6 before a crossover on the other diet in phase 4. Those diets were fed to cats for 14 days. Faecal hair excretion was quantified daily. Data were analysed using a generalized linear model procedure. The assessment of shedding showed that the study did not occur during moulting season. In the LH panel, diet 11 and diet 15 increased ($P < 0.001$) faecal hair excretion by 81% and 113% respectively, compared to the control diet. In the SH panel, no influence of the diets was observed. This study supports that fibre affects faecal hair excretion in LH cats, suggesting that a diet with psyllium and 11% or 15% TdF might

Citation: Mickael Weber, Laura Sams, Alexandre Feugier, Sandrine Michel, and Vincent Biourge, Influence of the dietary fibre levels on faecal hair excretion after 14 days in short and long-haired domestic cats, DOI: 10.1002/vms3.6

minimize hairball formation in 14 days and between shedding periods. In SH cats, 11% and 15% fibre levels had no effect on faecal hair excretion. This could be explained by the low quantity of hair ingested outside the shedding season or by the short duration of the study.

INTRODUCTION

A cat can spend 25% to 30% (Benjamin 1976; Panaman 1981) of its time on grooming. Grooming time may be greater than this for cats with limited outdoor access. Grooming behaviour may serve several functions for cats including cooling by coat moistening, removal of shed fur and ectoparasites and stress reduction (Willemse *et al.* 1994; Eckstein & Hart 2000a,b). Since the cat's tongue is covered with keratinous papilla, a large amount of hair is ingested while licking. On average, a short-haired (SH) cat loses approximately 28 g of hair per kg of body weight per year, with two-thirds of this loss being ingested and found in excrement (Hendriks *et al.* 1998). Usually ingested hair is eliminated in faeces however large quantities can accumulate in the digestive tract forming trichobezoars (or hairballs) that can cause digestive problems.

There is no previously published data regarding the incidence of hairballs in pet cats. An epidemiological survey of a large number of cats is necessary to shed more light on the topic. With this aim, a survey of cat owners was recently conducted in order to estimate how common it is for domestic cats to bring up hairballs (Cannon 2013). The survey, based on 48 SH cats, suggested that there was an overall incidence of hairball vomiting of approximately 10% in healthy SH cats. Vomiting, abdominal pain and constipation are the most frequent clinical signs, but hairballs can also result in severe consequences such as anorexia or intestinal obstruction, leading to surgery. This phenomenon is particularly noticeable in long-haired (LH) cats living indoors and during moulting (spring and autumn) but any cat may be affected.

For cats that regularly or intermittently suffer from hairballs, preventive treatment is indicated. Common suggestions include regular brushings (Cannon 2013), the use of petroleum-based laxatives or lubricants (Ryan & Wolfer 1978; Barrs *et al.* 1999; Agnello & Kantrowitz 2003) or specific dry products (Dann *et al.* 2004; Beynen *et al.* 2011).

Diets formulated to reduce the incidence of hairballs generally contain increased levels of soluble and/or insoluble fibre with the aim of increasing the passage of hair through the gastrointestinal tract and in faeces without causing obstruction or constipation, as well as minimizing formation of hairballs in the digestive tract.

A recent study reported that a diet enriched with insoluble fibre (cellulose) reduced the severity of clinical signs in cats with existing hairballs (Beynen *et al.* 2011). A chew enriched in slippery elm and psyllium husk, a gel-forming and soluble fibre source, has also been shown to reduce the severity of hairball clinical signs in cats by delaying the gastric content (Dann *et al.* 2004). However, the efficacy of these diets has been evaluated from questionnaires or surveys and hairball elimination was subjectively assessed by cat owners. There are no published studies measuring objectively the efficacy of hairball products on faecal hair excretion in cats. This could be due to the difficulty of precisely quantifying faecal hair excretion.

The aim of this study was therefore to assess the impact of psyllium husk and the influence of different levels of total dietary fibre (6% vs. 11% vs. 15% TdF) on faecal hair excretion in short and LH cats by directly measuring hair in their faeces.

MATERIALS AND METHODS

The present study was performed in summer (from July to September).

Animals

Twenty-one healthy adult research cats (4.8 ± 1.1 kg) participated in the study. One panel ($n = 7$) was used to assess fur shedding throughout the study: this panel (called 'shedding panel') was composed of three LH cats (two Birmans and one Maine coon) and four SH cats (four European domestic SH cats). Two collective panels ($n = 7$) were used to evaluate the impact of the diets on faecal hair excretion: a SH panel composed of six Chartreux and one British Short Hair, and an LH panel composed of five European domestic LH cats, one Ragdoll and one Birman.

Ten cats were female and 11 cats were male, and were matched across groups: three females and four males were used in SH and shedding panels and four females and three males in LH panel. All cats were neutered and the median age was 4 years (range 2–11 years). All cats remained healthy throughout the study, based on physical examination. They were treated monthly with a topical flea – tick product (Frontline®Plus; Merial, Dultuh, GA, USA). They were housed in closed indoor (13 m^2) and outdoor (14 m^2) runs with unlimited outdoor access. Every morning, the cattery was cleaned. In order to prevent cats from being disturbed by external noises, music was played inside the cattery during the day. Temperature remained constant at 22–23°C in the cattery and cats were exposed to normal day length and natural lighting throughout the study.

Housing and management protocols adhered to European regulatory guidelines for animal welfare, whilst all experimental protocols complied with European Union guidelines on animal welfare and were approved by the Royal Canin Committee for Animal Ethics and Welfare.

Diet and food intake

Three experimental dry, expanded, complete and balanced maintenance diets designed for adult cats were used in the present study (Table 1). The diets varied in TdF and psyllium contents. The control diet (diet 6) contained a low-fibre level (6% TdF) and no psyllium. The first test diet (diet 11) presented moderate fibre content (11% TdF) and 0.5% psyllium husk. The second test diet (diet 15) contained a high fibre level (15% TdF) and 0.5% psyllium husk. The increase in TdF was obtained by supplementation of cellulose: 0% for diet 6, 5.17% for diet 11 and 9.68% for diet 15. During the study, all cats were fed *ad libitum* and the diet was given once a day, in the morning. All food consumptions were measured out using electronic scales (XS4001S; Mettler Toledo, Columbus OH, USA) accurate to within 0.1 g.

Table 1: Dietary composition of the three diets used in the study

	Units	Diet 6	Diet 11	Diet 15
Dry matter	g 100 g^{-1}*	94.2	94.7	94.4
Crude protein	g 100 g^{-1}	33.8	34.7	34.8
Fat	g 100 g^{-1}	14.4	14.1	13.6
Ash	g 100 g^{-1}	7.3	7.3	7.3
Crude fibre	g 100 g^{-1}	1.2	4.6	7.2
TdF	g 100 g^{-1}	6.0	11.2	14.9
Nitrogen free extract	g 100 g^{-1}	43.2	39.3	37.1
Metabolizable energy†	kJ kg^{-1}	16 565	15 963	15 336

TdF, total dietary fibre. Ingredients: dehydrated poultry protein, maize, vegetable protein isolate, rice, wheat, cellulose (only for diet 11 and 15), animal fats, hydrolysed animal proteins, soya oil, beet pulp, minerals, fish oil, yeasts, fructo-oligosaccharides, psyllium (*Plantago ovata*) husks (>95%) and seeds (<5%) (only for diet 11 and 15), borage oil. *g 100 g^{-1} = grams per 100 g diet on an as fed basis; †Metabolizable energy is calculated with NRC 2006. NRC = National Research Council.

Protocol design

Study #1: assessment of shedding throughout the study in the shedding panel

Three times a week, each cat of the shedding panel received 24 brush strokes: six on the back, four on the neck, the head and the breast and two on the tail and the hind legs. For each cat, the hair collected was weighed carefully to quantify shedding over the study (a total of 8 weeks divided into four 14 day long phases designated phases 1–4).

Study #2: impact of the diets on faecal hair excretion in SH and LH cats

One week before starting the study, SH and LH panels underwent a purge for 3 days to eliminate accumulated hair in the digestive tract (Savorial, MSD Santé animale, Beaucouzé, France). Then they were fed diet 6 for 14 days during phase 1. In phase 2 (14 days), both panels were fed either diet 11 or diet 15. In phase 3, all cats returned to diet 6 for 14 days before crossing over to the other experimental diet (diet 15 or diet 11) in phase 4 (14 days). In order to avoid digestive disorders, 3 days of gradual food transition were made at the beginning of each phase (Fig. 1).

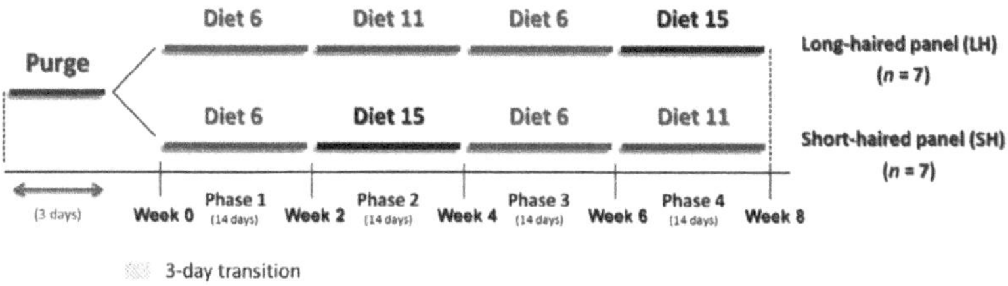

Figure 1: Study design 2: impact of the diets on faecal hair excretion.

Faecal hair excretion was quantified daily for each collective panel fed each diet according to the modified method of Hendriks *et al.* (1998) and Tournier *et al.* (2005). All faeces excreted were collected every morning, pooled and stored at −20°C. Pooled faeces were then dried in an oven (70°C, 24 h) then ground carefully in a blender (GM200; Retsch Grindomix, Haan, Germany) for 12 s at medium speed. Through a sieve (1 mm), hair was then collected and washed using a solution of 20 mL of detergent (IDOS 2000; Elcopharma, Villeneuve s/Yonne, France), and 2 L of boiling water for 30 min. A second stage of sieving and washing (15 min) was then performed. After a third sieving process, hair samples were isolated by vacuum filtration, and then hair moisture was evaporated in an oven (110°C, 15 h). The hair sample obtained was finally weighed by a precision balance (XP504 DR; Mettler Toledo, OH, USA).

Statistical analysis

Statistical analyses were performed with the SAS version 9.3 software (SAS Institute Inc., Cary, NC, USA). Results were expressed as mean ± SEM.

Study #1

A mixed model was performed to evaluate the impact of the following fixed effects: hair length (long or short), phase (from 1–4) and the interaction hair length × phase on the quantity of hair brushed. The cat was defined as a random term considering that each cat was its own control through weekly measurements. False discovery rate method was used to avoid alpha risk inflation due to multiple comparisons. In this respect, *P*-values were adjusted to compare phase within hair length and hair length within phase.

Study #2

A generalized linear model was used to assess the effects of panel (SH/LH), diet (diet 6/diet 11/diet 15) and the interaction panel × diet on faecal hair excretion and energy consumption. For faecal hair excretion, food intake was added as covariate to this two-way analysis of variance.

Residuals of each model were checked for fit with normal distribution according to Kolmogorov–Smirnov, Cramer-von Mises and Anderson-Darling tests. Results are expressed as least square means ± SEM. Differences in Least-squares (LS) means were assessed using the Scheffe test to correct for the multiple comparisons. Significance level was set at 5%.

RESULTS

Study #1

The quantity of hair brushed in the shedding panel was impacted by hair length ($P = 0.013$) but not by phase ($P = 0.409$). Significant interaction was found (hair length × phase: $P < 0.001$). The quantities of hair collected were higher in LH cats than in SH cats in the second phase (519.3 ± 20.7 mg vs. 311.2 ± 30.2 mg, $P = 0.0155$), the third phase (552.5 ± 23.0 mg vs. 312.6 ± 33.4 mg, $P = 0.0055$) and the fourth phase (552.9 ± 23.5 mg vs. 316.7 ± 31.6 mg, $P = 0.006$). This effect was not significant during the first phase (338.2 ± 17.8 mg vs. 484.1 ± 65.2 mg, $P = 0.088$). No significant individual effect was observed on the quantity of hair brushed ($P = 0.061$).

Study #2

Energy consumption

Energy consumption results expressed in kJ day^{-1} are shown in Table 2. Energy consumption was influenced by diet and panel effects (diet effect: $P < 0.001$; panel effect $P < 0.001$; panel × diet: $P < 0.001$). Indeed diet effect depended on the panel considered. For LH panel, energy consumption did not vary between the different diets. For SH panel, no difference was found in energy intake during the phases 2, 3 and 4. However, significantly higher energy consumption was observed when cats were fed diet 6 in phase 1 ($P < 0.001$).

Table 2: Values (mean ± SEM) of the daily energy consumption (in kJ day^{-1}) and faecal hair excretion (in mg day^{-1}) for SH and LH panels

LH panel	Diet 6	Diet 11	Diet 6	Diet 15
Energy consumption (kJ day^{-1})	812.2 ± 91.3	824.4 ± 17.6	862.9 ± 15.1	826.5 ± 14.7
Faecal hair excretion (mg day^{-1})	1512 ± 185^{a}	2735 ± 254^{b}	1610 ± 177^{a}	3435 ± 164^{b}
SH panel	**Diet 6**	**Diet 15**	**Diet 6**	**Diet 11**
Energy consumption (kJ day^{-1})	1062.6 ± 18.0^{a}	916.5 ± 25.1^{b}	897.2 ± 13.4^{b}	903.5 ± 18.8^{b}
Faecal hair excretion (mg day^{-1})	1627 ± 156	1631 ± 105	1084 ± 107	1431 ± 109

LH, long-haired; SH, short-haired. Different superscript letters (a, b) in the same line are significantly different ($P < 0.05$).

Faecal hair excretion

On the day after the 3 days of purge, 2.45 and 6.31 g of hair were recovered in faeces of SH and LH panels respectively.

Faecal hair excretion data for LH and SH cats fed different diets are given in Table 2. Faecal hair excretion was influenced by diet only in LH panel (diet effect: $P < 0.001$;

panel effect $P < 0.001$; panel × diet: $P < 0.001$). Indeed in LH cats, faecal hair excretion significantly increased by 81% in diet 11 and by 113% in diet 15 compared to diet 6 ($P < 0.001$). The cumulative amounts of hair excreted during the 14-day period were 40.5 and 48.1 g when LH panels were fed diet 11 and diet 15 respectively but only 22 g when fed diet 6. No significant differences in faecal hair excretion were observed between phases 1 and 3 when the cats were fed diet 6, and between diet 11 and 15 fed in phases 2 and 4. In SH cats, no difference was observed in faecal hair excretion when fed diet 6, 11 or 15.

DISCUSSION

The objective of the present study was to assess the influence of psyllium and different levels of TdF (6% vs. 11% vs. 15%) on faecal hair excretion in short and LH cats.

The predisposition of cats to forming hairballs following hair ingestion could be due to their digestive physiological particularities. For example, it has been reported that cats lack interdigestive migrating myoelectric complexes (IMMCs). In other species, these motor complexes begin in the stomach during periods of fasting and result in powerful peristaltic waves which facilitate transportation of indigestible substances such as bone, fibre and hair from the stomach through the small intestine (De Vos 1993). In cats, activity resembling IMMCs has only been identified in the distal small intestine (Roche *et al.* 1982). This slow peristalsis in cats could thus explain both the accumulation of hair in their digestive tract and their slow total gastrointestinal transit time (around 35–40 h) (Fucci *et al.* 1995; Peachey *et al.* 2000) compared to small breed dogs (24 h) (Hernot *et al.* 2005).

Very few studies have been conducted to evaluate the efficacy of diets on the incidence of hairballs in cats (Cannon 2013; German & German2013). This is likely due to the difficulty of precisely quantifying hairballs. Among existing studies, most used questionnaires or surveys and the frequency of hairball vomiting (Cannon 2013) or clinical signs (vomiting, retching and coughing) (Dann *et al.* 2004; Beynen *et al.* 2011) were evaluated by cat owners, making the results quite subjective.

In the present study, hair was quantified directly in faeces. Faecal hair excretion was measured daily according to the modified method of Hendriks *et al.* (1998) and Tournier *et al.* (2005). Two washing and three sieving steps were needed to separate hair from faeces. Although this method was time consuming, it gave accurate and repeatable measurements (data not shown).

At the beginning of this study, a purge was performed for 3 days in SH and LH cats to eliminate hair accumulated in the digestive tract. Although these cats did not show any clinical signs of hairballs, large quantities of hair were recovered in their faeces within the few days after the purge. As expected, higher faecal hair elimination was observed in LH cats than in SH cats (2.5 times more). Hair accumulated in the digestive tract prior to commencing the study could have altered the results.

Shedding is a natural phenomenon which can have a strong impact on faecal hair excretion. It was therefore assessed throughout the study with a normalized brushing three times a week on all shedding panel cats. The quantity of hair brushed in all cats was not significantly different between 2 phases, indicating that the present study did not occur during a shedding season. The quantity of hair recovered per cat and per brush stroke (63 mg on average) was extremely close to that obtained by Tournier *et al.* (2005) outside the shedding season. This previous study showed that semi-long-haired cats lost on average 70 mg hair per brush stroke and that this quantity increased up to 140 mg during the shedding season.

The shedding panel lived in the same environment as SH and LH cats. It is therefore unlikely that the variations of faecal hair excretion observed in these cats were the consequence of a change in hair losses during the study. Because this study was performed during the summer (from July to September), the shedding period was probably finished.

Different factors such as gender, flea burdens or breed could have affected grooming behaviour and thus impacted on the faecal hair excretion results. To our knowledge, no data are available on the effect of gender on grooming behaviour in cats. However, balanced panels in terms of male and female cats were used in the present study to minimize this possible effect. Flea exposure can strongly increase grooming rate in cats (Eckstein & Hart 2000b). A flea treatment was thus used monthly in all cats and regular observations of hair and skin were made to detect any infestation.

Several pedigree cat breeds were used in SH and LH panels, which may have had an impact on the results. Indeed hair coat length and density, as well as the relative proportions of guard and undercoat hairs may vary with breed and this may have had an impact on the hair excretion. However, the majority of cats present in each panel ($n = 7$/panel) were of the same breed (six Chartreux in SH panel and five European domestic LH cats in LH panel), thereby limiting this potential effect.

Because food intake affects the quantity of fibre ingested, it was important to ensure that both panels consumed similarly diet 6, 11 and 15. In this study, cats surprisingly ingested similar quantities of energy, despite *ad libitum* access to food and differences in food composition. This supports previous studies demonstrating that cats regulate their energy intake when fed foods containing moderate fibre content (9% cellulose; 8.2% crude fibre) (Prola *et al.* 2006).

Higher energy consumption was only observed in SH cats when fed diet 6 in phase 1. Although not statistically significant, the higher faecal hair excretion observed in SH cats fed diet 6 in phase 1 (1627 ± 156 mg) compared with phase 3 (1084 ± 107 mg) could be explained by this larger consumption (+18%; $P < 0.001$).

The impact of fibre level on faecal hair excretion varied according to hair coat length. In LH panel, consumption of diets 11 and 15 induced significantly higher faecal hair excretion, compared to diet 6 ($P < 0.001$), indicating that the combination of psyllium and cellulose facilitate faecal hair elimination in those cats. This supports previous studies based on cat owner questionnaires showing that the supplementation of cellulose in a diet or of psyllium husks in a treat lowered the incidence of clinical signs of hairballs (Dann *et al.* 2004; Beynen *et al.* 2011).

The mechanism by which the ingestion of cellulose and psyllium depresses the clinical signs of hairballs and stimulates their excretion in faeces is not known. Psyllium husk is a source of gel-forming soluble fibre which has the property of increasing viscosity of the digestive content. Psyllium husk could thus promote the binding of hair to food particles and thereby increase the transfer of gastric hair into the duodenum and enhanced passage through the intestine. Cellulose is a dietary insoluble fibre source which enhances the intestinal transit rate of digesta (Burrows *et al.* 1982) and this may promote the excretion of hair in faeces.

The present study cannot determine which of the two fibre sources (psyllium or cellulose) presents the greatest capacity to stimulate hair excretion in cat faeces. The inclusion of a diet containing 6% fibre and 0.5% psyllium or diets with 11% or 15% fibre without psyllium would have been necessary and their lack is a limitation of this study.

Similar low faecal hair excretions were observed when diet 6 was fed in phases 1 and 3 in LH cats, confirming the weak effect of a low-fibre diet on hair transit. No significant difference was found between diet 11 and 15, suggesting that an 11% fibre level would be sufficient to stimulate faecal hair excretion or that the study was too short to observe significantly higher hair excretion in cats fed diet 15.

In SH cats, similar faecal hair excretions were observed when fed diet 6, 11 and 15. This lack of effect could be explained by insufficient ingestion of hair in this population outside the shedding season. Indeed the quantities of hair excreted by SH animals fed diets 11 and 15 were respectively 40 and 60% lower than those found in LH cats fed the same diets. Moreover, when fed diet 15, the highest daily faecal hair excretion observed was equivalent to the lowest faecal hair excretion in LH cats. The exposure to the diets (14 days) might also have been too short to obtain significant results.

CONCLUSIONS

The results of this study showed that dietary fibre significantly affects faecal hair excretion in LH cats over only 14 days, and outside shedding periods. Results obtained suggest that a diet containing psyllium husk and 11% or 15% TdF facilitates faecal excretion of hair in LH cats. Clinical studies are however required to determine whether such psyllium and TdF levels result in a significant reduction in hairball related clinical signs in cats.

In SH cats, 11% and 15% fibre levels combined with psyllium have no effect on faecal hair excretion. This could be explained by the low quantity of hair ingested by those animals outside the shedding season, by the relatively short duration of the study or by the small number of cats included in the study.

Therefore, future studies would be valuable to evaluate the effect of these diets during the shedding season in both short and LH cats, over a longer period of time and on a larger number of cats.

ACKNOWLEDGEMENT

The authors thank Sophie Clément for assistance in writing this manuscript.

CONFLICTS OF INTEREST

All authors were employees of Royal Canin at the time of writing the manuscript.

CONTRIBUTIONS

All authors were involved in the study design, in the collection, analysis and interpretation of data, in the writing of the manuscript and in the decision to sub-mit the manuscript for publication.

REFERENCES

1. Agnello K.A. & Kantrowitz L. (2003) Esophageal obstruction. Journal of the American Veterinary Medical Association 15, 1115–1116.
2. Barrs V.R., Beatty J.A., Tisdall P.L., Hunt G.B. & Gunew M. (1999) Intestinal obstruction by trichobezoars in five cats. Journal of Feline Medicine and Surgery 1, 199–207.
3. Benjamin L. (1976) Feline behavior. Feline Practice 7, 14–17.
4. Beynen A.C., Middelkoop J. & Saris D.H.J. (2011) Clinical signs of hairballs in cats fed a diet enriched with cellulose. American Journal of Animal and Veterinary Sciences 6, 69–72.
5. Burrows C.F., Kronfeld D.S., Banta C.A. & Merritt A.M. (1982) Effects of fibre on digestibility and transit time in dogs. Journal of Nutrition 112, 1726–1732.
6. Cannon M. (2013) Hair balls in cats, a normal nuisance or a sign that something is wrong. Journal of Feline Medicine and Surgery 15, 21–29.
7. Dann J.R., Adler M.A., Duffy K.L. & Giffard C.J. (2004) A potential nutritional prophylactic for the reduction of feline hairball symptoms. Journal of Nutrition 134, 2124S–2125S.
8. De Vos W.C. (1993) Migrating spike complex in the small intestine of the fasting cat. American Journal of Physiology 265, G619–G627.
9. Eckstein R.A. & Hart B.L. (2000a) The organization and control of grooming in cats. Applied Animal Behaviour Science 68, 131–140.
10. Eckstein R.A. & Hart B.L. (2000b) Grooming and control of fleas in cats. Applied Animal Behaviour Science 68, 141–150.
11. Fucci V., Pechman R.D., Hedlund C.S. & Venugopalan C.S. (1995) Large bowel transit times using radiopaque markers in normal cats. Journal of the American Animal Hospital Association 31, 473–477.
12. German A.J. & German A.C. (2013) Bad hair day. Journal of Feline Medicine and Surgery 15, 6–7.
13. Hendriks W.H., Tartellin M.F. & Moughan P.J. (1998) Seasonal hair loss in adult domestic cats (Felis catus). Journal of Animal Physiology and Animal Nutrition 79, 92–101.
14. Hernot D., Biourge V., Martin L., Dumon H. & Nguyen P. (2005) Relationship

between total transit time and faecal quality in adult dogs differing in body size. Journal of Animal Physiology and Animal Nutrition 89, 189– 193.

15. Panaman R. (1981) Behavior and ecology of free-ranging female farm cats (Felis catus L). Zeitschrift fur Tierpsy- € chologie 56, 59–73.
16. Peachey S.E., Dawson J.M. & Harper E.J. (2000) Gastrointestinal transit times in young and old cats. Comparative Biochemistry and Physiology Part A: Molecular & Integrative Physiology 126, 85–90.
17. Prola L., Dobenecker B. & Kienzle E. (2006) Interaction between dietary cellulose content and food intake in cats. Journal of Nutrition 136, 1988S–1990S.
18. Roche M., Bueno L., Vagne M. & Blourde C. (1982) Patterns of electrical activity in the digestive tract of the conscious cat. British Journal of Nutrition 48, 129–135.
19. Ryan C.P. & Wolfer J.J. (1978) Recurrent trichophytobezoar in a cat. Veterinary Medicine Small Animal Clinician 73, 891–893
20. Tournier C., Dumon H., Nguyen P., Biourge V. (2005) Dietary fiber stimulates fecal hair excretion in cats. Proceeding of the 9th European Society of Veterinary and Comparative Nutrition Congress 112, 27–28.
21. Willemse T., Mudde M., Josephy M. & Spruijt B.M. (1994) The effect of haloperidol and naloxone on excessive grooming behavior of cats. European Neuropsychopharmacology 4, 39–45.

4
CHAPTER

SEROPREVALENCE OF SCHMALLENBERG VIRUS INFECTION IN SHEEP AND GOATS FLOCKS IN GERMANY, 2012–2013

Carina Helmer[1], Regina Eibach[1], Esther Humann-Ziehank[1], Philip C. Tegtmeyer[1], Daniela Bürstel[2], Kathrin Mayer[3], Udo Moog[4], Sieglinde Stauch[5], Heinz Strobel[5], Katja Voigt[6], Philipp Sieber[6], Matthias Greiner[7,8], and Martin Ganter[1]

[1]Clinic for Swine and Small Ruminants, University of Veterinary Medicine Hannover, Foundation, Hannover, Germany

[2]Tierseuchenkasse (Animal Diseases Fund) Baden-Wuerttemberg, Fellbach, Germany

[3]Small Ruminant Health Service, Sächsische Tierseuchenkasse (Animal Diseases Fund), Dresden, Germany

[4]Animal Health Service Thuringia e.V., Thüringer Tierseuchenkasse (Animal Diseases Fund), Jena, Germany

[5]Schafpraxis (sheep veterinary practice) Stoffenried, Stoffenried, Germany

[6]Clinic for Ruminants, Ludwig Maximilians University (LMU) Munich, Oberschleißheim, Germany

[7]Federal Institute for Risk Assessment (BfR), Berlin, Germany

[8]University of Veterinary Medicine Hannover, Foundation, Hannover, Germany

SUMMARY

Schmallenberg virus (SBV) is a member of the family Bunyaviridae and mainly affects ruminants. It is transmitted by biting midges, first and foremost *Culicoides* spp., and causes congenital malformations reflected in arthrogryposis–hydranencephaly (AH) syndrome. The aim of this study was to collect data on the emergence of SBV as a new arthropod-borne disease introduced into Europe in 2011. Germany was located

---

Citation: Helmer, C., Eibach, R., Humann-Ziehank, E., Tegtmeyer, P. C., Bürstel, D., Mayer, K., Moog, U., Stauch, S., Strobel, H., Voigt, K., Sieber, P., Greiner, M. and Ganter, M. (2016), Seroprevalence of Schmallenberg virus infection in sheep and goats flocks in Germany, 2012–2013. Veterinary Medicine and Scienc, 2: 10–22. doi: 10.1002/vms3.14

in the core region of the 2011/2012 epidemic. Following two seroprevalence studies in the north-west of Germany in 2012, this study focused on the epidemiology and distribution of SBV throughout 130 small ruminant flocks in the whole country. Blood samples were obtained of 30 animals per flock and a SBV-specific questionnaire was used to collect operating data of the farms. The median within-herd seroprevalence for all 130 flocks tested was 53.3% with a total range from 0% to 100%. The median within-herd seroprevalence for goats was 30% [interquartile range (IQR): 40.3%] and 57% for sheep (IQR: 43.3%). Small ruminant flocks kept permanently indoors or housed overnight had a significantly lower seroprevalence than flocks kept permanently outdoors. In addition, this study revealed a significantly lower seroprevalence in the north-east of Germany. These results show that small ruminants in Germany are still at risk of contracting new SBV infections following incomplete seroconversion of flocks especially in the north-east of Germany. This might contribute to SBV becoming enzootic in central and northern Europe. Furthermore, the survey revealed that housing animals at least during mating and early pregnancy may reduce the risk of new SBV infections and may thus be an option to reduce losses as long as there is no licensed vaccine available on the German market.

INTRODUCTION

Schmallenberg virus (SBV) was first detected in Europe in autumn 2011. It was named after the place where the original isolate derived from, a town called Schmallenberg, located in the north-west of Germany. In autumn 2011, dairy cattle farmers from the Netherlands and Germany almost simultaneously reported disease outbreaks in their herds including mild fever, therapy-resistant diarrhoea and a reduction in milk yield (Hoffmann *et al.* 2012; Muskens *et al.* 2012). After ruling out several classical bovine endemic and emerging viruses as cause of these outbreaks, the Friedrich-Loeffler-Institute (FLI, Federal Research Institute for Animal Health, Germany) identified a new virus as causative agent utilising a meta-genomic approach with next-generation sequencing (Hoffmann *et al.* 2012). SBV belongs to the Simbu serogroup of the family Bunyaviridae, genus *Orthobunyaviruses* and is closely related to other arthropod-borne viruses, which are known to primarily infect ruminants such as Akabane, Sathuperi, Aino and Shamonda virus. All these viruses are transmitted by vectors such as mosquitoes and biting midges and can induce congenital malformations in neonates if a susceptible dam is infected during a vulnerable period in early pregnancy (Hoffmann *et al.* 2012).

In two real-time PCR (RT-PCR) studies on the occurrence of SBV-RNA in*Culicoides* subspecies (*C.* ssp.) performed in autumn 2011 in Belgium and Denmark, several *C.* ssp. (*C. obsoletus* complex, *C. dewulfi, C. chiopterus*) were tested positive for SBV, strongly suggesting that these species are relevant natural vectors for the virus (De Regge *et al.* 2012; Rasmussen*et al.* 2012).

Based on the pathogenesis of Akabane virus, it is believed that in small ruminants an infection between day 1 and 28 of gestation may lead to early embryonic death and abortion, followed by an increased rate of animals returning to oestrus. If infection takes place between day 28 and 56 of gestation, it might result in birth of congenitally malformed or stillborn lambs. Thus, this period represents the most critical period in pregnancy. After day 56 of gestation, the foetus becomes immunocompetent and has the ability to fight the virus with its matured immune system (The Center for Food and Security and Public Health, Iowa State University 2009). So far there is no evidence to refute the assumption that SBV infection induces a long-term immunity in affected animals, so that clinical signs can only be observed in ruminants infected for the first time [The European Food Safety Authority (EFSA), 2013]. Elbers *et al.* (2014) found that 80% of adult dairy cows still had measurable antibodies against SBV at least 24 months after the estimated introduction of the virus into the herd. This field study supports the assumption that natural SBV infection in adult cows induces a long-term immunity of at least 2 years. Whether these assumptions can be completely transferred to small ruminants remains to be clarified.

Typical congenital malformations can be summarised by the arthrogryposis–hydranencephaly (AH) syndrome, reflected in stiffening of the joints and cranial distension, spinal malformations (scoliosis, lordosis, kyphosis and torticollis) and brachygnathia or agnathia. Frequent pathomorphological findings are malformations of the central nervous system such as hydranencephaly, anencephaly, porencephaly, cerebellar hypoplasia and brain stem hypoplasia besides several musculoskeletal and vertebral malformations which are most likely a result of failures in the development of the central nervous system. True skeletal defects could not be observed in malformed neonates (Herder *et al.* 2012).

Two studies on the zoonotic potential of SBV conducted in Germany and in the Netherlands in 2012 revealed a lack of evidence for transmission of SBV to humans (Ducomble *et al.* 2012; Reusken *et al.* 2012).

From September 2011 until April 2013 more than 8000 holdings with laboratory confirmed SBV cases were recorded in 22 European countries [The European Food Safety Authority (EFSA), 2013]. The FLI provided case numbers and maps of the distribution and spread of approved SBV cases in Germany which were monthly updated from January 2012 until today. These maps revealed that the core region of the 2011/2012 epidemic was located in the north-west of Germany. First cases of SBV infection were not reported until winter 2012/2013 of federal states located more southerly or easterly. To date, 2504 SBV cases have been proven in Germany by RT-PCR with 1478 cattle herds, 973 sheep flocks and 53 goat flocks being SBV positive with a high estimate of unreported cases (FLI, Federal Research Institute for Animal Health, 24 March 2014). So far SBV has been detected by RT-PCR in cattle, sheep, goats, bison, deer, moose, buffalos, alpacas [The European Food Safety Authority (EFSA), 2013] and dogs (Sailleau *et al.* 2013).

Germany was located in the core region of the 2011/2012 epidemic. After two seroprevalence studies performed in the north-western parts of Germany (Helmer *et al.* 2013a,b) and another survey based on 462 sheep and 125 goat sera gained from 14 different German federal states (Wernike *et al.* 2014), this study focused on the epidemiology and distribution of SBV in small ruminant flocks throughout the entire German country. The main objectives were to possibly detect regional differences in inter-herd and within-herd prevalences and to check for the potential influence of certain variables on the within-herd prevalence [e.g. species, flock size, production type, location, type of wool (coarse wool, crossbred wool, fine wool, hair sheep/goats), treatment with repellents, housing management, exposure to wet- and/or woodland, other species kept on the farm with special focus on cattle].

MATERIALS AND METHODS

Germany is divided into 16 federal states whereof three states are free cities (Free Hanseatic City of Bremen, Free and Hanseatic City of Hamburg and Berlin). The total population size of small ruminants (sheep and goats) in Germany is 2,023,500 animals kept on 33,492 farms in March 2013 (Federal Statistical Office of Germany, 2013). In detail, 130,200 goats were housed on 10,800 farms and 1,893,300 sheep were housed on 20,000 farms with an average flock size of 12.06 in goats and 94.7 in sheep (Federal Statistical Office of Germany, 2013). The three free cities were not taken into consideration for this serosurvey as the sheep and goat population in these areas are extremely low (in total 200 goats and 3600 sheep). With an assumed true prevalence of 10%, an assumed test sensitivity of 90% and specificity of 99.75% (according to the manufacturer's instructions), a confidence level of 95% and a desired precision of 20%, the sample size to estimate the true prevalence was 10 flocks per federal state (AusVet. Animal Health Services: EpiTools – epidemiological Calculators, 2013). One hundred and thirty small ruminant holdings were therefore tested from the 13 remaining federal states. These comprised 27 goat and 103 sheep flocks. Herd size ranged from 10 to 2200 in goats and 15 to 2100 in sheep. Venous blood samples were taken from 30 animals per flock (population size: 2,238,477, confidence level: 95%, assumed true prevalence: 10%). If there were less than 30 animals on the farm all adult females were tested. A SBV-specific questionnaire was used to collect information on potential risk factors (RFs) at the time of blood sampling. The questionnaire had been pre-tested and adapted after previous studies (Helmer *et al.* 2013a,b).

Ethic statement

The samples were taken in accordance with the principles outlined by the European Convention for the Protection of Vertebrate Animals used for experimental and other scientific purposes. Most of the blood samples were taken by veterinarians of the University of Veterinary Medicine Hannover, Foundation with help of veterinarians of the Clinic for Ruminants, LMU Munich (Bavaria) and of the Small Ruminant Health Services of the federal states of Baden-Wuerttemberg, Saxony and Thuringia, as well as by veterinarians of a private practice (Schafpraxis Stoffenried, Bavaria, Germany).

Samples

Between January and the beginning of October 2013, a total of 3779 serum samples were obtained from female sheep and goats (>1 year) in 13 German federal states. One hundred and fifteen of the 130 tested sheep and goat holdings were visited between January and May 2013 representing the vector season 2012. The remaining 15 farms were visited during the summer period representing the vector period 2013. The 15 flocks sampled during the summer months were evenly distributed over the study area. Blood samples were taken from the *vena jugularis externa* or the *vena cava cranialis*

(Ganter*et al.* 2001). The blood was centrifuged at 10,000 *g* for 10 min and the serum was stored at −18°C until analysis.

ELISA

Serum samples were analysed for the presence of antibodies against SBV using a commercial ELISA (ID Screen®, SBV Indirect; IDvet Laboratories, Montpellier, France) according to the manufacturer›s instructions. The test can be used with individual bovine, ovine and caprine serum or plasma.

SBV-specific questionnaire (Supplementary Material)

Participating farmers were interviewed to complete a SBV-specific questionnaire to collect information on potential RFs at the time of blood sampling. The questionnaire was filled in by the veterinarian who visited the flock and obtained the blood samples which was in >75% of the cases the first author herself. The evaluation of the questionnaire data was performed by the first author only. The questionnaire had been pre-tested and adapted following previous studies (Helmer *et al.* 2013a,b). Information was gathered on species, flock size, location, breed, type of wool, production type, clinical signs of SBV infection, RT-PCR results (if existing), treatment with repellents, deworming management, vaccinations, additional treatments, other known health problems, housing conditions, exposure to wetland/woodland, other animals kept on the farm (e.g. cattle), mating period, number of lambs per ewe, number of lambs born alive, number of abortions, number of stillbirths, number of malformed lambs and clinical signs in adult animals during the possible time of first SBV infection (fever, languor, reduced milk yield, diarrhoea).

Statistical analysis

Explorative statistical analyses were performed using SAS 9.1 (SAS Institute Inc, Cary, NC, USA). Putative RF for infection were investigated using the herd-level serological response (*k* out of *n* animals tested positive) as outcome by means of a fixed effects logistic regression for grouped (i.e. flocks) binomially scaled observations (R command glm, R) (R Core Team, 2014). The final model was obtained after stepwise backwards elimination of variables based on the Akaike's information criterion (AIC) (compared to a chi-squared statistic). This final model was also fitted with a random effects term on the level of the flock (R command glmmML) (Broström 2014). Multilevel RF where introduced into the model by choosing a suitable reference category. Statistical significance was assumed if the *P*-values were 5% or below.

RESULTS

Clinical signs

Forty-nine per cent of the farmers ($n = 66$) reported higher than usual proportions of abortions and stillbirths as well as lambs born with congenital malformations consistent with intrauterine SBV infection. Forty-eight per cent of these ($n = 31$) only reported individual cases of malformed neonates (1–5 cases per flock). Twenty-eight per cent ($n = 18$) reported 5–20 cases of congenital malformation, 11.5% ($n = 7$) reported 20–50 cases per flock and 12.5% ($n = 8$) of the farmers reported massive losses due to intrauterine SBV infections with more than 50 lambs showing typical signs of AH syndrome. The congenital malformations observed in the flocks can mainly be summarised as AH syndrome with lambs showing stiffening and deformation of the joints and of the vertebral column as well as cranial distension. Brachygnathia and agnathia were also frequently observed. In many cases the malformed foetuses led to dystocia resulting in higher numbers of caesarean sections and fetotomies. Some ewes died or had to be euthanised due to dystocia. These problems during parturition often resulted in endometritis followed by reduced fertility in the next mating season. None of the farmers reported clinical signs in adult small ruminants during viremia as described for cattle (mild fever, languor, reduced milk yield and diarrhoea) (Muskens*et al.* **2012**). Only a small number of flocks ($n = 9$) suffered from losses due to SBV infections in two consecutive years. None of these farmers repeatedly observed malformed offspring from one and the same animal. These statements were derived from the answers to the questionnaire and could not be followed up by the veterinarians.

Serological response

The median within-herd prevalence for all 130 flocks tested was 53.3% with a range from 0% to 100%. A significantly lower median within-herd prevalence of 30% (IQR: 40.3%) was observed in goat flocks ($n = 27$) compared to sheep flocks ($n = 103$), where a median of 57% (IQR: 43.3%) of the animals were seropositive (Fig. 1). Two sheep and four goat flocks were seronegative for SBV antibodies. Both sheep flocks were located in the north-eastern state of Brandenburg, administrative district Maerkisch-Oderland. The four goat flocks were located in the eastern German federal states Brandenburg, Mecklenburg Western-Pomerania, Saxony and Saxony-Anhalt. All seronegative goat flocks were dairy goats and were either kept indoors all year round or stabled during the night. On one goat and two sheep farms all animals sampled for this survey tested positive for SBV antibodies (seroprevalence of 100%). All three of these farms were located in the Western part of the country, in the Saarland ($n = 2$) and North Rhine-Westphalia ($n = 1$). All these flocks were kept outdoors all year round with only a shed for shelter. The calculated median within-herd prevalences for the different federal states are as follows (listed from north to south): Schleswig-Holstein (SH) 40%, Mecklenburg Western-Pomerania (MV) 36%, Lower Saxony (NI) 42%, Brandenburg (BB) 10%, Saxony-Anhalt (ST) 23%, North Rhine-Westphalia (NRW) 67%, Hesse (HE) 73%, Thuringia (TH) 48%, Saxony (SN) 59%, Rhineland-Palatinate (RP) 52%, Saarland (SL) 65%, Baden-Wuerttemberg (BW) 70% and Bavaria (BY) 68% (Fig. 2). We divided the Federal Republic of Germany into the four regions northeast (NE: BB, MV, ST), northwest (NW: NI, NRW, SH), southeast (SE: BY, SN, TH) and southwest (SW: BW, HE, RP, SL) for a more illustrative presentation. According to Eurostat, 12,685,990 heads of livestock were kept on German farms in December 2013 (European Commission: Eurostat Data Explorer, 2013), 5,234,050 of these animals are kept on farms in the NW of Germany (41.4%), 4,088,290 are kept on farms in the SE of

Germany (32.3%), 1,880,890 are kept on farms located in the SW of Germany (14.8%) and 1,465,410 heads of livestock are kept on farms located in the NE of Germany (11.5%). Regarding sheep and goats 657,900 (34%) are kept in the SE, 565.300 (28%) are reared in the NW, 521,000 (25%) sheep and goats are kept in the SW and 269,100 (13%) in the NE of Germany (Federal Statistical Office of Germany, **2013**). The calculated median within-herd prevalences for these regions are given in Figure 3.

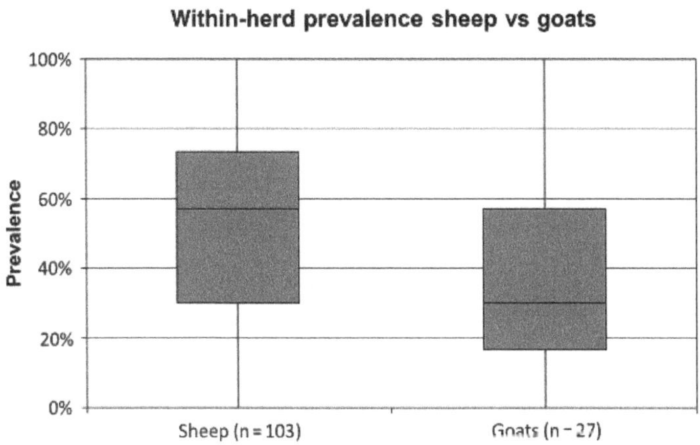

Figure 1: Comparison of the median within-herd prevalence of sheep and goats; the difference concerning the median within-herd prevalence was statistically significant in a regression model without random effect on flock basis ($P = 0.00308$).

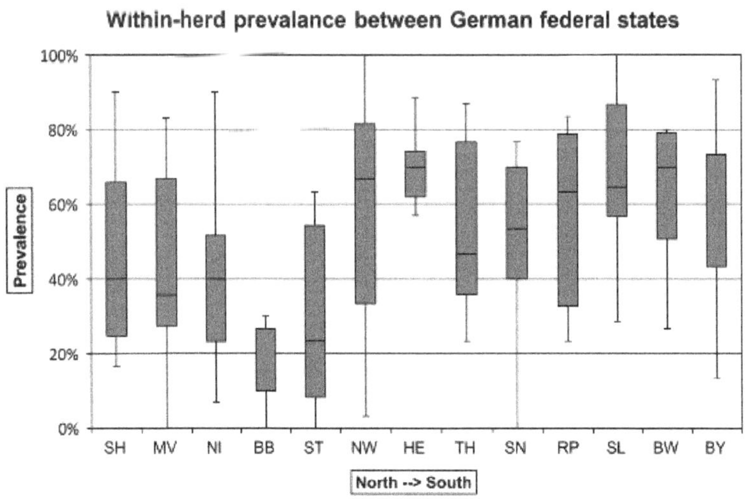

Figure 2: Comparison of the median within-herd prevalences of the different federal states of Germany listed from north to south. SH, Schleswig-Holstein; MV, Mecklenburg Western-Pomerania; NI, Lower Saxony; BB, Brandenburg; ST, Saxony-Anhalt; NW, North Rhine-Westphalia; HE, Hesse; TH, Thuringia; SN, Saxony; RP, Rhineland-Palatinate; SL, Saarland; BW, Baden-Wuerttemberg; BY, Bavaria.

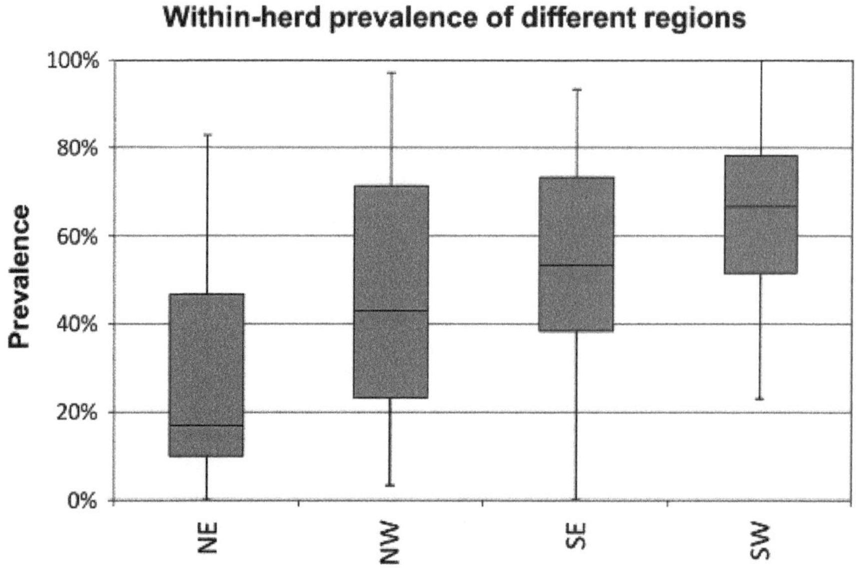

Figure 3: Comparison of regional differences in the distribution of Schmallenberg virus (SBV) infection throughout Germany. NE, north-east; NW, north-west; SE, south-east; SW, south-west; the NE of Germany is significantly less affected by SBV infection than the other regions of Germany in both logistic regression models (P-value without random effect on flock basis = 9.3×10^{-8}; P-value with random effect on flock basis = 0.005).

Questionnaire results

Sixty per cent of the flocks (n = 77) included in this survey are kept for environmental grazing projects and meat production. Twenty per cent are kept for milk production (n = 27) or as hobby breeding animals (n = 26), respectively. Roughly 60% of the farmers treated their flocks against external parasites (n = 77). More than 80% of these used products containing deltamethrin as active agent (n = 64). Ten farmers used products containing phoxim as active agent and four farmers used alternative treatments such as neem oil or garlic compounds. Only 4% (n = 5) of the farmers treated their animals during the mating period or early gestation. On most farms the animals were treated after shearing which is generally performed in spring. RT-PCR results were available for 19 flocks. Lambs of 15 of these were tested positive for SBV by RT-PCR, while lambs submitted from the other four were tested negative despite all submitted foetuses showing evident clinical signs of congenital malformations consistent with SBV infection. Eighty per cent of the flocks (n = 102) included in the study were kept permanently outdoors and were only housed for lambing, whereas 5% were kept permanently indoors throughout the entire year (n = 8). The remaining 15% were regularly housed during the night (n = 20). Thirty per cent of the farmers interviewed stated that their farms and pastures were located in dry areas not adjacent to stagnant water or woodland (n = 40). Another 30% reported that their farm and pastures were located close to wetland (n = 36), while 20% responded that their farm area and pastures were located close to woodland ($n = 27$). The remaining 20% stated that their farms and pastures were surrounded by both wet- and woodland ($n = 27$). The presence of other ruminant species was also of interest. Forty per cent of the farmers interviewed stated that their sheep and goats did not have any contact with other animals, except wildlife such as deer and wild boar or companion animals such as cats and dogs ($n = 51$). Of the remaining farms, 40% also kept cattle ($n = 33$) and 22% of the sheep farmers also kept goats ($n = 17$). Four of the 103 sheep flocks came into contact with transhumance flocks. One sheep farmer kept a herd of bison on his farm. In addition, several small ruminant flocks, especially the hobby flocks, were kept together with horses, donkeys, swine and poultry.

Risk analysis of RFs of SBV infection

The final fixed effect and random effect logistic regression models, denoted as FEM (residual deviance 731.49 on 114 degrees of freedom; AIC: 1185) and REM (residual deviance of 369 on 111 degrees of freedom; AIC: 407), respectively, contained seven explanatory variables (Table 1). Sheep flocks showed a higher level of SBV infection than goat flocks (significant in FEM but not in REM). Flock sizes of 1–56, 57–255, 251–500 and >500 animals were categorised into the quartiles Q1, Q2, Q3 and Q4, respectively. Large flocks (third and fourth quartiles) displayed a lower level of SBV infections than small (first quartile) flocks (significant in FEM, but not in REM). Flocks located in the north-east of Germany showed a lower level of SBV infections than flocks located in the north-west of Germany (significant in both FEM and REM). Flocks located in the south-east (SE) and the south-west (SW) of Germany displayed a higher risk of SBV infections than flocks located in the north-west of Germany (SE: significant in FEM, but not in REM; SW: significant in both FEM and REM). The production type was not included in the final model due to lack of significance. The type of wool showed no statistically significant differences in the final models. Farms using deltamethrin pour on treatments revealed a lower level of SBV infection compared to flocks where deltamethrin was not used against external parasites (significant in both FEM and REM). Flocks kept permanently indoors or housed overnight showed a lower level of SBV infection than those kept permanently outdoors (significant in both FEM and REM). Flocks exposed to both wetland and forest/woodland and those exposed to forest/woodland only displayed a higher level for SBV infection than those without any exposure (wetland and woodland: significant in both FEM and REM; forest/woodland: significant in FEM, but not in REM). No significant effects were found for exposure to wetlands only. The presence of cattle on the premises was not included in the final models due to lack of significance.

Table 1: Results of the fixed effects (FEM) and random effects (REM) logistic regression models to investigate risk factors for SBV infection in German goat and sheep flocks

Risk factor (reference)	FEM		REM	
	Estimate	*P*-value	Estimate	*P*-value
Intercept	−0.16	0.350	−0.29	0.530
Species (goat)				
Sheep	0.58	0.002**	0.77	0.110
Flock size (Q1)†				
Q2	0.21	0.067	0.31	0.290
Q3	−0.47	0.000***	−0.42	0.180
Q4	−0.35	0.007**	−0.28	0.420
Location (NW)				
NE	−0.66	0.000***	−0.91	0.003**
SE	0.46	0.000***	0.52	0.091
SW	0.56	0.000***	0.66	0.025*
Type of wool (hair)				
Coarse	−0.24	0.253	−0.37	0.520
Crossbred	0.14	0.398	0.02	0.960
Fine	−0.19	0.296	−0.44	0.370
Treatment (none)				
Butox	−0.56	0.000***	−0.62	0.014*
Other	−0.11	0.283	−0.10	0.710
Housing (no)				
Night	−0.86	0.000***	−0.95	0.005**
Yes	−1.66	0.000***	−2.09	0.000***
Exposure (none)				
Forest and wetland	0.73	0.000***	0.85	0.005**
Forest	0.36	0.001***	0.51	0.069
Wetland	−0.08	0.446	−0.01	0.960

$^*P \leq 0.05$, $^{**}P \leq 0.01$, $^{***}P \leq 0.001$. †Flock size has been categorised into four quartiles (Q1–Q4).

DISCUSSION

While most conducted seroprevalence studies on SBV focused on cattle, the focus of this serosurvey was on the distribution and epidemiology of the disease in small ruminants which were more affected by SBV infection than cattle. Dominguez *et al.* (2014) found that congenital SBV morbidity was on average moderate, although higher in sheep than in other ruminant species. They estimated typical congenital SBV deformities of 8% in lambs, 3% in calves and 2% in goat kids, respectively. A study focusing on the impact of SBV on British sheep farms found a mortality of 10.4% for lambs born on farms where SBV infection was confirmed. Moreover, they found that 25% of farmers where SBV was confirmed or suspected perceived a high impact of SBV on emotional well-being and that 13% of these farmers believed that the disease would have a large impact on flock welfare and financial performance (Harris *et al.* 2014). Two previous seroprevalence studies focusing on small ruminants were performed in north-western parts of Germany in 2012 (Helmer *et al.* 2013a,b). Moreover, the FLI conducted a seroprevalence study in cattle and small ruminants for which 462 sheep and 125 goat sera were obtained from 14 different federal states in 2012 (Wernike *et al.* 2014). The study area for this seroprevalence study was extended to the entire German country with the aim of gaining additional insight into the developments of SBV infection in small ruminants in the north-west as well as to ascertain whether and how much the infection had spread to southern and eastern parts of Germany in 2013. In addition, the present study focused on potential RFs for SBV infection which were assessed by questionnaire.

The estimated seroprevalence of antibodies against SBV in dairy cows in the Netherlands was 72.5% (Elbers *et al.* 2012) and 90.8% for cattle in Belgium (Garigliany *et al.* 2012) in 2012. A serosurvey conducted in France in winter 2011–2012 revealed seroprevalences of 90% for cattle herds and 30% for sheep flocks in highly affected areas (Gache *et al.* 2014). A seroprevalence study focusing on ruminants performed in Germany in 2012 revealed an average seroprevalence among German cattle, sheep and goats of 61%, 24.7% and 26.4%, respectively. In the core region of the epidemic in north-western Germany up to 98% of the animals tested positive for SBV antibodies (Wernike *et al.* 2014). The median within-herd prevalence calculated for German small ruminant holdings in this seroprevalence study was 30% (IQR: 40.3%) for goats and 57% for sheep (IQR: 43.3%) (Fig. 1). Small ruminant flocks seem therefore to be less exposed to SBV than cattle during the recent SBV outbreak in Europe.

This seroprevalence study confirmed earlier findings (Helmer *et al.* 2013a,b; Veldhuis *et al.* 2013a) revealing that goat flocks have a lower risk of contracting SBV infection than sheep flocks. This species-specific statistically significant difference in within-herd prevalence of sheep and goat flocks is, however, no longer sustainable in a logistic regression model with random effect on flock basis. The within-herd seroprevalence for SBV in Belgium was estimated at 84.3% for sheep and 40.7% for goats (Méroc *et al.* 2013), showing similar results for goat flocks to those observed in the current survey, whereas the within-herd prevalence for sheep was much higher in Belgium than in Germany. Veldhuis *et al.* (2013a) found a within-herd prevalence of 89% in sheep and 50.8% showing that a sheep flock had a 13.7 times higher odds to be seropositive than a goat herd. The aforementioned study of Wernike *et al.* (2014) revealed an average seroprevalence of 24.7% in sheep and 26.4% in goats, not showing any difference concerning the within-herd prevalence of these two small ruminant species. The difference in seroprevalence between sheep and goat flocks found in this survey is probably due to the fact that 74% of the goat flocks tested were dairy herds (20 out of 27) and were therefore kept permanently indoors or at least housed overnight (18 out of 27). Both models used for statistical analyses of the obtained data revealed a significantly lower risk of SBV infection for small ruminants permanently stabled or at least housed overnight. This finding is statistically confirmed using a fixed effects model (FEM), but not using a random effects model (REM). The application of a REM has been recommended for studying RFs in farmed animals to account for the clustering of animals in herds or flocks (McDermott & Shukken 1994). The results of the FEM can be regarded as indicative while conclusions should be based on the REM. Thus, the present study does not provide conclusive evidence for a differential risk of seropositivity between sheep and goats. The lower seroprevalence in goat flocks compared to sheep flocks is therefore probably due to the housing system rather than a species-specific factor. This is supported by the observation that several goat flocks which were permanently kept outdoors throughout the entire year showed seroprevalences for SBV antibodies of 70% and more (n = 3). The four goat flocks that were serologically negative for SBV were all dairy goat flocks and therefore kept permanently indoors or housed overnight. In the Belgian seroprevalence study the housing management is not reported so the possible influence of housing on seroprevalence could not be addressed (Méroc *et al.* 2013). According to a personal communication of Stephen Valas and Anses Niort cited by Wernike *et al.* (2014), the between-herd seroprevalence of goats located in the central–western parts of France was 62%. Differences between extensive and intensive goat farming was noticed in this study as well.

As reported by other groups, cattle seem to be more exposed to biting midges than small ruminants even when they are kept permanently indoors. The reasons for these differences concerning the within-herd prevalences of cattle and small ruminants might be explained as follows:

- Different host preferences of the vectors: Most *Culicoides* (*C.*) spp. prefer to feed on cattle if present (Bartsch *et al.* 2009; Lassen*et al.* 2011, 2012; Ninio *et al.* 2011). The thick fleece of sheep makes the reachable surface for midge bites fairly small as only non-woollen areas of the skin or those with a short hair coat such as the udder, the inner shank and thigh, the interdigital skin, the head and the bottom side of the tail are approachable for bites by *C.* spp. Possibly the species-specific odour of goats might be a reason for the lower attractiveness for biting midges compared to cattle and sheep.
- Different housing conditions and uses: Most small ruminant flocks in Germany are kept extensively on pasture day and night. The main reasons for sheep farming are landscape protection, meat production and breeding, while the main reasons for goat farming are milk production and breeding. The only time of year when animals are stabled is during the lambing period. Exceptions are dairy sheep and goats, which are mainly kept indoors on deep litter year round or are at least housed during the night. It is expected that animals kept outdoors are more exposed to vectors than animals kept indoors, which could also be shown by Baylis *et al.* (2010). In addition, grazing has been identified as a potential RF for bluetongue disease, which is another vector-borne disease transmitted by *C.* spp. (Santman-Berends *et al.* 2010). This study confirmed findings of a previous survey (Helmer *et al.* 2013a) revealing that permanently housed sheep and goat flocks were considerably less affected by SBV infection than flocks kept permanently outdoors. Thus, housing of animals, at least during the night, is an adequate method to reduce SBV infection in small ruminants. In contrast to most small ruminant flocks, German cattle herds are mainly kept indoors year round on slatted floors with cesspools below for the storage of dung. Although most cattle are permanently housed throughout the entire year, the reported

seroprevalences are much higher for cattle than for sheep and goats (Elbers *et al.* 2012; Garigliany *et al.* 2012; Gache *et al.* 2014; Wernike *et al.* 2014). This is most probably due to the storage of the liquid and nutrient-rich manure which provides perfect conditions for the reproduction and development of *C.* spp. Several studies outlined that *C.* spp. breed in cattle manure and may even use it for hibernation (Meiswinkel *et al.* 2008; Zimmer *et al.* 2008). In contrast, no larval stages of biting midges could be found in sheep manure or soil inside sheep barns (Gonzáles *et al.* 2013). Veldhuis *et al.* (2013b) found that cattle herds that were grazed in 2011 had increased odds of a high seroprevalence for SBV compared to cattle herds that were kept indoors. Moreover, when animals were grazed in 2011, the odds of malformations in newborn calves tended to be 2.6 times higher compared to herds in which cattle was kept indoors. However, the study also revealed that keeping cattle indoors year round did not prevent SBV infection as an average within-herd prevalence of 63.9% was found in herds that stated not to have been grazed in 2011.

The presence of other animals on the same farm area, namely cattle, could not be identified as a RF for SBV infection. Several authors indicated that *C.* spp. prefer to feed on cattle rather than on small ruminants (Bartsch *et al.* 2009; Lassen *et al.* 2011, 2012; Ninio *et al.* 2011). Nevill (1978) stated that keeping cattle near sheep appear to have appreciably reduced the incidence of bluetongue disease in sheep. This could not be confirmed for SBV in our study.

This study found that large sheep and goat flocks (third and fourth quartiles) displayed a lower level of SBV infections than small (first quartile) flocks. These findings could be confirmed by Veldhuis *et al.* (2013a) who also found a significantly lower mean seroprevalence in large sheep and goat flocks compared to small ones.

The logistic regression models indicated a lower level of SBV infections in the NE of Germany compared to the NW, SW and SE, putting them at greater risk of infection in the future season. First outbreaks of the new viral disease were reported almost simultaneously in the NW of Germany and in the Netherlands in autumn 2011 (Hoffmann *et al.* 2012; Muskens *et al.* 2012). The core region of the epidemic during the lambing season 2011/2012 was also located in the north-western parts of Germany. Due to an incomplete infection of small ruminant flocks in this first season, the viral disease spread to southern and eastern parts of Germany in 2012/2013 which can be monitored on the homepage of the FLI, which provides case numbers and maps of the spread of SBV throughout Germany from January 2011 until today (FLI, Federal Research Institute for Animal Health, 24 March 2014). As this serosurvey shows, small ruminant flocks in north-eastern parts of Germany [Brandenburg (BB), Mecklenburg Western-Pomerania (MV) and Saxony-Anhalt (ST)] had significantly lower median within-herd prevalences (17%) than the other regions (NW: 46.5%, SE: 58%, SW: 67%) and are therefore still at risk of SBV outbreaks during the next lambing seasons. BB had the lowest median within-herd prevalence of all federal states with 10%. Two sheep flocks and one goat flock tested in BB were seronegative for SBV antibodies. Both sheep flocks were located in the administrative district Maerkisch-Oderland close to the Polish border. Both flocks were kept permanently outdoors close to dykes of the river

Oder and were only stabled during the lambing period. Several seroprevalence studies performed in small ruminants, cattle and elk in Poland showed that SBV had already entered Poland (Kaba *et al.* 2013; Larska *et al.* 2013a,b). Even more Eastern countries such as Turkey had reported cases of SBV infections (Azkur *et al.* 2013; Yilmaz *et al.* 2014). The seronegative goat flock was a dairy flock which was kept indoors overnight. This might explain why the flock did not come into contact with the virus-transmitting vectors. It seems that SBV did not occur in the NE of Germany at such a high level as in the other regions although there are many large woods, rivers and lakes located in these federal states. Similar observations were made during the bluetongue epidemic, which hit Germany in 2006/2007, when the north-eastern parts of Germany were less affected by bluetongue virus (BTV) than the other parts of the country [Friedrich-Loeffler-Institute (FLI), Federal Research Institute for Animal Health, Germany 2009]. Hesse (HE), which is located in the middle of Germany, had the highest median within-herd prevalence of all German federal states with 73%, followed by Baden-Wuerttemberg with 70% and Bavaria with 68%. It seems that especially the SE (58%) and the SW (67%) of Germany were affected by this new emerging disease. A possible explanation for these findings might be the livestock density of the individual federal states. On the basis of the livestock density, we would expect the lowest within-herd prevalence in the NE of Germany as this region has the lowest livestock density and should therefore not be as attractive for biting midges as other regions of the country. Moreover, we would expect the other regions to be affected in the following order (from low to high): SW, SE and NW. On the basis of the numbers of sheep and goats reared in these regions, we would expect the SE to be most affected, followed by the NW and SW. However, the serology results revealed that the SW of Germany has the highest median within-herd prevalence throughout the country. Hence, livestock density might have an influence on the within-flock prevalence as seen in the NE of Germany, but other factors must also be involved. Wernike*et al.* (2014) obtained 462 sheep and 125 goat sera from 14 different federal states for their serosurvey conducted in 2012. They found the lowest seroprevalence for goats in MV which is also located in the north-east of Germany. The highest within-herd prevalence for goats was found in Schleswig-Holstein which is located in the North of the country. No data are available for goat holdings located in the states Bavaria, Hamburg, Hesse and Thuringia. For sheep, the lowest within-herd prevalence was also found in MV and the highest seroprevalence was found in Rhineland-Palatinate followed by North Rhine-Westphalia. No data are available for sheep holdings located in Hamburg or Thuringia. Thus, the survey of Wernicke *et al.* confirms findings revealed in the current study showing that the lowest seroprevalences for sheep and goat holdings could be found in north-eastern parts of Germany.

None of the models revealed a significant difference regarding the production type of the flocks. We would have expected a lower risk for dairy sheep and goats compared to the other production types, as most dairy flocks are kept permanently indoors or are at least housed overnight. They should therefore be better protected against *C.* spp. due to the housing management. However, this effect might be masked by the housing variable in the multivariable model.

Both models showed a statistically significant difference regarding the treatment with repellents. Farms with flocks treated with products containing deltamethrin as an active agent against external parasites were at a lower risk for SBV infection than flocks that were treated with other pharmaceutical products or that were not treated at all. Deltamethrin is a pyrethroid ester insecticide and a neurotoxin, which induces paralysis and convulsions resulting in death of the insects after absorption. It needs to be mentioned that none of the farmers treated their flocks during the mating period or during early pregnancy so that protection against SBV due to treatment with repellents is not absolutely proven.

As most small ruminants are kept out on pasture day and night with only a shed for shelter against adverse weather conditions, they are not protected against biting midges during the main flight time. Exceptions are dairy sheep and goats which are mainly kept permanently indoors or at least housed indoors overnight. Both logistic regression models revealed a higher risk of SBV infection for flocks that were exposed to both wet- and woodland. Due to the fact that *C.* spp. develop aquatically and are dependent on humid substrate, it is hardly surprising that flocks with an exposure to wet- and woodland have a higher risk of contracting SBV infection than flocks without any exposure to wet- and/or woodland. In summary, this study shows that German sheep and goat flocks are still at risk of contracting new SBV infections due to incomplete seroconversion of flocks especially in the north-eastern parts of Germany. This might contribute to establishing an enzootic situation in central and northern Europe for SBV. Furthermore, this survey showed that small ruminant flocks that are housed permanently or at least kept indoors overnight have a lower risk of contracting SBV infection than flocks kept permanently outdoors. Housing animals at least during mating and early pregnancy might therefore reduce the risk of new SBV infection during the critical time of early gestation. Housing might therefore be a valuable tool to protect small ruminants against SBV, while there is no vaccine available in the German market.

Since SBV very recently entered Europe in autumn 2011, further studies are needed to understand the pathogenesis of the disease and to find possible routes of entry into central and northern Europe. Further studies are also needed to ascertain the so far assumed hypothesis of long-term immunity in adults. The field study of Elbers *et al.* (2014) revealed a persistence of SBV-specific antibodies in adult cows for at least 24 months. Whether these findings can be extrapolated to small ruminants remains to be clarified. Furthermore, it would be useful to investigate after which time specific antibodies against SBV start to decline. Since two vector-borne diseases have hit Europe in recent years (BTV and SBV), more studies on the biology and distribution of biting midges are needed to gain more detailed knowledge about these species which might be potential carriers of not only animal pathogens, but also their potential role in transmission of human pathogens.

ACKNOWLEDGEMENTS

The authors are very grateful for the excellent laboratory technical assistance given by the laboratory staff of the Clinic for Swine and Small Ruminants of the University of Veterinary Medicine Hannover, Foundation. Special thanks go to Christina Boss. Furthermore, we would like to use this opportunity to thank the Small Ruminant Health Services, the Chambers of Agriculture and the Tierseuchenkassen (animal diseases fund) of the following federal states: BW, MV, SN, ST, TH and RP for helping us collect blood samples and establish contact to sheep and goat farms in their states. Moreover, we wish to thank Frances Sherwood-Brock for reading the English manuscript. We also use this opportunity to thank all farmers of the 130 flocks investigated for the study for their support.

CONFLICT OF INTEREST

The authors declare that they have no competing interests.

REFERENCES

1. AusVet. Animal Health Services: EpiTools – epidemiological Calculators (2013) Available at: http://epitools.ausvet.com.au/content.php?page=PrevalenceSS (accessed 15 January 2013).
2. Azkur A.K., Albayarek H., Risvanli A., Pestil Z., Ozan E., Yilmaz O. *et al.* (2013) Antibodies to Schmallenberg virus in domestic livestock in Turkey. *Tropical Animal Health and Production* 45, 1825–1828.
3. Bartsch S., Bauer B., Wiemann A., Clausen P.H. & Steuber S. (2009) Feeding patterns of biting midges of the *Culicoides obsoletus* and *Culicoides pulicaris* groups on selected farms in Brandenburg, Germany. *Parasitology Research* 105, 373–380.
4. Baylis M., Parkin H., Kreppel K., Carpenter S., Mellor P.S. & McIntyre K.M. (2010)Evaluation of housing as a means to protect cattle from *Culicoides* biting midges, the vectors of bluetongue virus. *Medical and Veterinary Entomology* 24, 38–45.
5. Broström G. (2014) Package 'glmmML': Generalized linear models with clustering. Available at: http://cran.r-project.org/web/packages/glmmML/glmmML.pdf (accessed 5 July 2014).
6. De Regge N., Deblauwe I., De Deken R., Vantieghem P., Madder M., Geysen D. *et al.* (2012) Detection of Schmallenberg virus in different *Culicoides ssp.* by real-time RT-PCR. *Transboundary and Emerging Diseases* 59, 471–475.
7. Dominguez M., Gache K., Touratier A., Perrin J.B., Fediaevsky A., Collin E. *et al.* (2014)Spread and impact of the Schmallenberg virus epidemic in France 2012–2013. *BMC Veterinary Research* 10, 248.
8. Ducomble T., Wilking H., Stark K., Takla A., Askar M., Schaade L. *et al.* (2012) Lack of evidence for Schmallenberg virus infection in highly exposed persons, Germany, 2012.*Emerging Infectious Diseases* 18, 1333–1335.
9. Elbers A.R.W., Loeffen W.L.A., Quak S., De Boer-Luijtze E., Van Der Spek A.N., Bouwstra R. *et al.* (2012) Seroprevalence of Schmallenberg virus antibodies among dairy cattle, the Netherlands, Winter 2011–2012. *Emerging Infectious Diseases* 18, 1065–1071.
10. Elbers A.R.W., Stockhofe-Zurwieden N. & van der Poel W.H.M. (2014) Schmallenberg virus antibody persistence in adult cattle after natural infection

and decay of maternal antibodies in calves. *BMC Veterinary Research* 10, 103.

11. European Commission: Eurostat Data Explorer (2013) Lifestock Holding in December after NUTS-2-regions: Available at http://appsso.eurostat.ec.europa.eu/nui/show.do?dataset=agr_r_animal&lang=de (accessed 30 May 2014).
12. Federal Statistical Office of Germany (2013) Livestock Holding of farms – survey of agricultural structure fachserie 3 reihe 2.1.3 – 2013. Available at:https://www.destatis.de/DE/Publikationen/Thematisch/LandForstwirtschaft/ViehbestandTierischeErzeugung/Viehhaltung2030213109004.pdf?_blob=publicationFile (accessed 15 January 2014).
13. Friedrich-Loeffler-Institute (FLI), Federal Research Institute for Animal Health, Germany (2015) Schmallenberg virus. Available at:http://www.fli.bund.de/de/startseite/aktuelles/tierseuchengeschehen/schmallenberg-virus.html (accessed 24 March 2015).
14. Friedrich-Loeffler-Institute (FLI), Federal Research Institute for Animal Health, Germany (2009) Qualitative risk assessment to the abolition of the mandatory vaccination against bluetongue disease, serotype 8, in 2010. Available at:http://www.fli.bund.de/fileadmin/dam_uploads/tierseuchen/Risikobewertung_Impfung_BTV-8_091007.pdf (accessed 25 June 2014).
15. Gache K., Dominguez M., Pelletier C., Petit E., Calavas D., Hendrikx P. & Touratier A.(2014) Schmallenberg virus: a seroprevalence survey in cattle and sheep, France, winter 2011–2012. *The Veterinary Record* 173, 141.
16. Ganter M., Hermann J. & Waibl H. (2001) Blood sampling from the vena cava cranialis in sheep and goat using sampling systems armed by canula. *Tierarztl Prax Ausg G Grosstiere Nutztiere* 29, 37–40.
17. Garigliany M.M., Bayrou C, Kleijnen D, Cassart D, Desmecht D, 2012. Schmallenberg virus in domestic cattle, Belgium, 2012. *Emerging Infectious Diseases* 18, 1512–1514.
18. Gonzáles M., López S., Mullens B.A., Baldet T. & Goldarazena A. (2013) A survey of*Culicoides* developmental sites on a farm in northern Spain, with a brief review of immature habitats of European species. *Veterinary Parasitology* 191, 81–93.
19. Harris K.A., Eglin R.D., Hayward S., Milnes A., Davies I., Cook A.J.C. & Downs S.H. (2014)Impact of Schmallenberg virus on British sheep farms during the 2011/2012 lambing season. *The Veterinary Record* 175, 16–23.
20. Helmer C., Eibach R., Tegtmeyer P.C., Humann-Ziehank E. & Ganter M. (2013a) Survey of Schmallenberg virus (SBV) infection in German goat flocks. *Epidemiology and Infection* 141, 2335–2345.
21. Helmer C., Eibach R., Tegtmeyer P.C., Humann-Ziehank E., Runge M., Ganter M.,2013b: Serosurvey of Schmallenberg virus infections in sheep and goat flocks in Lower Saxony, Germany. *Transboundary and Emerging Disease* 62, 425–436.
22. Herder V., Wohlsein P., Peters M., Hansmann F. & Baumgärtner W. (2012) Salient lesions in domestic ruminants infected with the emerging so-called Schmallenberg

virus in Germany. *Veterinary Pathology* 49, 588–591.

23. Hoffmann B., Scheuch M., Höper D., Jungblut R., Holsteg M., Schirrmeier H. *et al.* (2012) *Orthobunyavirus* in cattle. *Emerging Infectious Diseases* 18, 469–472.
24. Kaba J., Czopowicz M. & Witkowski L. (2013) Schmallenberg virus antibodies detected in Poland. *Transboundary and Emerging Disease* 60, 1–3.
25. Larska M., Polak M.P., Grochowska M., Lechowski L., Zwiazek J.S. & Zmudzinski J.F.(2013a) First report of Schmallenberg virus in cattle and midges in Poland.*Transboundary and Emerging Disease* 60, 97–101.
26. Larska M., Krzysiak M., Smreczak M., Polak M.P. & Zmudzinski J.F. (2013b) First detection of Schmallenberg virus in elk (*Alces alces*) indicating infection of wildlife in Bialwoieza National Park in Poland. *Veterinary Journal* 198, 279–281.
27. Lassen S.B., Nielsen S.A., Skovgard H. & Kristensen M. (2011) Molecular identification of blood meals from midges *(Diptera: Ceratopogonidae: Culicoides Latreille)* in Denmark. *Parasitology Research* 108, 823–829.
28. Lassen S.B., Nielsen S.A. & Kristensen M. (2012) Identity and diversity of blood meal hosts of biting midges *(Diptera: Ceratopogonidae: Culicoides latreille)* in Denmark.*Parasites and Vectors* 5, 143.
29. McDermott J.J. & Shukken Y.H. (1994) A review of methods used to adjust for cluster effects in explanatory epidemiological studies of animal populations. *Preventive Veterinary Medicine* 18, 155–173.
30. Meiswinkel R., Baldet T., De Deken R., Takken W., Delécolle J.C. & Mellor P.S. (2008)The 2006 outbreak of bluetongue in northern Europe – the entomological perspective.*Preventive Veterinary Medicine* 87, 55–63.
31. Méroc E., De Regge N., Riocreux F., Caij A.B., Van den Berg T., Van der Stede Y., 2013:Distribution of Schmallenberg virus and seroprevalence in belgian sheep and goats.*Transboundary and Emerging Diseases* 61, 425–431.
32. Muskens J., Smolenaars A.J., Van Der Poel W.H., Mars M.H., Van Wuijckhuise L.,Holzhauer M. *et al.* (2012) Diarrhoea and loss of production on Dutch dairy farms caused by the Schmallenberg virus. *Tijdschrift voor Diergeneeskunde* 137, 112–115.
33. Nevill E.M. (1978) The use of cattle to protect sheep from bluetongue infection. *Journal of the South African Veterinary Association* 49, 129–130.
34. Ninio C., Augot D., Delecolle J.C., Dufour B. & Depaquit J. (2011) Contribution to the knowledge of *Culicoides (Diptera: Cerapogonidae)* host preferences in France.*Parasitology Research* 108, 657–663.
35. R Core Team (2014) The R project for statistical computing. Available at: http://www.R-project.org/ (accesses 15 April 2014).
36. Rasmussen L.D., Kristensen B., Kirkeby C., Rasmussen T.B., Belsham G.J., Bodker R. &Botner A. (2012) *Culicoides* as vectors of Schmallenberg virus. *Emerging Infectious Diseases* 18, 1204–1206.
37. Reusken C., Van Den Wijngaard C., Van Beek P., Beer M., Bouwstra R., Godeke G.J.*et al.* (2012) Lack of evidence for zoonotic transmission of Schmallenberg

virus.*Emerging Infectious Diseases* 18, 1746–1753.

38. Sailleau C., Boogaerts C., Meyrueix A., Laloy E., Bréard E., Viarouge C. *et al.* (2013)Schmallenberg virus infection in dogs, France, 2012. *Emerging Infectious Diseases* 19,1896–1898.
39. Santman-Berends I.M.G.A., Bartels C.J.M., van Schaik G., Stegeman J.A. & Vellema P.(2010) The increase in seroprevalence of bluetongue virus (BTV) serotype 8 infections and associated risk factors in Dutch dairy herds, in 2007. *Veterinary Microbiology* 142,268–275.
40. The Center for Food and Security and Public Health, Iowa State University (2009)Akabane disease. Available at:http://www.cfsph.iastate.edu/Factsheets/pdfs/akabane.pdf (accessed 5 May 2012).
41. The European Food Safety Authority (EFSA) (2013) "Schmallenberg" virus: analysis of the epidemiological data (May 2013). Available at:http://www.efsa.europa.eu/en/supporting/pub/429e.htm (accessed 15 June 2013).
42. Veldhuis A.M.B., Van Schaik G., Vellema P., Elbers A.R.W., Bouwstra R., Van der heijden H.M.J.F., Mars M.H., 2013a: Schmallenberg virus epidemic in the Netherlands: spatiotemporal introduction in 2011 and seroprevalence in ruminants. *Preventive Veterinary Medicine* 112, 35–47.
43. Veldhuis A.M.B., Carp-van Dijken S., Wuijckhuise L., Witteveen G. & van Schaik G.(2013b) Schmallenberg virus in Dutch dairy herds: potential risk factors for high within-herd seroprevalence and malformations in calves, and its impact on productivity. *Veterinary Microbiology* 168, 281–293.
44. Wernike K., Conraths F., Zanella G., Granzow H., Gache K., Schirrmeier H. *et al.* (2014)Schmallenberg virus – Two years of experiences. *Preventive Veterinary Medicine* 116,423–434.
45. Yilmaz H., HoffmannB, TuranN, CizmecigilUY, RichtJA, Van der PoelWHM, 2014:Detection and partial sequencing of Schmallenberg virus in cattle and sheep in turkey.*Vector Borne Zoonotic Diseases* 14, 223–225.
46. Zimmer J.Y., Haubruge E., Francis F., Bortels J., Simonon G., Losson B. *et al.* (2008)Breeding sites of bluetongue vectors in northern Europe. *The Veterinary Record* 162,700.

5
CHAPTER

ASSESSMENT OF PRACTICES, CAPACITIES AND INCENTIVES OF POULTRY CHAIN ACTORS IN IMPLEMENTATION OF HIGHLY PATHOGENIC AVIAN INFLUENZA MITIGATION MEASURES IN GHANA

Paa Kobina Turkson[1] and Iheanacho Okike[2]

[1]Department of Animal Science, School of Agriculture, University of Cape Coast, Cape Coast, Ghana

[2]International Livestock Research Institute, Nigeria, Ibadan, Nigeria

ABSTRACT

The animal health services-seeking behaviour of animal owners related to prevention and control of animal diseases may influence their decisions as to whether or not to use services provided by the public or private sectors. The specific objective of this paper was to assess the practices, capacities and incentives of actors involved in highly pathogenic avian influenza (HPAI) control to provide information for prevention and control in Ghana. Questionnaires were designed based on specific practices, incentives and capacities associated with each mitigation measure that was being assessed. Two peacetime preventive mitigation measures (biosecurity and reporting) and two outbreak containment measures (culling with compensation and movement control) were selected for evaluation. Supply chain actors were characterised based on baseline information. Tables were generated showing proportions of respondents in the various response categories in Likert-scale type itemised questionnaire. Mean scores (and their standard deviations) for the various actors with regard to mitigation measures were calculated. Pair-wise comparisons were done using *t*-ratio statistic and significance of differences were determined at a Bonferroni adjusted *P*-value of 0.0024. The study found statistically significant differences between certain actors for practices (biosecurity, reporting, culling and compensation and movement controls), incentives (reporting and movement

Citation: Turkson, P. K. and Okike, I. (2016), Assessment of practices, capacities and incentives of poultry chain actors in implementation of highly pathogenic avian influenza mitigation measures in Ghana. Veterinary Medicine and Scienc, 2: 23–35. doi: 10.1002/vms3.15

control) and capacities (reporting and movement control). The findings provide lessons to help improve education and messages on HPAI and to help provide technical assistance targeted at specific actors to prevent and control future HPAI H5N1 outbreaks in Ghana.

INTRODUCTION

Ghana experienced three outbreaks of highly pathogenic avian influenza (HPAI) H5N1 in 2007. The mitigation measures instituted by the Veterinary Services Directorate (VSD) included a ban on the movement and sale of poultry and poultry products in and out of infected areas; closure of wet poultry markets in infected areas; quarantine of infected farms; active search/surveillance of the disease in the outbreak area and beyond and disinfection of infected premises and farm machinery and equipment. Other measures were promotion of biosecurity measures and procedures; culling of affected and in-contact birds on the infected farms; culling of all poultry within a 3-km radius which was extended in one case to 5 km and then 8 km; destruction of eggs and feed present on affected premises and compensation for culled birds (Turkson *et al.* **2010**). These were in accordance with Food and Agriculture Organisation (FAO) recommendations on the prevention, control and eradication of HPAI (FAO **2004**). All the control measures reduce risk but none used in isolation is sufficient (FAO**2004**).

According to de Rooij *et al.* (**2007**), governments are not the only actors in animal disease control as the private sector actors are normally the implementers, beneficiaries and risk-takers in control measures and have core strategies and roles to play if HPAI control measures are to be effective. Disease control and prevention is a shared responsibility between government and the private sector as the private sector tends to be the main investor in livestock enterprises and will need to be engaged by government to ensure that it manages the risk of disease and reports of any disease outbreak to the government (Interministerial Conference on Animal and Pandemic Influenza. Ha Noi (IMCAPI) **2010**). It has been suggested that individual farmers have better information about their own preferences, disease risks and responsiveness to various incentives than policy makers, presenting difficulties when public actions alone are used to try to control HPAI efficiently (Beach *et al.* **2006**).

The behaviour of actors involved in HPAI control is influenced by factors related to the interaction between the nature of their poultry-related activities, the nature of the disease and risk of its transmission, and the nature of mitigation measures and how they are implemented (Turkson *et al.* **2010**). This behaviour is also influenced by the practices, incentives and capacities of actors. Studies in many countries have shown that practices and attitudes for prevention and control of HPAI disease spread and outbreaks have not changed, even though there is some level of awareness or knowledge about HPAI (Fielding *et al.* **2005**; Maton *et al.* **2007**; Di Giuseppe *et al.* **2008**; Leslie *et al.* **2008**). Understanding a person's knowledge, attitude, practices and perceptions of and towards risk is a necessary step in determining which cost-effective measure(s) ought to be adopted (Yakhshilikov *et al.* **2009**). Beach *et al.* (**2006**) noted that knowledge of farm behaviour is critical in understanding the distribution of impacts, the extent and cost of private disease prevention behaviour, the spread of HPAI and the effectiveness of public disease control programmes. National Academy of Sciences (NAS) (**2009**) suggested that capacity assessment information for animal health is critical as it is useful in devising national and local incentives, in establishing a disease surveillance system and in timely disease reporting by local and national stakeholders to protect human and animal health and livelihoods.

The effectiveness of public disease prevention and control measures on the spread of a disease have been shown to depend on how much private prevention behaviour responds to disease prevalence, disease impacts and the economic incentives created by public policy measures (Philipson **2000**), as depicted in cases of infectious animal diseases (McCarthy*et al.* **2003**). Animal health measures are often influenced by private strategies set at farm level by individuals, at company level by vertically integrated operations or nationally by stakeholders (national associations including traders and processors) (de Rooij *et al.* **2007**). The key to success in controlling disease is often the collective decisions of these actors to participate in mitigation measures. Across the value chain, dominant actors may set strategies that essentially govern how these chains operate as found in situations where dominant market actors aim for bigger market share and sustainable growth (de Rooij *et al.* **2007**).

A study was done in Ghana in 2009 to assess factors that influence the behaviour of various poultry value chain actors expected to comply with, or be responsible for implementing HPAI control measures in backyard and small-scale broiler and layer chicken production and marketing systems in Ghana (Turkson *et al.* **2010**). The objective of this paper, an offshoot of the study, was to assess the practices, capacities and incentives of actors involved in HPAI control in Ghana. This, it was hoped, would provide information to stakeholders to improve the implementation of mitigation measures for HPAI prevention and control in Ghana. The lessons learnt could be useful in future control or used for the control and prevention of other infectious diseases.

METHODOLOGY

The study used a supply chain as the unit of analysis rather than individual actors. This was to address the difficulty of designing a sampling strategy that provided a representative distribution numerically and spatially of all relevant poultry supply chain actors. Live bird supply chains were used with producers as primary and fixed sampling units based on which other more mobile actors, particularly transporters, traders and retailers were identified. The study focused on backyard, small-scale broiler and layer live-bird supply chains because live birds represent the greatest risk of H5N1 HPAI virus transmission through virus shedding and contamination of inanimate materials. Four regions out of ten in the country were selected purposively because these contribute significantly to commercial poultry production (Greater Accra 36%, Brong Ahafo 16% and Ashanti 36%) and to backyard poultry production (Northern Region).

Questionnaires were designed based on specific socioeconomic factors (practices, incentives and capacities) associated with each mitigation measure that was being assessed (Kelemework *et al.* **2010**; Onkundi *et al.* **2010**). Two peacetime preventive mitigation measures (biosecurity and reporting) and two outbreak containment measures (culling with compensation and movement control) were selected for evaluation

(Kelemework *et al.* **2010**; Onkundi *et al.* **2010**). The questionnaires were divided into sections. At the end of each set of questions for each mitigation measure, two open-ended questions were asked for each actor or mitigation agent to state reasons why they could or could not implement a measure. This information helped to explain some of the attitudes measured using the Likert-scale type items. The details of the dimensions representing practices, capacities and incentives influencing actors' compliance from which questions were framed for the questionnaire were similar to those reported by Onkundi *et al.* (**2010**) in Kenya and Kelemework *et al.* (**2010**) in Ethiopia.

The study used the FAO Poultry Farm categories identified in 2004 where a Sector 3 (S3) farm was defined as a commercial poultry production system with low to minimal biosecurity and with birds/products entering live bird markets, whereas a Sector 4 (S4) farm was a village or backyard production with minimal biosecurity and birds/products were consumed locally (FAO **2008**).

The sampling sites for the S4 producers were generated randomly using GIS software and are shown in Figure 1.

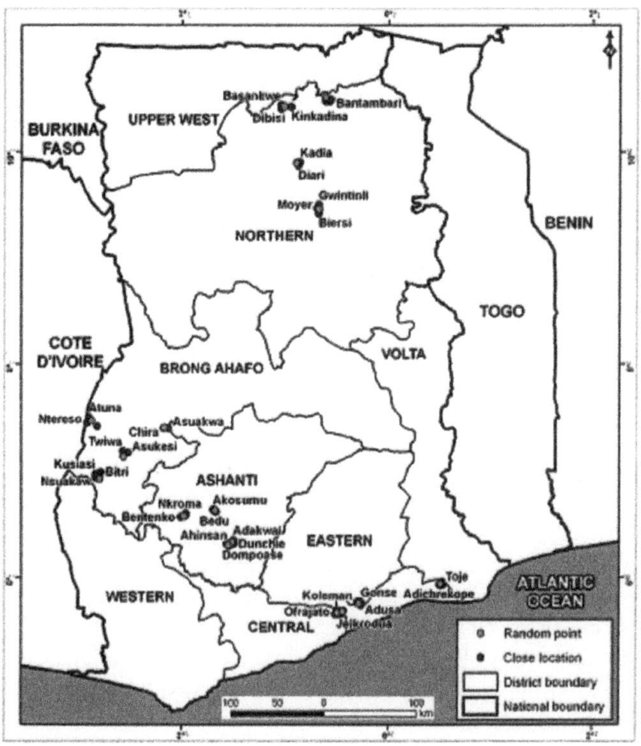

Figure 1: Map of Ghana showing selected points for sampling of S4 producers.

Four points per selected region were generated randomly and for each point, the names of three communities nearest to such points were provided along with their latitudes and longitudes. The enumerators used GPS to locate the community closest to the selected point and the first poultry producer/keeper encountered in that community was chosen for questionnaire administration. The other actors in the poultry value chain who had recent transactions linked to this producer were followed using the snowball method and appropriate actor-specific questionnaires administered.

For the S3 producers, lists of layer and broiler producers in the regions were obtained from the Ghana National Poultry Farmers Association office and the Regional Offices of the Ministry of Food and Agriculture. Random numbers were generated using a random number generator and based on the number of members per region. Those producers in the list whose numbers were chosen were selected for questionnaire administration. Here also, after the initial selection of the S3 producers, the snowball method was used in locating the other actors in the value chain who had recent transactions linked to them. For the implementing agents, five veterinarians from the VSD in the 4 regions (one each from a region except Greater Accra which had two representatives) were purposively selected and questionnaires administered to them. Altogether, there were 16 S4 producers, 16 S3 broiler producers, 16 S3 layer producers, 48 traders, 48 transporters, 48 retailers and 5 implementing agency respondents.

Data were entered into a database designed using spss version 17.0 (SPSS, Inc., Chicago, IL, 2007) and analysed using the same software. Supply chain actors were characterised based on baseline information and simple descriptive statistics. Tables were generated showing proportions of respondents in the various combined response categories of always and often; seldom and never; strongly disagreed and disagreed; agreed and strongly agreed; very likely and likely; or unlikely and very unlikely as determined by the questionnaire. Details of the response categories may be obtained from the first author. Mean scores and standard deviations of the Likert-scale items for the various actors for the mitigation measures were calculated in spss. The responses to the open-ended questions were transcribed, summarised and grouped.

Multiple comparisons between levels of the same effect were calculated in Microsoft Excel using a *t*-ratio statistic (mean A − mean B/standard error of difference between means), referred to a *t*-distribution with t degrees of freedom, where t = degrees of freedom at the actor level (Kelemework *et al.* **2010**; Onkundi *et al.* **2010**). The degrees of freedom in a *t*-ratio is $[(n_1 - 1) + (n_2 - 1)]$ where n_1 is the total number of sample A and n_2 is total number of sample B. A Bonferroni adjustment (significance level = alpha/n where$n$ = number of comparisons) was used to adjust the significance level to reduce the false-positive error rate caused by multiple comparisons (Kelemework *et al.* **2010**; Onkundi *et al.***2010**). In our case, the chosen alpha was 0.05 and the number of comparisons, n, was 21 giving an adjusted P-value of 0.0024.

RESULTS

Table 1 shows the mean scores (±SD) for practices, capacities and incentives of poultry chain actors in Ghana for various mitigation measures (biosecurity, reporting, culling and compensation and movement control). In general, when the mean score for a mitigation measure was higher for an actor compared with another, it meant that the actor with the higher mean score was of the opinion that that measure was more likely to influence compliant with the dimension than the other actor with a lower mean score.

Table 1: Mean scores (±SD) for practices, capacities and incentives of poultry chain actors for mitigation measures

Actor	Biosecurity	Reporting	Culling and compensation	Movement control
Practices				
S4 producer	2.8 (±0.6)	2.2 (±0.5)	2.9 (±0.5)	2.5 (±0.9)
S3 broiler producer	2.7 (±0.8)	3.1 (±0.6)	2.7 (±0.7)	4.2 (±0.4)
S3 layer producer	2.4 (±0.4)	3.0 (±0.4)	2.9 (±0.8)	4.1 (±0.4)
Trader	3.1 (±0.5)	3.0 (±0.5)	3.2 (±0.8)	3.2 (±0.8)
Transporter	2.3 (±0.6)	2.5 (±1.0)	n.a	3.2 (±0.7)
Retailer	3.1 (±0.4)	3.0 (±0.7)	2.9 (±0.6'	2.6 (±0.8)
Implementing Agency	3.0 (±0.5)	4.4 (±0.4)	2.0 (±0.7)	2.8 (±0.4)
Total	2.8 (±0.6)	2.9 (±0.8)	3.0 (±0.7)	3.1 (±0.9)
Capacities				
S4 Producer	3.0 (±0.8)	2.7 (±0.6)	2.9 (±0.8)	3.3 (±0.6)
S3 broiler producer	3.2 (±0.6)	3.1 (±0.7)	3.0 (±0.9)	3.1 (±0.6)
S3 layer producer	3.1 (±0.5)	2.8 (±0.8)	3.2 (±0.6)	3.1 (±0.6)
Trader	3.0 (±0.7)	2.9 (±0.8)	2.7 (±0.7)	2.6 (±0.9)
Transporter	2.9 (±0.9)	2.6 (±0.9)	n.a	2.9 (±0.5)
Retailer	3.1 (±0.8)	3.1 (±0.7)	2.7 (±0.7)	2.8 (±0.8)
Implementing Agency	3.6 (±0.5)	2.7 (±0.4)	2.9 (±0.5)	3.1 (±0.3)
Total	3.0 (±0.7)	2.9 (±0.8)	2.9 (±0.7)	2.9 (±0.7)
Incentives				
S4 Producer	3.3 (±0.5)	2.8 (±0.7)	3.2 (±0.9)	2.7 (±0.8)
S3 broiler producer	3.2 (±0.4)	3.2 (±0.7)	2.9 (±1.0)	3.4 (±0.5)
S3 layer producer	2.9 (±0.6)	3.3 (±0.4)	2.9 (±0.8)	3.3 (±0.5)
Trader	2.9 (±0.7)	2.8 (±0.6)	3.1 (±0.9)	3.0 (±0.6)
Transporter	3.0 (±0.5)	2.8 (±0.5)	n.a.	2.5 (±0.7)
Retailer	2.8 (±0.8)	3.0 (±0.5)	3.0 (±1.1)	3.2 (±0.6)
Implementing Agency	2.5 (±0.7)	2.6 (±0.4)	2.5 (±0.4)	2.8 (±0.2)
Total	2.9 (±0.6)	2.9 (±0.6)	3.0 (±1.0)	3.0 (±0.7)

n.a., not applicable.

Biosecurity scores among actors for practices ranged from 2.3 for transporters to 3.1 for retailers. For capacities, the biosecurity scores ranged from 2.9 (transporters) to 3.6 (implementing agencies) whereas for incentives the biosecurity scores ranged from 2.5 (implementing agencies) to 3.3 (S4 producers).

Reporting scores among actors for practices ranged from 2.2 (for S4 producers) to 4.4 for implementing agencies, while those for capacities ranged from 2.6 (transporter) to 3.1 (S3 producers and retailers). The reporting scores for incentives ranged from 2.6 for implementing agency to 3.2 for S3 layer producer.

For culling and compensation, the scores for practices among actors ranged from 2.0 (Implementing agency) to 3.2 (trader). The scores for capacities ranged from 2.7 (trader and retailer) to 3.2 (S3 layer producer) while those for incentives ranged from 2.5 (implementing agency) to 3.2 (S4 producer).

Movement control scores for practices ranged from 2.5 (S4 producer) to 4.2 (S3 broiler producer). The scores for capacities ranged from 2.6 (trader) to 3.3 (S4 producer) whereas those for incentives ranged from 2.5 (transporter) to 3.4 (S3 broiler producer.

Table 2 presents results of pair-wise comparisons of poultry chain actors where the *P*-values were significant at Bonferroni adjusted value of 0.0024.

Table 2: Pair-wise comparisons of mean scores with *P*-values significant at Bonferroni adjusted *P*-value of 0.0024

	m1	m2	*t*-statistic	df	*P*-value
Practice					
Biosecurity					
Trader vs. layer	3.1	2.4	5.54	62	0.0000
Retailer vs. layer	3.1	2.4	5.90	62	0.0000
Trader vs. transporter	3.1	2.3	7.02	94	0.0000
Retailer vs. transporter	3.1	2.3	7.61	94	0.0000
Reporting					
Broiler vs. S4	3.1	2.2	4.46	30	0.0001
Layer vs. S4	3	2.2	4.84	30	0.0000
Trader vs. S4	3	2.2	5.40	62	0.0000
Retailer vs. S4	3	2.2	4.86	62	0.0000
I agency vs. S4	4.4	2.2	9.24	19	0.0000
I agency vs. broiler	4.4	3.1	5.14	19	0.0000
I agency vs. layer	4.4	3	6.22	19	0.0000
Trader vs. transporter	3	2.5	3.07	94	0.0014
I agency vs. trader	4.4	3	6.58	51	0.0000
I agency vs. transporter	4.4	2.5	7.68	51	0.0000
I agency vs. retailer	4.4	3	6.23	51	0.0000
Culling					
Trader vs. I agency	3.2	2	3.25	51	0.0010
Movement control					
Broiler vs. S4	4.2	2.5	6.69	30	0.0000
Layer vs. S4	4.1	2.5	6.29	30	0.0000
Broiler vs. trader	4.2	3.2	6.42	62	0.0000
Broiler vs. transporter	4.2	3.2	6.89	62	0.0000
Broiler vs. retailer	4.2	2.6	10.27	62	0.0000
Broiler vs. I agency	4.2	2.8	6.22	19	0.0000
Layer vs. trader	4.1	3.2	5.78	62	0.0000
Layer vs. transporter	4.1	3.2	6.20	62	0.0000

Layer vs. retailer	4.1	2.6	9.63	62	0.0000
Layer vs. I agency	4.1	2.8	5.78	19	0.0000
Trader vs. retailer	3.2	2.6	3.64	94	0.0002
Transporter vs. retailer	3.2	2.6	3.87	94	0.0001
Capacities					
Reporting					
Broiler vs. transporter	3.1	2.6	3.01	94	0.0017
Retailer vs. transporter	3.1	2.6	3.01	94	0.0017
Movement control					
S4 vs. trader	3.3	2.6	3.45	62	0.0005
Incentives					
Reporting					
Layer vs. trader	3.3	2.8	3.69	62	0.0002
Layer vs. transporter	3.3	2.8	3.95	62	0.0001
Movement control					
Broiler vs. transporter	3.4	2.5	5.47	62	0.0000
Broiler vs. I agency	3.4	2.8	3.67	19	0.0008
Layer vs. transporter	3.3	2.5	4.86	62	0.0000
Trader vs. transporter	3	2.5	3.72	94	0.0002
Retailer vs. transporter	3.2	2.5	5.21	94	0.0000
Retailer vs. I agency	3.2	2.8	3.01	51	0.0020

m1, mean score A; m2, mean score B; df, degrees of freedom; S4, Sector 4 producer; broiler, S3 broiler producer; layer, S3 layer producer; I. agency, implementing agency agent.

DISCUSSION

The animal health services-seeking behaviour of livestock owners related to prevention and control of animal diseases may influence their decisions as to whether or not to use services provided by the public or private sectors. In poultry production de Rooij *et al.* (**2007**) observed that in backyard systems (FAO poultry classification Sector 4), poultry health has been the domain of the individual producer because providing animal health services is not very profitable for the private sector and is very difficult for the public sector. On the other hand, for Sectors 3 and 2, whereas the integrated commercial poultry systems are well covered by private animal health providers, a large number of poultry are in production systems that are neither covered by public nor private animal health services. These may have serious implications for practices, incentives and capacities of poultry chain actors for disease prevention and control.

The practice of biosecurity is critical in efforts to prevent and control HPAI H5N1. Otte *et al.* (**2008**) noted that the effect of biosecurity measures is not only restricted to lowering the risk of HPAI introduction but also to decreasing the risk of other contagious diseases getting to the farm/flock. FAO (**2008**) recognised biosecurity as vital to the control of HPAI, based on the needs for segregation, cleaning and disinfection. Biosecurity, also, requires people adopting a set of attitudes and behaviours to reduce the risk of introduction and spread of disease agents in all activities involving domestic, captive exotic and wild birds and their products (FAO **2008**). The mean scores for biosecurity practices were higher for traders and retailers compared with producers (Table 1). This means that the traders and retailers were more likely to be influenced to comply with these biosecurity dimensions than the producers. The practice of biosecurity should be paramount on the farms because farms have been identified as the most critical control points in Ghana (Mensah Bonsu **2010**). The VSD of the Ministry of Food and Agriculture in Ghana provided biosecurity training in all ten regions and also developed a biosecurity manual targeted at poultry producers after the initial outbreak of HPAI H5N1 in 2007. The relatively lower mean scores for biosecurity practice for the producers, compared with others except transporters, may point to the lack of effectiveness of these trainings or low/poor adoption/uptake of the procedures and processes of biosecurity. Mensah Bonsu **2010**) noted that even though biosecurity practices were established and enforced during the outbreak period in Ghana, these were not accompanied by incentives for the farms. Commercial poultry producers in this study explained that although the measures were supposed to be normal operational practices their enforcement had increased the farms' operational costs and were, therefore, most often ignored.

FAO (**2008**) noted that the details of how biosecurity is applied depend on the type of poultry production unit in question; the emphasis being placed on 'bioexclusion' for farms and villages, and 'biocontainment' for markets. The FAO observed that many known biosecurity measures currently in place have been developed mostly for large-scale commercial production systems in developed countries with few of the commonly recommended measures being appropriate for small-scale commercial systems or for rural (free-range) poultry and that biosecurity measures have not been designed for other actors in the chain and service providers. The FAO recommended that where they do not exist, appropriate biosecurity measures must be designed and implemented; where they do exist, they may not be sufficiently effective or implemented widely enough requiring re-evaluation of their effectiveness.

In Ghana, even though some biosecurity procedures were established and a manual was produced during the HPAI outbreak in 2007, the adoption of these procedures was and is very limited or perfunctory. The poultry farmers' associations advocated the adoption and use of levels of biosecurity as a classification system for farms in an effort to encourage adoption of such procedures and processes. A Delphi study in 2010 revealed that the efficacies of six private and nine public control strategies were significantly higher in the commercial than in the non-commercial/semi-commercial producers in Ghana (Birol *et al.* **2010**). Biosecurity training and surveillance were identified in the Delphi study as two very effective strategies that might be undertaken by VSD to control HPAI risk in non-commercial/semi-commercial and among small-scale producers in five countries including Ghana. Movement control, on the other hand, was not considered as effective as biosecurity training and surveillance.

FAO (**2008**) has advised that planning for biosecurity must include socioeconomic analysis to help determine the social and cultural acceptability of proposed measures, the level of cost that people can and are willing to pay and the regulations, incentives and penalties that may be appropriate to induce the change in behaviour necessary in many situations. The decision to invest in biosecurity measures may be influenced by the perception of poultry owners of the risk of disease introduction into their flocks, the economic scale of expected losses once their flock is infected and the additional costs that would be incurred (Otte *et al.* **2008**). These are yet to be investigated in Ghana.

Beach *et al.* (**2006**) noted that Sectors 3 and 4 are generally considered to be more susceptible to infection because of their low levels of biosecurity, as in these systems poultry are usually not confined and may come into contact or mingle freely with wild birds, greatly increasing the risk of spread of HPAI to poultry. Our study found that 75% of S4 producers never confined their chickens during the day and 69% allowed their chickens to mix with their neighbours' flock, increasing the risks for spread of disease. FAO (**2008**) recommended that biosecurity for S4 producers should emphasise creation of physical barriers against infection and to control access, if need be through public funding; cleaning of inanimate objects and using participatory fieldwork to establish which measures are feasible and sustainable, to produce and disseminate extension messages and to monitor and report on uptake and impact of these messages. Alhaji & Odetokun (**2011**) from studies in Nigeria advocated community-led initiatives to create physical barriers against infection for free-range poultry keepers because these cannot act alone. They reported that free-range flocks were at lower risk compared with small-scale commercial operators. FAO (**2007**) advised on the need to find a balance between biosecurity requirements and livelihood demands of affected producers.

Biosecurity improvements in sectors 3 and 4 are difficult to impose and enforce due to the sectors' internal diversity and low investment capacities (FAO **2007**). Recommendations for improvement in animal husbandry practices that recognise local constraints and capacities have a higher chance of success and sustainability. Further, any efforts to deal with the complexity of sectors 3 and 4 by imposing strict regulations and restrictions should be undertaken with a good understanding of both epidemiological risk and the sectors' operations. This is because these producers and traders have little incentives to cooperate with authorities and often try to find illegal ways to move birds' outside restricted areas to avoid regulations (FAO **2007**). These illegal movements are difficult to monitor and may represent high risks of disease transmission. IMCAPI (**2010**) recommended that biosecurity measures at the smallholder and village level need to be simple, cheap and cost effective, taking into consideration the existing production systems or else farmers would not be able to implement them or the costs of the measures might outweigh the benefits to the farmer.

The lowest mean score for biosecurity practice in this study (2.3) was for transporters (Table 1) meaning that they were the group least likely to institute biosecurity measures.

These, generally, asserted in their responses to open-ended questions that it was not their responsibility to institute certain biosecurity procedures. Even where there were disinfection dips to be used before entering farms, 60% of the transporters said they often or always avoided these. These transporters will need to be educated on their role in the use of biosecurity as mitigation measures for HPAI control and should in future be targeted to be part of the biosecurity training programmes organised by VSD. FAO (**2004**) recommended that cages for carrying birds from farms to markets should be constructed of materials such as plastic or metal, easy to clean and disinfect. Also measures should be implemented during transport to reduce the risk of faecal contamination of the area around markets when cages were off-loaded. Further, facilities for cleaning and disinfection of transport cages before being taken back to the farms were necessary together with an official system for monitoring their effectiveness. These should be considered in the training of transporters in Ghana.

According to the Canadian Food Inspection Agency (**2006**), the key considerations for greater biosecurity include preventing exposure of poultry to wild birds by keeping poultry in closed housing and ensuring that wild birds cannot access poultry feed and water supplies; preventing exposure to potentially infected new poultry introduced into existing flocks by isolating new birds or avoiding their introduction into existing flocks; and preventing exposure to infectious agents transported by people or equipment by limiting access to poultry houses and thoroughly cleaning all clothing, shoes, and equipment before and after coming into contact with birds. These should be stressed during biosecurity training.

On reporting practices, S4 producers had the lowest mean score compared with the other actors (Table 1). This meant that they were the group least likely to comply with biosecurity practices. In open-ended questions, these producers said that there was no need to report poultry diseases or mortalities neither was it their business to report diseases. They also claimed that the process and procedures for reporting was expensive. FAO (**2008**) observed that a widespread perception that poultry sickness and death were natural has led to lack of reporting of sick and dead birds. According to IMCAPI (**2010**), other diseases that cause high mortality in poultry (including New Castle disease) occurred regularly in the past so such 'expected' losses of poultry in low-input systems may not always result in disease outbreak being reported to authorities as these are seen by poultry owners as normal, seasonal events. Also, there is a perception that promptly reporting disease outbreaks may negatively impact trade or public confidence in products resulting in incurring costs (Cash & Narasimhan **2000**). NAS (**2009**) recommended that local authorities need effective disease surveillance to identify local outbreaks and to contain them before spreading to animals and humans, if zoonotic.

Padmawati & Nichter (**2008**) posited that small holder poultry farmers avoided reporting disease incidents to authorities because of fear of losing their own animals through culling and also the social risk of angering neighbours whose birds would be subject to culling within a 2–5 km radius of an outbreak location. In our study, the proportions of producers who agreed or strongly agreed that reporting would result in their chickens being killed were relatively low (31% of S4 producers, 31%

of S3 broiler producers and 25% of S3 layer producers). The proportions agreeing or strongly agreeing that other poultry producers would be angry if a disease outbreak was reported were 44% of S4 producers, 44% of S3 broiler producers and 31% of S3 layer producers. These findings do not seem to suggest that producers were averse to reporting disease. IMCAPI (**2010**) noted that culling inhibited disease reporting because of the consequences of such reports on local communities. Trust and technical skills of government animal health workers were important in determining whether or not local stakeholders reported poultry mortalities in Asia (Kleinman *et al.* **2008**). These involved trust that authorities would provide adequate and timely compensation for culled birds and trust that animal health officers would conduct appropriate diagnostic tests to ascertain HPAI H5N1 and not just act on the basis of suspicion because signs and symptoms of Newcastle disease could mimic those of HPAI H5N1. These may also be relevant in Ghana.

Reporting takes place at various levels: local (producers, traders, retailers, transporters, animal health workers, consumers), district, provincial, national, regional and global with various degrees of responsibilities. NAS (**2009**) stated that early reporting of a disease outbreak, even if it brings sanctions also provides opportunities for formal early intervention in containing the outbreak and thus reduce the costs of eradication. Further, providing incentives for local participation in timely disease detection and reporting could encourage farmers or other actors to declare early emergence of a disease which could, in turn, reduce the cost of containment or control. Also, to avoid problems of concealment of outbreaks, it was necessary to provide incentives for outbreak reporting by designing appropriate control measures and providing adequate compensation schemes.

FAO (**2007**) noted that the level of compensation was a determining factor for the rate of reporting. Too low levels induce producers to hide animals from culling and too high levels would encourage the introduction of animals from outside the region (NAS **2009**). Beach*et al.* (**2006**) said that the level of compensation is very important as a policy lever influencing producer behaviour because if compensation is set too low producers are likely to conduct less disease surveillance and may attempt to hide the disease rather than report it. On the other hand, if it is set too high then producers will have little incentive to invest in costly control measures. The World Bank has recommended compensation rates between 75% and 90% of market value before the disease outbreak for live animals and lower rates for dead animals. In Ghana, compensation rates ranged from 50% for table eggs to 90% for broilers, layers and day-old chicks (Aning *et al.* **2008**). NAS (**2009**) reported that farmers, at the farm level, may delay reporting because of fears of economic sanctions or inadequate or delayed compensation so it is important especially for smallholders not only to address the rate of compensation but also the timeliness and reliability of payment.

From Table 2, the mean score for culling practices for traders (3.2) was significantly higher than that for implementing agencies (2.0) which was surprising, but could be expected. This is because traders were more likely to benefit from cheaper producer prices (because producers would want to get rid of their birds) or higher retail prices (due to scarcity of products as a result of enforcement of control measures). FAO (**2007**) noted that culling results in loss of livelihoods, discourages reporting and encourages panic selling. In our study, various actors identified prevention of diseases as a reason why they would be willing and able to cooperate with the culling of chickens during a disease outbreak. As to why they would not be willing or able to cooperate, the major reasons cited were no/inadequate compensation or economic/financial losses. Beach *et al.* (**2006**) observed that low or no compensation for culled birds was a major barrier to disease reporting necessary to identify outbreaks and producer cooperation with depopulation of infected and exposed birds. Further, the absence of adequate veterinary expertise to aid in proper culling was a key factor affecting the effectiveness of the depopulation programmes. The implementing agents, in our study, cited inappropriate culling process/procedures or disposal facilities as a reason why agents would not do a good job implementing culling during disease outbreaks. Schiffer *et al.* (**2009**) reported that the actual destruction of thousands of birds with limited technical infrastructure and in hot tropical climate took a toll on the veterinary staff members in Ghana charged with the culling process. In addition, there was no well thought-out plan for culling and disposal of carcasses raising questions about its effectiveness.

For movement control practice, the mean scores for S3 producers (layer and broiler) were statistically significantly higher than those for the rest of the actors (Table 2). These producers are most at risk to lose economically when there is disease outbreak and may be more amenable to compliance than others. FAO (**2007**) noted that sector 3 producers are those especially hard hit by HPAI regulations because the sector combines low biosecurity with relatively larger flock sizes and may be considered a high risk sector. Therefore, complying with movement control to stem disease spread may be better welcomed by S3 producers. Birol *et al.* (**2010**) reported that movement control was considered to be a more effective strategy among commercial producers than among non-commercial/semi-commercial producers in 5 countries including Ghana. The S4 producers in our study had the lowest scores for movement control practice (Table 1) because they were least inclined to confine birds as their practice is to allow birds to roam freely (free-range). FAO (**2007**) observed that confinement to enclosed spaces, which is an essential aspect of movement control, has been found to be most difficult implementing by S4 producers as what is attractive and cost effective for S4 producers is the free-range nature of the production system. Otte *et al.* (**2008**) noted that S4 producers will require special consideration in national HPAI control programme because they are used to recurring poultry losses, have little incentives to comply with disease control programmes or to invest in biosecurity and cannot be effectively policed by public animal health agencies. VSD will have to target these producers for extension purposes.

VSD (**2007**) stated that because of the artificial boundaries and the mix of socio-cultural relations that exist in the West African sub-region, it is almost impossible enforcing quarantine measures in one country in the event of the outbreak of trans-boundary diseases and uncontrolled movement of live poultry and poultry products within and across borders in the sub-region posed a serious threat to animal health. Furthermore, producers of poultry products (eggs and spent layers) on S3 farms often sell their products to traders moving from farm to farm in hired vehicles in search of poultry products to buy and may oftentimes introduce infection onto healthy farms.

In Ghana, even though the movement of poultry requires movement permit by law (Diseases of Animal Act 1961), it is common to see poultry being moved without permit or the law on movement not being enforced. The proportions of producers in our study who agreed or strongly agreed that even if they did not comply with movement ban, no action would be taken against them were 44% of S4 producers, 50% of S3 broiler producers and 44% of S3 layer producers. This points to a worrying situation where people may flout the law knowing very well that they would escape punishment. The transporters said it was not their responsibility to obtain permits when moving poultry but rather that of the poultry owners (the producers, traders or retailers). The various actors in the study cited bribery or corruption and lack of or low motivation as major reasons why government workers might not want or be able to do a good job in ensuring that movement controls were fully enforced. These claims may need to be investigated further if movement control measures are to be effective.

Our study found statistically significant differences among certain actors for capacities for reporting (between mean scores for broiler producers and transporters and between transporters and retailers) and movement controls (between mean scores for S4 producers and traders)(Table 2). Whether or not the capacities were adequate for preventing or mitigating HPAI H5N1 outbreaks were not ascertained. At the producer level, 69% of the S4 producers indicated that they could get credit if they thought it was important to build better housing for their poultry, implying that they had capacity to confine their birds if they so wished. A high proportion (75%) of the layer producers were of the opinion that it was not difficult to control vehicles in and out of their premises, compared with 50% of broiler producers. Thus, they had some capacity to institute certain biosecurity measures. A larger proportion (75%) of S4 producers said they could provide feed and water during confinement of chickens. The capacity to store chickens till movement restrictions were lifted were limited in the broiler producers compared with layer producers. Traders (75%) and retailers (69%) were unlikely or very unlikely to have other sources of income to rely on when trade in chicken was suspended during movement control. It is necessary to identify and address the shortfalls in capacities of the various actors for the mitigation measures if their effectiveness is to be improved.

With regard to capacity for mitigation measures at the implementing agency level, FAO (**2004**) noted that official veterinary services are key players in the definition and implementation of control measures and their extent and efficiency do have a major bearing on the capacity of countries to deal with HPAI. The outbreak of Avian Influenza in Ghana in 2007 resulted in some major investments by government and donors to improve the quality of veterinary services. Many animal health staff members at district, regional and national levels were trained in areas related to disease control, reporting and investigation whereas selected poultry farmers and stakeholders were trained in biosecurity at all the regional capitals. There were also major investments in laboratory facilities, diagnostic equipment, reagents and training of personnel, with funding from international agencies and donors resulting in enhancement of the capacities and capabilities of the laboratories. As noted by IMCAPI (**2010**) for Vietnam, which could also be true for Ghana, these investments built on a relatively low base and may not have immediate impact but may contribute over many years to VSD meeting the quality standards for veterinary services defined and measured in OIE's veterinary assessment process (PVS). FAO (**2004**) recommended a strong chain of command and scientific capabilities and infrastructure to deal with disease diagnosis, surveillance, data analysis, reporting and disease control which must be continually reinforced and augmented, in partnership with industry, the private sector, the veterinary profession and other stakeholders.

On incentives, Beach *et al.* (**2006**) observed that farmers play a key role in implementing control measures and may need technical and financial support as incentives to adopt prevention and control measures at socially optimal levels. FAO (**2007**) stated that compensation schemes provide incentives to report disease outbreaks and at the same time reduce the economic damage caused to producers by culling. However, farmers in Sector 3 and 4 may not benefit much from such schemes because their record keeping is minimal; birds may be indigenous with different market values; and farmers often need immediate cash compensation. Anecdotal information from Ghana during the outbreaks seems to support these observations (Aning *et al.* **2008**).

Otte *et al.* (**2008**) noted that depending on incentives or disincentives for disease reporting such as compensation or culling, the real incidence and impact of HPAI may be under or over-reported. In the absence of proper incentives in place for reporting suspected cases of disease to authorities, producers may hide suspected cases due to concerns about their economic losses in the face of quarantine or culling of their flock, as evidenced by reports of low or no compensation being a significant impediment to disease reporting in some Asian countries (Beach *et al.* **2006**). Further, some sick birds were likely to be consumed or sold rather than destroyed while producers might try to sell exposed birds that appear healthy before signs of illness appear. Beach *et al.* (**2006**) said these actions were likely to delay public response to an outbreak, allowing the disease time to spread or potentially contribute directly to disease spread if sick birds were transported or sold. This made it more difficult and costly to bring the outbreak under control, hence the development of endemicity. In our study, a high proportion (81%) of S4 producers was of the opinion that farmers often or always took chickens to market when birds were sick or dying. This finding has serious implications for disease spread and prevention. There is the need for intensive education to reduce this practice to stem disease spread.

IMCAPI (**2010**) observed that farmers have to see the benefits in making changes and if they do not, no changes will occur. Recommendations which may be technically sound but result in dramatic change in production system may not be attractive, as at the moment 'many farmers do not see AI as a significant threat in part because the disease has been contained which also makes communicating the need for behavioural change challenging' (IMCAPI **2010**). This needs to be considered in designing and implementation of mitigation measures.

In conclusion, our study found some significant differences between poultry chain actors in practices for biosecurity, reporting and movement controls and in capacities and incentives for reporting and movement control. These findings may be used to enable targeting of classical epidemiological investigations, strengthening linkages in the value chain and providing valuable insights to help tailor future interventions as suggested by other authors (Azhar *et al.* **2010**; Catley *et al.* **2012**.).

ACKNOWLEDGEMENTS

We thank Dr Tom Randolph and Dr Bernard Bett of ILRI, Nairobi, Kenya for the assistance in the development of the questionnaires and methodology. We are grateful to all the enumerators and respondents for their contribution.

CONFLICT OF INTEREST

The authors declare that there is no conflict of interest.

REFERENCES

1. Alhaji N.B. & Odetokun I.A. (2011) Assessment of biosecurity measures against highly pathogenic avian influenza risks in small-scale commercial farms and free-range poultry flocks in the North-central Nigeria. *Transboundary end Emerging Diseases* **58**, 157–161.
2. Aning K. G., Turkson P. K. & Asuming-Brempong S. (2008) Pro-poor HPAI Risk Reduction Strategies in Ghana - Background Paper. Africa/Indonesia Region Report, IFPRI, Washington, DC, USA. 104p.http://www.hpai-research.net/working-papers.html
3. Azhar M., Lubis A.S., Siregar E.S., Alders R.G., Brum E., McGrane J. *et al.* (2010) Participatory disease surveillance and response in Indonesia: strengthening veterinary services and empowering communities to prevent and control highly pathogenic avian influenza. *Avian Diseases* **54**(s1), 749–753.
4. Beach R.H., Poulus C. & Pattanayak S.K. (2006) Prevention and control of Avian Influenza: a view from the farm household. Presentation at the CAES-FLP-CATPRN Joint workshop. Crises in Agricultural and Resource Sector Workshop: Analysis of Policy Responses. October 15–17, 2006.
5. Birol E., Asare-Marfo D. & Yakhshilikov Y. (2010) Efficacy and adoption of strategies for Avian Flu control in developing countries- A Delphi study. IFPRI Discussion paper 001023 IFPRI Washington, DC, 33 pp.
6. Canadian Food Inspection Agency (2006) Avian Influenza: Biosecurity. Available athttp://www.inspection.gc.ca/english/anima/heasan/disemala/avflu/bacdoc/prevente.shtml (accessed 21 May 2010)
7. Cash R.A. & Narasimhan V. (2000) Impediments to global surveillance of infectious diseases: Consequences of open reporting in a global economy. *Bulletin of World Health Organisation* **78**,1358–1367.
8. Catley A., Alders R.G. & Woods J. (2012) Participatory epidemiology: approaches, methods, experiences.*The Veterinary Journal* **191**, 151–160.
9. Di Giuseppe G., Abbate R., Albano L., Marinelli P., Angelillo I.F. (2008) A survey of knowledge, attitudes, and practices towards avian influenza in an adult population of Italy. *BMC Infectious Diseases* **8**: 36. Available at http://www.biomedcentral.com/1471-2334/8/36 (accessed 20 May 2010).

10. FAO (2007) HPAI and sustainable livelihoods: managing risk and development options. Livelihoods Support Programme Brief. Food and Agriculture Organisation, Rome, Italy.

11. FAO (2008) Biosecurity for Highly Pathogenic Avian Influenza: Issues and options. FAO Animal Production and Health paper 165. Food and Agriculture Organisation, Rome, Italy.

12. Fielding R., Lam W.W.T., Ho E.Y.Y., Lam T.H., Hedley A.J. & Leung G.M. (2005) Avian influenza risk perception, Hong Kong. *Emerging Infectious Diseases* **11**, 677–682.

13. Food and Agriculture Organisation (FAO) (2004) Recommendations on the prevention, control and eradication of Highly Pathogenic Avian Influenza (HPAI) in Asia. September 2004. Food and Agriculture Organisation, Rome, Italy.

14. IMCAPI (Interministerial Conference on Animal and Pandemic Influenza. Ha Noi) (2010). Avian Influenza and Pandemic: Vietnam›s experience: Available at http://www.imcapi-hanoi-2010.org/fileadmin/templates/imcapi/documents/imcapi_book_small-1.pdf (accessed 15 November 2010).

15. Kelemework F., Belay B., Bett B., Randolph T. (2010) Alignment of poultry sector actors with avian influenza control measures in Ethiopia. Africa/Indonesia Team Working Paper 32, IFPRI, Washington DC, USA. 43p

16. Kleinman A.M., Bloom B.R., Saich A, Mason K.A., Aulino F. (2008) Avian and pandemic influenza: a biosocial approach. *Journal of Infectious Diseases* **197**(Suppl. 1):S1–S3.

17. Leslie T., Billaud J., Mofleh J., Mustafa L. & Yingst S. (2008) Knowledge, attitudes, and practices regarding avian influenza (H5N1), Afghanistan. *Emerging Infectious Diseases* **14**, 1459–1461.

18. Maton T., Butraporn P., Kaewkangwal J. & Fungladda W. (2007) Avian influenza protection knowledge, awareness, and behaviors in a high-risk population in Suphan Buri province, Thailand. *Southeast Asian Journal of Tropical Medicine and Public Health* **38**, 560–568.

19. McCarthy N., McDermott J. & Coleman P. (2003) Animal Health and the Role of Communities: An Example of Trypanasomosis Control Options in Uganda. EPTD Discussion Paper No. 103. Washington, DC: International Food Policy Research Institute.

20. Mensah Bonsu A. (2010) Ghana's poultry sector value chains and the impacts of HPAI. Draft Report. Pro-poor HPAI Risk Reduction Project International Food Policy Research Institute, Washington, DC.

21. National Academy of Sciences (NAS) (2009) Sustaining global surveillance and response to emerging zoonotic diseases. The National Academy of Sciences Press. Available athttp://www.books.nap.edu/openbook.php?record_id=126258. page=165 (accessed 20 May 2010).

22. Onkundi D., Bett B., Omore A., Randolph T. (2010) Alignment of poultry sector actors with avian influenza control measures in Kenya. Africa/Indonesia Working Paper 31 Report, IFPRI, Washington DC USA. 57p

23. Otte J., Henrichs J., Rushton J., Roland Hoist D., Zilberman D. (2008) Impacts of avian influenza virus on animal production in developing countries. CAB Reviews: Perspective in Agriculture, Veterinary Science, Nutrition and Natural Resources 3 No 080. Available at http://www.cababstractsplus.org/cabreviews(Accessed on 15 November 2010).

24. Padmawati S. & Nichter M. (2008) Community response to avian flu in Central Java, Indonesia.*Anthropology & Medicine* **15**, 31–51.

25. Philipson T. (2000) Economic epidemiology and infectious diseases. In: Handbook of Health Economics volume 1 (eds A.J. Culyer & J.P. Newhouse), pp 1761–1799. Elsevier Science, Amsterdam.

26. de Rooij R., Rushton J., McLeod A., Domenech J. (2007) Public and private sector roles in addressing animal health issues. Background paper. Technical meeting on Highly Pathogenic Avian Influenza and Human H5N1 infection. 27-29 June 2007. FAO Rome.

27. Schiffer E., Narrod C., von Grebner K. (2009) Surveillance and control of highly pathogenic avian influenza (HPAI) in Ghana. An assessment of institutions and actors. Pro-poor HPAI Risk Reduction Africa/Indonesia Team Working paper 18.

28. Turkson P.K., Okike I., Bett B., Randolph T. (2010) Alignment of poultry sector actors with avian influenza control measures in Ghana. Africa/Indonesia Region Report, IFPRI, Washington, DC, USA.

29. VSD (Veterinary Services Directorate, Ghana) (2007). Document on "Fund request to support prevention and control of avian and human influenza (Ghana) through the Support Programme to Integrated National Action Plans for Avian and Human Influenza (SPINAP-AHI)" submitted to the African Union/Inter-African Bureau for Animal Resources (AU-IBAR), Nairobi, Kenya.

30. Yakhshilikov Y., Tiongco M., Narrod C., Friedman J. (2009) Knowledge and practices of Indonesian rural communities and poultry farmers toward Avian Flu. Controlling Avian Flu and protecting people›s livelihoods in Africa and Indonesia. HPAI Research Brief No 1.

6
CHAPTER

GRAPIPRANT: AN EP4 PROSTAGLANDIN RECEPTOR ANTAGONIST AND NOVEL THERAPY FOR PAIN AND INFLAMMATION

Kristin Kirkby Shaw[2], Lesley C. Rausch-Derra[1], and Linda Rhodes[1]

[1]Aratana Therapeutics, Inc., Kansas City, Kansas, USA

[2]Animal Surgical Clinic of Seattle, Seattle, Washington, USA

ABSTRACT

There are five active prostanoid metabolites of arachidonic acid (AA) that have widespread and varied physiologic functions throughout the body, including regulation of gastrointestinal mucosal blood flow, renal haemodynamics and primary haemostasis. Each prostanoid has at least one distinct receptor that mediates its action. Prostaglandin E_2 (PGE_2) is a prostanoid that serves important homeostatic functions, yet is also responsible for regulating pain and inflammation. PGE_2 binds to four receptors, of which one, the EP4 receptor, is primarily responsible for the pain and inflammation associated with osteoarthritis (OA). The deleterious and pathologic actions of PGE_2 are inhibited in varying degrees by steroids, aspirin and cyclo-oxygenase inhibiting NSAIDs; however, administration of these drugs causes decreased production of PGE_2, thereby decreasing or eliminating the homeostatic functions of the molecule. By inhibiting just the EP4 receptor, the homeostatic function of PGE_2 is better maintained. This manuscript will introduce a new class of pharmaceuticals known as the piprant class. Piprants are prostaglandin receptor antagonists (PRA). This article will include basic physiology of AA, prostanoids and piprants, will review available evidence for the relevance of EP4 PRAs in rodent models of pain and inflammation, and will reference available data for an EP4 PRA in dogs and cats. Piprants are currently

Citation: Kirkby Shaw, K., Rausch-Derra, L. C. and Rhodes, L. (2016), Grapiprant: an EP4 prostaglandin receptor antagonist and novel therapy for pain and inflammation. Veterinary Medicine and Scienc, 2: 3–9. doi: 10.1002/vms3.13

in development for veterinary patients and the purpose of this manuscript is to introduce veterinarians to the class of drugs, with emphasis on an EP4 PRA and its potential role in the control of pain and inflammation associated with OA in dogs and cats.

INTRODUCTION

Prostanoids are metabolites of arachidonic acid (AA) and have been the target of medicinal therapies for centuries (Appelboom **2002**). However, until recently, preparations aimed at inhibiting the action of prostanoids have, with varying degrees of prostanoid specificity, prevented their production and thus impacted both pathologic and homeostatic activity (Curry *et al.* **2005**; KuKanich *et al.* **2012**). The evolution of pain management has entered a new era – that of selectively blocking the single prostanoid receptor that is primarily responsible for pain and inflammation, thereby preserving the production and activity of homeostatic prostanoids (Nakao *et al.* **2007**; Kawabata **2011**).

This manuscript reviews the mechanism of action of anti-inflammatory drugs for use in animals and introduce the first-in-class drug for managing pain and inflammation associated with osteoarthritis (OA) in veterinary patients: grapiprant, an EP4 prostaglandin receptor antagonist (PRA).

AA cascade revisited

Arachidonic acid is an omega 6 polyunsaturated lipid that is an integral part of cell membranes and is liberated from the cell membrane by the enzyme phospholipase A_2 (PLA_2) as part of normal cellular metabolism and following cell injury (Curry *et al.* **2005**; KuKanich*et al.* **2012**). The freed AA molecule is then shuttled into one of three pathways that generate three groups of molecules: prostanoids, leukotrienes and epoxides (Curry *et al.* **2005**; KuKanich *et al.* **2012**). This manuscript will focus on the prostanoid group.

The enzymes cyclo-oxygenase 1 and 2 (COX-1 and COX-2) convert AA into prostaglandin H_2(PGH_2), and PGH_2 is subsequently converted, via tissue-specific isomerases and oxidoreductases, to five active prostanoid molecules: thromboxane (TXA), PGD_2, PGI_2(prostacyclin), PGF_2 and PGE_2 (Simmons *et al.* **2004**; Ricciotti & FitzGerald **2011**). COX-1 is expressed constitutively in most cells and is the dominant source of prostanoids that are involved in gastric epithelial cytoprotection and homeostasis. COX-2 is constitutively expressed in some tissues, but is also inducible by inflammatory stimuli, and is an important source of prostanoid formation in periods or locations of inflammation. In inflammation, the profile of prostanoid production is determined by the differential expression of these enzymes within cells at the site of inflammation (Ricciotti & FitzGerald **2011**). Production of PGE_2 and PGI_2 predominates in sites where COX-2 is activated (Simmons *et al.* **2004**).

In the mid-1990s, prostanoid receptors were identified and continue to be characterized (Woodward *et al.* **2011**). These receptors have varying distributions throughout the body and mediate the activities of each prostanoid. Each prostanoid interacts with at least one distinct receptor to mediate specific physiological effects, and in some cases this includes specific receptor subtypes for a particular prostanoid.

Inhibiting prostanoid production: the good and the bad

Prostanoids are responsible for a wide range of homeostatic functions in mammals including regulation of renal haemodynamics and ion transport, gastrointestinal cytoprotection and motility, vascular and bronchial smooth muscle activity, immune function and platelet aggregation (Woodward *et al.* **2011**; KuKanich *et al.* **2012**). Pain and inflammation are also mediated by prostanoids, in particular PGE_2, and thus therapeutic drugs are often used to decrease the production and activity of this molecule (Curry *et al.* **2005**; KuKanich *et al.* **2012**). Steroids and cyclo-oxygenase inhibiting drugs have until now been the primary options for treating pain and inflammation, and because of their mechanism of action, these approaches have some drawbacks that are discussed below (Stahn *et al.* **2007**; KuKanich*et al.* **2012**).

Corticosteroids inhibit the enzyme PLA_2, acting up-stream of the COX enzymes in inhibiting the metabolism of AA (Stahn *et al.* **2007**). Corticosteroids prevent the synthesis of prostanoids, leukotrienes and epoxides, and thus have broad anti-inflammatory action, but also inhibit the production of many homeostatic AA metabolites. Short-acting corticosteroids can be important therapeutics in the management of acute allergic reactions, and while they may also provide some degree of pain relief, the untoward side effects make them a poor choice for long-term treatment of pain in veterinary patients.

Salicylic acid is a natural product derived from plants such as willow bark and meadowsweet, and its medicinal properties of pain relief and fever reduction have been utilized for centuries (Vane **1971**). Aspirin, or acetylsalicylic acid, is a synthetic drug made from salicylic acid. Aspirin irreversibly binds to the COX enzymes and inhibits the formation of all prostanoids (Flower **2003**; KuKanich *et al.* **2012**). While aspirin is effective in reducing fever, pain and inflammation, there are significant adverse effects of treatment with aspirin that are well-recognized in humans and animals, in particular gastrointestinal irritation and ulceration. Furthermore, irreversible inhibition of platelet TXA by aspirin leads to reduced aggregation that lasts up to 7–10 days (the life span of the affected platelets). This anti-thrombotic property can be useful in clinical conditions where reducing blood clotting is called for, but should also be recognized as a potentially significant unwanted side effect of aspirin administration.

Cyclo-oxygenase inhibiting non-steroidal anti-inflammatory drugs (COX inhibiting NSAIDs) decrease inflammation through inhibition of COX enzymes and subsequent inhibition of prostaglanoid production (Curry *et al.* **2005**; KuKanich *et al.* **2012**). This class includes aspirin, as described above, as well as other non-selective COX inhibitors (i.e. drugs that inhibit both COX 1 and COX 2 enzymes) such as ketoprofen and indomethacin. In addition, drugs have been developed that preferentially inhibit COX-2, such as carprofen, meloxicam, deracoxib, firocoxib and robenacoxib.

The two cyclo-oxygenase isoenzymes, COX-1 and COX-2, were isolated in the 1980s and shortly thereafter it was discovered that COX-2 is induced in response to tissue injury and is associated with inflammation and pain (Vane **1971**; KuKanich *et al.* **2012**).

Drug development then concentrated on molecules that preferentially inhibited this enzyme in the hope of sparing the so-called 'house-keeping' prostaglandins produced by COX-1. The coxib class of drugs, or selective COX-2 inhibitors, were first marketed in human medicine in 1999. In humans, COX-2 selective products such as rofecoxib (Vioxx® Merck & Co., Inc. Kenilworth, NJ USA) and celecoxib (Celebrex® Pfizer Inc. New York, NY USA) did show improved GI tolerability; however, in some cases, the FDA reviewed evidence leading the agency to conclude that their use was related to significant cardiovascular side effects and thus, all but one product have been removed from the US market (Harirforoosh *et al.* **2013**). The underlying cause for these adverse cardiovascular events may be attributed to inhibition of COX-2 synthesis of PGI_2 (prostacyclin). PGI_2 is a potent vasodilator and has anti-thrombotic properties (an endogenous antagonist of TXA), thus decreased production of PGI_2 by coxib-inhibiting NSAIDs may lead to increased thrombosis and vasoconstriction, two methods of potentiating cardiovascular disease (Harirforoosh *et al.* **2013**). The cardiovascular adverse events associated with COX-2 selective NSAIDs in humans have not been observed in dogs taking COX-2 selective NSAIDs. However, severe gastrointestinal, renal and hepatic adverse events have been reported in dogs taking these products (Lascelles *et al.* **2005**; KuKanich*et al.* **2012**; Monteiro-Steagall *et al.* **2013**).

Both COX-1 and COX-2 activity are important in maintaining gastrointestinal integrity and renal haemodynamics in dogs, primarily through the actions of PGE_2 and PGI_2 (Wilson *et al.* **2004**; KuKanich *et al.* **2012**). COX-2 is expressed in the canine kidney and involved in regulation of vessel tone and salt and water balance via synthesis of PGE_2 and PGI_2. In the stomach and intestinal tract, COX-1 is the primary mediator of gastro-protective prostanoid (PGE_2 and PGI_2) production in the healthy animal. COX-2 is up-regulated in areas of gastrointestinal irritation and it is important in promoting the healing of gastrointestinal ulcerations (KuKanich *et al.* **2012**). This suggests that administration of a selective COX-2 inhibitor drug in the face of gastrointestinal ulceration, such as due to stress or administration of corticosteroids or a non-selective cyclo-oxygenase-inhibiting NSAID such as aspirin, may reduce healing and potentiate ulceration and perforation (Lascelles *et al.* **2005**). Another potential mechanism for gastrointestinal injury secondary to cyclo-oxygenase inhibiting NSAID administration is the increased production of inflammatory leukotrienes (Curry *et al.* **2005**). Inhibition of the COX pathways may result in increased AA that must be metabolized by the lipo-oxygenase enzyme (LOX) pathway.

The four FDA approved COX inhibitor NSAIDs for use in dogs, unless contra-indicated, are considered to be effective treatments for the pain associated with OA. However, these COX-inhibiting NSAIDs, as a class, carry the potential for adverse effects including gastrointestinal ulceration and perforation and renal insufficiency (Lascelles *et al.* **2005**; Monteiro-Steagall*et al.* **2013**). While COX-2 selective and preferential NSAIDs are associated with fewer side effects compared to aspirin and older, non-selective COX inhibitor NSAIDs, many dogs do not tolerate these drugs, and alternative pharmacologic pain relief is indicated. Currently, no other class of pharmaceuticals is approved by the FDA for the treatment of pain and inflammation associated with OA in dogs. Thus, it is evident that an FDA approved product that demonstrates targeted pain relief with improved tolerability is needed.

THE PIPRANT CLASS: PRA

After the identification of prostanoid receptors in the 1990s, significant research ensued into methods of targeting each receptor with synthetic agonists and antagonists (Woodward*et al.* **2011**). In October 2013, the World Health Organization defined a newly recognized class of drugs that act as PRAs as the piprant class (World Health Organization, **2013**).

EP4 PRAs and anti-inflammatory effects: experimental models

Prostaglandin E_2 (PGE_2) is a key mediator of swelling, redness and pain, the classic signs of inflammation, with pain resulting from PGE_2-mediated sensitization of sensory neurons and swelling and redness resulting from PGE_2-mediated vasodilation and increased vascular permeability (Ricciotti & FitzGerald **2011**). PGE_2 exerts its effects via four receptors, EP1, EP2, EP3 and EP4 (Woodward *et al.* **2011**). The EP4 receptor is the primary mediator of the PGE_2-elicited sensitization of sensory neurons and PGE_2-elicited inflammation (Southall & Vasko **2001**; McCoy *et al.* **2002**; Lin *et al.* **2006**; Nakao *et al.* **2007**; Clark *et al.* **2008**; Chen *et al.* **2010**; Boyd *et al.* **2011**). Grapiprant (AT-001) is a new analgesic and anti-inflammatory drug in the piprant class that functions as a selective EP4 PRA (Nakao *et al.* **2007**). The following is a review of the literature and studies that demonstrate the anti-inflammatory effects of EP4 PRAs and of grapiprant in particular.

The use of receptor knockout mice has been helpful in understanding the roles of the specific EP receptors in inflammation. Collagen antibody-induced arthritis (CAIA) in mice is a model for the human inflammatory disorder rheumatoid arthritis (RA). The individual PGE_2receptors were evaluated by inducing CAIA in mice which were genetically modified to knock out the EP1, -2, -3, or -4 receptors and measuring the clinical, histopathological and cellular markers of disease (McCoy *et al.* **2002**). When mice with one of these four receptors knocked out were evaluated for signs of pain and inflammation, the EP4 receptor knock-out mice, but not the EP1, EP2 or EP3 receptor knock-out mice, had decreased incidence and severity of disease, decreased histopathological deterioration associated with arthritis and decreased levels of inflammatory markers, implicating EP4 as a key mediator of inflammation. In a mouse model of acute inflammation, EP1, 2, 3 or 4 receptor knock-out mice were subjected to UV irradiation of the skin. EP4 and EP2 knock-out mice, but not EP1 or EP3 knock-out mice, had significantly decreased ear swelling compared to control mice. The reduction in swelling was also seen when the wild-type mice were treated with an EP4 PRA (Kabashima *et al.* **2007**).

The anti-inflammatory effects of EP4 receptor antagonism have also been investigated in animal models of inflammation. In a study by Clark *et al.* (**2008**), joint inflammation (as measured by paw swelling) was created using an adjuvant-induced arthritis (AIA) model in rats. Rats treated with an EP4 PRA (MF498), but not an EP1 or an EP3 PRA, demonstrated reduced paw swelling. The reduction in swelling was similar to that seen in mice treated with a cyclo-oxygenase-2 (COX-2) inhibitor. In a study by Murase *et al.* (**2008**), the selective EP4 PRA, CJ-042,794, caused decreased paw swelling in a complete Freund's adjuvant model of chronic inflammatory pain in rats. The reductions in paw swelling in the CJ-042,794 treated rats were again similar to those seen with rofecoxib (a COX-2 inhibitor) treated rats. Using a complete Freund's adjuvant administration as a rodent model for pain and inflammation, treatment with an EP4 PRA, identified as 1a, also demonstrated reduced swelling of the paw (Boyd *et al.* **2011**). In a series of experiments reported by Chen *et al.* (**2010**), an EP4 PRA, ER-819762, suppressed inflammatory cytokine production, suppressed disease and slowed disease progression in collagen and GPI-induced arthritis in mice. These data support the anti-inflammatory role of EP4 receptor antagonism in rodents. Indeed, these results demonstrated that EP4 PRAs can reduce inflammation as effectively as COX-2 inhibitors.

Several studies have been conducted examining the anti-inflammatory and analgesic effects of grapiprant (AT-001, referred to as CJ-023,423 in the publications) in rats (Nakao *et al.* **2007**). Studies using rat models have demonstrated grapiprant's ability to reduce acute and chronic pain and inflammation (Nakao *et al.* **2007**; RaQualia **2007a,b**). The anti-inflammatory effect of grapiprant on paw swelling, inflammatory biomarkers in the serum and synovial inflammation was examined in the tarsal joint in AIA in rats (RaQualia **2007b**). Grapiprant exhibited dose-dependent and significant anti-inflammatory effects on all parameters tested. The efficacy of grapiprant on paw swelling was comparable to those of rofecoxib and piroxicam (COX-inhibiting drugs). In another study, the anti-inflammatory activity of grapiprant on rat carrageenan-induced foot swelling was investigated (RaQualia **2007a**). Grapiprant inhibited foot swelling in a dose-dependent manner compared to rats treated with placebo control. Nakao *et al.* (**2007**) investigated three different models of pain in rats: mechanical hyperalgesia, thermal hyperalgesia and weight bearing deficit. Oral administration of CJ-023,423 significantly reduced hyperalgesia in rodents in all three models, including significantly reversing complete Freund's adjuvant-induced chronic inflammatory pain.

Not only is the EP4 receptor prominently involved in inflammation and pain, but importantly this receptor may mediate central sensitization and play a role in chronic pain. Lin *et al.* (**2006**) reported that in rodents, the EP4 receptor is expressed by sensory neurons, and the level of EP4 receptors increased following peripheral inflammation. Administration of an EP4 PRA decreased pain and hypersensitivity in rodents.

EP4 PRA in veterinary medicine: targeted pain management

The EP4 receptor in mice, humans and dogs has been cloned and characterized. The canine EP4 receptor has approximately 90% homology to the human receptor (Castleberry *et al.* **2001**). Grapiprant is a PRA that selectively blocks the EP4 receptor in rodents, humans, and dogs (RaQualia **2007c**). Grapiprant has undergone experimental and pilot studies in laboratory and client-owned dogs. A multi-site, masked, placebo-controlled, randomized field trial for the control of pain and inflammation associated with OA in dogs was recently completed and was submitted to and accepted by the FDA in support of regulatory approval (www.aratana.com). The results of these studies in client-owned dogs demonstrate that this drug provides control of the pain associated with OA. Studies are currently underway investigating the use of grapiprant in cats, and at this time data are not yet available.

As part of development of grapiprant for FDA approval for dogs with OA, a safety study in healthy Beagles investigated the effects of daily orally administered doses up to 50 mg kg^{-1} day^{-1} oral suspension (equivalent to approximately 30.5 mg kg^{-1} day^{-1} of the tablet formulation) for nine consecutive months (Rausch-Derra *et al.* **2015a**,**b**). There were no drug-related effects on liver enzyme values, BUN/creatinine, or platelet function. Mild and reversible dose- and time-dependent decreases in total protein, albumin and calcium were seen. Clinical signs were also dose dependent and restricted to mild gastrointestinal signs including soft stool, occasional stool with mucus or blood, and sporadic vomiting. There were no histopathological changes to any tissues, including the stomach, kidneys or liver except in one dog in the 50 mg kg^{-1} group had mild mucosal regeneration of the ileum seen on histopathology.

The relative lack of toxic effects with grapiprant compared to those that have been reported in dogs treated with COX-inhibiting NSAIDs is not surprising. Grapiprant is a targeted approach to pain management – it selectively blocks the EP4 receptor, does not interfere with the production of prostanoids, and therefore does not affect the other PG receptor pathways that are affected in animals treated with COX inhibitor NSAIDs.

CONCLUSION

PGE_2 is a key mediator of pain and inflammation and has its effect through binding to the EP4 receptor. Grapiprant directly and specifically blocks the EP4 receptor, and therefore blocks PGE_2-elicited pain and inflammation. An EP4 PRA, such as grapiprant, which has been demonstrated to provide relief from arthritic pain in canine clinical patients, acts without affecting the synthesis and widespread activity of PGE_2 and other prostanoids.

Safety studies in laboratory dogs have demonstrated an excellent safety profile, and a wide safety margin, and this has been confirmed in two large field effectiveness studies in dogs with OA (Rausch-Derra *et al.* **2015a**,**b**). The relative lack of toxic effects with grapiprant compared to those that have been reported in dogs treated with COX-inhibiting NSAIDs is consistent with grapiprant's unique mechanism of action, although until FDA review and approval, claims of safety and effectiveness cannot be made. Grapiprant may offer a more targeted, and potentially better tolerated, method of pain management in dogs with OA.

ACKNOWLEDGEMENT

We would like to acknowledge the scientists at RaQualia who pioneered basic research and development of EP4 PRAs.

CONFLICTS OF INTEREST

At the time of writing, all authors were employees of Aratana Therapeutics, Inc., Kansas City, KS, USA At the time of publication, KK Shaw will be a full time employee of

Animal Surgical Clinic of Seattle; Seattle, WA, USA and a paid consultant for Aratana Therapeutics, Inc.

REFERENCES

1. Appelboom T. (2002) Arthropathy in art and the history of pain management – through centuries to cyclooxygenase-2 inhibitors. *Rheumatology* 41, 28–34.
2. Boyd M.J., Berthelette C., Chiasson J.F., Clark P., Colucci J., Denis D. *et al.* (2011) A novel series of potent and selective EP4 receptor ligands: facile modulation of agonism and antagonism. *Bioorganic & Medicinal Chemistry Letters* 21, 484–487.
3. Castleberry T.A., Lu B., Smock S.L. & Owen T.A. (2001) Molecular cloning and functional characterization of the canine prostaglandin E_2 receptor EP4 subtype. *Prostaglandins & Other Lipid Mediators* 65,167–187.
4. Chen Q., Muramoto K., Masaaki N., Ding Y., Yang H., Mackey M. *et al.* (2010) A novel antagonist of the prostaglandin E(2) EP(4) receptor inhibits Th1 differentiation and Th17 expansion and is orally active in arthritis models. *British Journal of Pharmacology* 160, 292–310.
5. Clark P., Rowland S. E., Denis D., Mathieu M. C., Stocco R., Poirier H. *et al.* (2008) MF498 [N-{[4-(5,9-Diethoxy-6-oxo-6,8-dihydro-7H-pyrrolo[3,4-g] quinolin-7-yl)-3-m ethylbenzyl]sulfonyl}-2-(2-methoxyphenyl)acetamide], a selective E prostanoid receptor 4 antagonist, relieves joint inflammation and pain in rodent models of rheumatoid and osteoarthritis. *The Journal of Pharmacology and Experimental Therapeutics* 325, 425–434.
6. Curry S.L., Cogar S.M. & Cook J.L. (2005) Nonsteroidal anti-inflammatory drugs: a review. *Journal of the American Animal Hospital Association* 41, 298–309.
7. Flower R. (2003) What are all the things that aspirin does? *BMJ* 327, 572–573.
8. Harirforoosh S., Asghar W. & Jamali F. (2013) Adverse effects of nonsteroidal anti-inflammatory drug: an update of gastrointestinal, cardiovascular and renal complications. *Journal of Pharmacy and Pharmaceutical Sciences* 16, 821–847.
9. Kabashima K., Nagamachi M., Honda T., Nishigori C., Miyachi Y., Tokura Y., Narumiya S. (2007)Prostaglandin E2 is required for ultraviolet B-induced skin inflammation via EP2 and EP4 receptors.*Laboratory Investigation* 87, 49–55.
10. Kawabata A. (2011) Prostaglandin E2 and pain–an update. *Biological and Pharmaceutical Bulletin* 34,1170–1173.
11. KuKanich B., Bidgood T. & Knesl O. (2012) Clinical pharmacology of nonsteroidal ant-inflammatory drugs in dogs. *Veterinary Anaesthesia and Analgesia* 39, 69–90.
12. Lascelles B.D.X., Blikslager A.T., Fox S.M. & Reece D. (2005) Gastrointestinal tract perforation in dogs treated with a selective cyclooxygenase-2 inhibitor: 29 cases (2002–2003). *Journal of the American Veterinary Medical Association* 227, 1112–1117.

13. Lin C. R., Amaya F., Barrett L., Wang H., Takada J., Samad T. A., Woolf C. J. (2006) Prostaglandin E2 receptor EP4 contributes to inflammatory pain hypersensitivity. *Journal of Pharmacology and Experimental Therapeutics* 319, 1096–1103.

14. McCoy J.M., Wicks J.R. & Audoly L.P. (2002) The role of prostaglandin E2 receptors in the pathogenesis of rheumatoid arthritis. *The Journal of Clinical Investigation* 110, 651–658.

15. Monteiro-Steagall B.P., Steagall P.V.M. & Lascelles B.D.X. (2013) Systematic review of nonsteroidal anti-inflammatory drug-induced adverse effects in dogs. *Journal of Veterinary Internal Medicine* 27,1011–1019.

16. Murase A., Okumura T., Sakakibara A., Tonai-Kachi H., Nakao K., Takada J. (2008) Effect of prostanoid EP4 receptor antagonist, CJ-042,794, in rat models of pain and inflammation. *European Journal of Pharmacology* 580, 116–121.

17. Nakao K., Murase A., Ohshiro H., Okumura T., Taniguchi K., Murata Y. *et al.* (2007) CJ-023,423, a novel, potent and selective prostaglandin EP4 receptor antagonist with antihyperalgesic properties. *Journal of Pharmacology and Experimental Therapeutics* 322, 686–694.

18. RaQualia (2007a) Determination of the Dose Response Relationship of CJ-023423 in the Rat Carrageenin-Induced Foot Edema Model. SR_DB1_CJ-023423_RAT_CFE_1_2007.

19. RaQualia (2007b) Investigation of the Inhibitory Effects of CJ-023423 on Inflammation and Bone Destruction in Adjuvant-Induced Arthritis Rats. SR_DB1_CJ-023423_AIA_1_2007.

20. RaQualia (2007c) Determination of the Binding Affinity of CJ-023423 for the Cloned Dog EP4 Receptor. SR_PPL_CJ-02423_dog_EP4BD_2007.

21. Rausch-Derra L., Rhodes L., Freshwater L. (2015a) Pharmacokinetic Comparison of Oral Tablet and Suspension Formulations of Grapiprant, a Novel Therapeutic for the Pain and Inflammation of Osteoarthritis in Dogs. Presented at AAVPT Biennial Symposium, Fort Collins, CO.

22. Rausch-Derra L., Huebner M. & Rhodes L. (2015b) Evaluation of the safety of long-term, daily oral administration of grapiprant, a novel drug for treatment of osteoarthritic pain and inflammation, in health dogs. *American Journal of Veterinary Research* 76, 853–859.

23. Ricciotti E. & FitzGerald G.A. (2011) Prostaglandins and inflammation. *Arteriosclerosis, Thrombosis, and Vascular Biology* 31, 986–1000.

24. Simmons D.L., Botting R.M. & Hla T. (2004) Cyclooxygenase isozymes: the biology of prostaglandin synthesis and inhibition. *Pharmacological Reviews* 56, 387–437.

25. Southall M.D. & Vasko M.R. (2001) Prostaglandin receptor subtypes, EP3C and EP4, mediate the prostaglandin E2-induced cAMP production and sensitization of sensory neurons. *The Journal of Biological Chemistry* 276, 16083–16091.

26. Stahn C., Lowenberg M., Hommes D.W. & Buttgereit F. (2007) Molecular mechanisms of glucocorticoid action and selective glucocorticoid receptor agonists. *Molecular and Cellular Endocrinology* 275, 71–78.

27. Vane J.R. (1971) Inhibition of prostaglandin synthesis as a mechanism of action for aspirin-like drugs.*Nature: New Biology* 231, 232–235.

28.

29. Wilson J.E., Chandrasekharan N.V., Westover K.D. *et al.* (2004) Determination of expression of cyclooxygenase-1 and -2 isozymes in canine tissues and their differential sensitivity to nonsteroidal anti-inflammatory drugs. *American Journal of Veterinary Research* 65, 810–818.

30. Woodward D.F., Jones R.L. & Narumiya S. (2011) International Union of basic and clinical pharmacology. LXXXIII: classification of prostanoid receptors, updating 15 years of progress. *Pharmacological Reviews*63, 471–538.

31. World Health Organization (2013) Pre-stems: Suffixes Used in the Selection of INN.

7

CHAPTER

COMPARATIVE ASPECTS OF CANINE MELANOMA

Adriana Tomoko Nishiya [1], Cristina Oliveira Massoco [1], Claudia Ronca Felizzola [1,2], Eduardo Perlmann [3], Karen Batschinski [1], Marcello Vannucci Tedardi [1], Jéssica Soares Garcia [1], Priscila Pedra Mendonça [3], Tarso Felipe Teixeira [4], and Maria Lucia Zaidan Dagli [1]

[1]Department of Pathology, School of Veterinary Medicine and Animal Science, University of São Paulo, Av. Prof. Dr. Orlando Marques de Paiva, 87, CEP 05508-270, São Paulo, Brazil

[2]Surgical Oncology Rua Antônio Alves Magan, 124, CEP 01251-150, São Paulo, Brazil

[3]Department of Surgery, School of Veterinary Medicine and Animal Science, University of São Paulo, CEP 05508-270, São Paulo, Brazil

[4]Pathology Veterinary Medicine, FEPI Itajubá University Center, Dr. Antonio Braga Filho Street, 687, Itajubá, 37.501-002 Minas Gerais, Brazil

ABSTRACT

Melanomas are malignant neoplasms originating from melanocytes. They occur in most animal species, but the dog is considered the best animal model for the disease. Melanomas in dogs are most frequently found in the buccal cavity, but the skin, eyes, and digits are other common locations for these neoplasms. The aim of this review is to report etiological, epidemiological, pathological, and molecular aspects of melanomas in dogs. Furthermore, the particular biological behaviors of these tumors in the different body locations are shown. Insights into the therapeutic approaches are described. Surgery, chemotherapy, radiotherapy, immunotherapy, and the outcomes after these treatments are presented. New therapeutic perspectives are also depicted. All efforts are geared toward better characterization and control of malignant melanomas in dogs, for the benefit of these companion animals, and also in an attempt to benefit the treatment of human melanomas.

Citation: Adriana Tomoko Nishiya, Cristina Oliveira Massoco, Claudia Ronca Felizzola, Eduardo Perlmann, Karen Batschinski, Marcello Vannucci Tedardi, Jéssica Soares Garcia, Priscila Pedra Mendonça, Tarso Felipe Teixeira, and Maria Lucia Zaidan Dagli, Comparative Aspects of Canine Melanoma, doi:10.3390/vetsci3010007

INTRODUCTION

Melanoma is a malignant neoplasm originating from melanocytes. Melanocytic neoplasms have been described in men and in most domesticated animal species, including dogs, cats, horses, and also in wild terrestrial and marine animals [1].

Since dogs live in close proximity to humans, they are influenced by similar environmental factors that may lead to chronic diseases and cancer. In fact, the domestic dog (*Canis familiaris*) reportedly presents more naturally inherited chronic diseases than any other animal species. Hence, those aspects have to be considered in the selection of an animal model for a multifactorial human disease, and the dog appears to be the one with the best characteristics [2,3,4]. Dogs are considered recommended models due to their relatively high susceptibility to cancers, including melanomas, and many behavioral similarities [5].

While many genetic alterations of melanomas have recently been discovered and studied, control of this disease is still challenging in both humans and animals, particularly in dogs and cats. The aim of this review is to report a comparative approach of the etiological, epidemiological, pathological, and molecular aspects of melanomas in dogs.

CANINE MELANOMA EPIDEMIOLOGY

Melanoma is one of the most devastating types of cancer, killing around 50,000 people worldwide every year [6,7]. In 2015, according to the American Cancer Society, it is estimated that about 73,870 new melanoma cases will be diagnosed (about 42,670 in men and 31,200 in women), and 9940 people are expected to die of melanoma (about 6640 men and 3300 women).

Human malignant mucosal melanoma of the head and neck is increasing rapidly in incidence in the United States. It is an uncommon and fatal malignancy that does not appear to have the same etiologic basis as cutaneous melanoma. In 452 observed cases, the majority of patients had sino-nasal location (72.6%) and white women ages 70 or older were most affected [8]. This kind of human malignant melanoma is uncommon and has aggressive behavior with increasing rates of recurrence and regional and distant metastasis [9]. Regional lymphatic metastasis occurred in 57.9% to 21% of patients and recurrence rates were 57.9% to 26.3% for patients treated with surgery alone and for those treated with surgery and radiotherapy, respectively. Distant metastases occurred in 52.6% receiving surgery alone and in 47.3% receiving both therapies [10].

Canine oral malignant melanomas in dogs accounted for 0.99% of all (338/33826) canine pathology cases received from 1992 through 1999 at the University of Missouri—Veterinary. The most common sites are the gingiva and labial mucosa [11].

In a retrospective study of neoplasms in domestic animals (data collected between 1993 and 2002 at the School of Veterinary Medicine and Animal Science of the University of São Paulo, Brazil), of 1813 cases of neoplasms in dogs, 58 were melanocytic neoplasms, accounting for 3% of the total in this species [12]. In another retrospective study, 2154 neoplasms were diagnosed at the University of São Paulo between 2000 and 2006. A total of 193 cases (8.9%) were melanocytic neoplasms, of which 186 cases occurred in dogs (96.4%), and only seven in cats (3.6%). Male mixed-breed dogs with black hair coats, with ages varying from 8 to 11 years, were the most commonly affected animals [13].

Canine malignant melanomas are located at different anatomical sites, such as the mouth (Figure 1A,B), lips, skin (Figure 1C), eyes, and digits (Table 1). Studies are controversial about the most common location for this disease in dogs; however, most studies point to the oral cavity and skin as the most common sites [14,15,16,17]. In a survey of 384 melanocytic canine tumors, oral, cutaneous, lips/feet, and eye sites comprised 19%, 59%, 19%, and 3%, respectively [18]. In another study considering malignant melanomas, oral cavity and cutaneous localization were the most common in 40%–62% and 27%–31%, respectively [13,19].

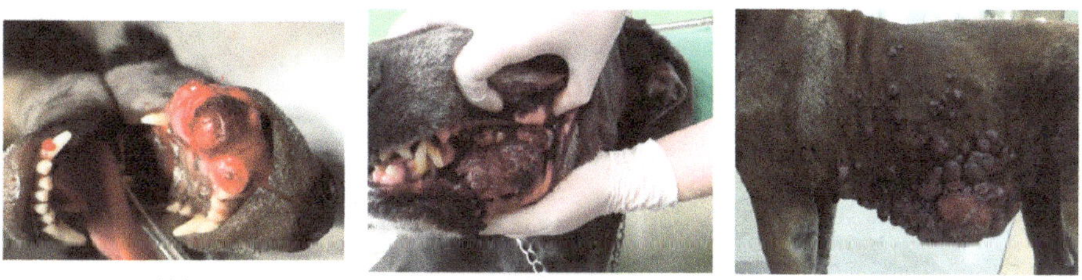

(A) (B) (C)

Figure 1: Clinical aspect of malignant oral melanomas (**A**) in maxilla; (**B**) in mandible. Clinical aspect of malignant cutaneous melanoma (**C**) in thoracic and abdominal wall (*Adriana Nihiya*).

Table 1: Common sites of malignant melanomas in dogs.

Sites/Total Number of Cases	n = 1652	n = 143	n = 209
Oral	1026	57	67
Cutaneous	448	44	88
Scrotum	-	4	-
Digit	94	21	-
Ungual	60	-	-
Ocular	24	17	-
Lips/Feet	-	-	54
Reference	Gillard *et al.*, 2014 [19]	Teixeira *et al.*, 2010 [13]	Spangler and Kass, 2006 [18]

Data obtained from historical studies indicated that the following breeds of dogs are considered at risk to develop melanocytic tumors: Airedale Terrier, Boston Terrier, Boxer, Chihuahua, Chow Chow, Cocker Spaniel, Doberman Pinscher, English Springer Spaniel, Golden Retriever, Irish Setter [20], Miniature Schnauzer, Scottish Terrier [19,20], Poodles, Beauce Shepherds, Rottweilers, and Labrador Retrievers [19]. Some breeds of dogs, specifically the Schnauzer family (miniature and standard), Scottish Terriers, and Irish Setters are at risk for developing digital malignant melanomas [21,22].

Malignant melanomas typically occur in middle-aged to older dogs, as Miller *et al.* [23] found an average age of nine years, and with no gender predilections.

Teixeira *et al.* [24] studied 25 canine oral melanomas, including 16 melanotic and nine amelanotic specimens. In this study, 25% of the melanotic melanoma-bearing dogs were eight-year old animals, and 22.2% of amelanotic melanoma-bearing group were younger, with ages varying from four to eight years.

Most information on animal cancer epidemiology in the literature comes from laboratories or hospitals, usually from a unique center and using non-standard coding protocols. This may lead to epidemiological bias, and the data rarely generate reliable information useful to establish comparisons. Cancer registries are the most important source of epidemiological data for neoplasms [25]. There are some animal cancer registries around the world, situated mostly in Europe and the USA. In 2013, the São Paulo Animal Cancer Registry was created at the University of São Paulo, Brazil, serving as the first animal cancer registry in Latin America [25,26]. This system will allow for better and more accurate epidemiologic studies in domestic animals in this region.

CANINE MALIGNANT MELANOMA ETIOLOGY

In humans, malignant melanoma is the most aggressive, therapy-resistant, and deadly form of skin cancer [27]. The major risk factors for human melanoma include family history, skin and mucosal pigmentation characteristics, sun exposure, particularly to UVB light, and skin reactions to sun exposure. Another type of melanoma, oral malignant melanoma, is a rare aggressive neoplasm usually seen in middle-aged adults.

Several etiological factors are supposed to be involved in canine malignant melanomas, including consanguinity, trauma, chemical exposure, hormones, and genetic susceptibility [28]. However, there is no consensus regarding the etiology of malignant melanomas in dogs [29]. Sunlight may be involved in the development of this disease in the sun-exposed skin areas of the body, such as the face and pinnae; however, sunlight probably is not involved in mucosal melanomas, like the ones found in the canine buccal cavity. Other factors, like the presence of pigmented cells, trauma, chemical agents, or even the buccal microbiota, and inflammation may be associated with the etiology of these tumors [30].

Although melanomas can arise in any dog, the prevalence of this disease is higher in purebred dogs, especially Standard and Miniature Schnauzers, Doberman Pinschers, Scottish Terriers, Irish and Gordon Setters, and Golden Retrievers. This fact supports the theory that melanomas in dogs could have a genetic basis [28]. Genetic and epigenetic modifications in melanocytes that lead to alterations in expression or function of genes and proteins involved in cell cycle control and apoptosis are certainly involved in the development of melanomas.

CANINE MELANOMA PATHOLOGICAL ASPECTS AND PROGNOSIS

Melanocytic neoplasms can be classified as benign or malignant tumors [31]. Malignant melanomas are considered malignant neoplasms arising from melanocytes, while melanocytomas are the benign counterparts [31].

Melanocytes, which are dendritic cells derived from the neuroectoderm and melanoblasts of the neural crest, migrate during embryogenesis to the dermis and epidermis, mucous membranes, and eyes [29,32]. These dendritic cells in melanoma development have demonstrated altered expression of cell–cell adhesion molecules, such as decreased expression of E-cadherin and V-CAM 1 and increased expression of N-cadherin, Mel-CAM 1, ICAM 1, and α β integrins [33]. The development of malignant melanoma is generally characterized by a series of transitions that are outlined in [34], and arises from melanocytes that normally reside within the basal layer of epidermis [35].

According to Head *et al.* [36], a melanocytoma is a benign tumor composed of melanocytes in the basal region of the epithelium and extending into the submucosa (junctional melanocytoma) or in the sub-epithelial connective tissue under normal epithelium (dermal melanocytoma). Malignant melanoma can be subdivided into three patterns on the basis of cell shape [36]:

- epithelioid—round and polygonal cells (Figure 2)

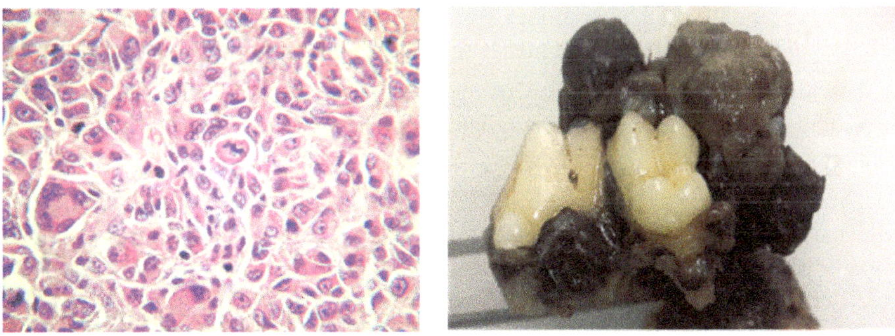

(A) (B)

Figure 2: Photomicrograph of the most common histopathology type of malignant melanoma (epithelioid), showing formation of cell nests, with the presence of multinucleated giant cells and atypical mitotic figures, HE, Objective 40 × (**A**). Canine oral malignant melanoma, pigmented, exophytic mass protruding from the gingiva (**B**). Formalin-fixed tissue. Photographs are courtesy of Professor Dr. José Guilherme Xavier.

- spindle cell—tumor resembles fibroblasts
- mixed tumors—show both cell types

Malignant melanoma histologically can be the highly melanotic type or the highly anaplastic amelanotic type. Anaplastic melanocytes can be large with abundant cytoplasm with one or more oval or elongated nuclei, with obvious nucleoli. These are frequently characterized to form nests in the submucosa by a mixed structure of epithelial-like cells and fusiform cells and junctional infiltration between basal cells and in the submucosa [36] (Figure 3).

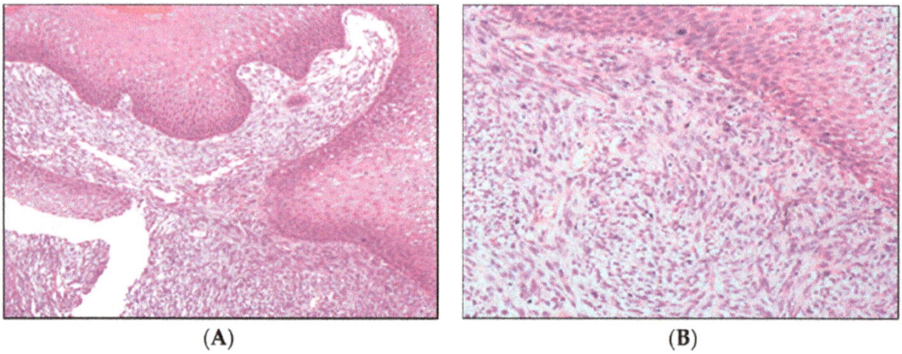

Figure 3: Photomicrograph of oral amelanotic melanoma ((**A**), Objective 10 ×; (**B**), Objective 20 ×). Hematoxylin and eosin.

The most prominent biological property of melanoma cells is the ability to produce melanin [37]. The disruption of homeostasis of close association between melanocytes and basal keratinocytes may trigger a continuous proliferation of the melanocytes, which may lead to the development of a malignant melanoma [7]. Once malignant melanoma cells have escaped from the keratinocyte control, they become able to invade the tissue by the degradation of extracellular matrix through the action of metalloproteinases [38].

The histopathological diagnosis of melanoma may be difficult if the tumor does not contain melanin. Amelanotic malignant melanomas may represent one third of all melanoma cases in dogs.

Their histopathological aspect may resemble carcinomas, sarcomas, lymphomas, and osteogenic tumors. For this reason, the diagnosis of malignant melanoma should be made with the use of immunohistochemistry [11,39,40]. Teixeira *et al.* [13] used two different antibodies to confirm the diagnosis of malignant melanoma in amelanotic cases: HMB 45 (Mouse monoclonal anti-human HMB45, from Dako) and Melan A (Monoclonal mouse anti-human Melan-A, from Dako), and both were considered suitable to immunostain canine melanocytes. Ramos-Vara *et al.* [11] considered Melan A as a specific and sensitive marker for malignant melanomas. Smedley *et al.* [41] evaluated 49 amelanotic melanomas and created a cost-effective and efficient immunodiagnostic cocktail panel containing antibodies against PNL2, Melan-A, TRP-1, and TRP-2 that had 100% specificity and 93.9% sensitivity in identifying canine oral amelanotic melanocytic neoplasms. In addition, malignant melanomas are positive for vimentin and variably positive for S-100 protein and neuron-specific enolase (NSE) [42].

In order to use immunohistochemical techniques to study melanoma cell characteristics, it is frequently necessary to remove melanin from the histopathological specimen. There are several methods to do bleaching in melanoma cells, but the one described by Silva *et al.* [43] is one of the most effective, in which slides were immersed only in 10% hydrogen peroxide in pH 7.4 0.2 mol/L Tris-HCl buffer solution for 24 h in the dark at room temperature.

CANINE MELANOMA: MOLECULAR ASPECTS

Melanomas in humans seem to arise from normal melanocytes that suffer a number of molecular events that lead to their transformation. The progression from normal melanocytes to melanoma sometimes involves its transformation to melanocytic nevus. The genetic alterations involved in this progression are still under study. Several genes/genetic pathways were identified in human melanomas, and these are important for the diagnosis, establishment of prognosis, and drug targeting [44]. Some of these genes are described below:

- CDKN2A Locus—about 70% of melanomas harbor mutations or deletions in this locus on chromosome 9p21.
- Genes that are altered when normal melanocytes generate a nevus: BRAF, NRAS, and INK4a/ARF.
- Genes that are mutated or deregulated when a nevus is transformed to a melanoma: BRAF, NRAS, INK4a/ARF, PTEN, c-kit, NEDD9, and MITF.

Genetic alterations in canine malignant melanomas from mucosal or acral sites have not been fully described. Activating mutations in BRAF exon 15 have not been found [6,45]. Activating mutations of NRAS and c-kit appear to be absent in canine mucosal melanoma, in contrast to human mucosal melanoma, where these genes are mutated in 15% of tumors [44,46,47]. Further studies are necessary to understand the molecular basis of canine malignant melanomas.

Genetic alterations in canine malignant melanomas from human mucosal melanomas have not been fully studied (Table 2). Mutations in exon 15 of BRAF are not found [6], similar to human mucosal malignant melanoma [48]. Activating mutations of NRAS are presented in three of 77 cases [19] and c-kit appears absent in canine mucosal melanomas [49], in contrast to human mucosal melanoma, where these genes are mutated in 4% and 14% of tumors, respectively [50].

Table 2: Genes altered by mutations in canine and human mucosal malignant melanomas

	Human	Dog
BRAF	4% [50], 2% [48], 6% [14]	0% [6,19]
C-KIT	12.5% [16], 4% [50]	0% [49]
NRAS	22% [15], 14% [50], 10% [14]	6% [19]
PTEN	48.1% [15]	4% [19]
GNAQ	0% [16]	0% [19]
CDK4	0% [17]	0% [19]

In 2014, Gillard *et al.* [19] compared the histopathology and genetic alterations of canine and human melanomas. They observed that dog malignant melanomas present cytological characteristics similar to human melanoma simulating "nevus" and "animal type," suggesting a new melanoma classification. They also studied six genes in canine melanomas that are recurrent mutations in human melanomas, BRAF, NRAS, PTEN, KIT, GNAQ, and CDK4. In total, out of the 95 cases (77 oral and 18 cutaneous melanomas), no mutations were found in BRAF, KIT, GNAQ, and CDK4 genes; only three had a positive NRAS mutation and two had a PTEN gene mutation, of which one case had both changes [19]. BRAF mutations were seen in 57% of human cutaneous melanomas and NRAS was mutated in 17% of samples. Both changes were seen in 15.4% [51].

The low frequency of BRAF mutations associated with UV-independent carcinogenesis and oral anatomical distribution of canine melanomas supports the dog as a spontaneous model for investigation of non-UV-associated human melanomas [52].

Human and canine melanoma share differential gene expression patterns of MAPK, but similar sensitivity in cell culture to therapeutic inhibitors of MAPK (AZD6244) and PI3K/AKT (rapamycin) [6].

Dog malignant melanomas share numerous immunohistochemistry similarities (KIT, PTEN, and phosphorylated forms of AKT and ERK1/2) with human melanoma subtypes; particularly with mucosal, digital and ungual localizations that usually show high growth and aggressive behavior [5].

CANINE ORAL MELANOMAS

Melanoma is considered the most common oral malignancy in dogs [53], accounting for 14.4% to 45.5% of all oral tumors [54,55,56,57,58,59]. Some studies describe melanomas as the second most frequent oral cancer in dogs [54,56]. Oral malignant melanoma may also occur in cats and humans, but it is infrequent [60,61].

Malignant melanoma can be located in any portion of the oral cavity, but the gingival mucosa is the most common site [54,62]. The mandibular labial mucosa was the most common area, affected in 53% of cases, as described by Ramos-Vara *et al.* [11]. Although malignant melanoma rarely affects the tongue, it is considered the most common tumor type of this anatomic site as described by Dennis *et al.* [63], and large-breed dogs, particularly Chow Chow and Shar Pei, are at increased risk for malignant lingual melanoma [62,63].

Small-breed dogs and dogs with pigmented oral mucosa appear to be at increased risk for the development of oral malignant melanoma [61,62]. Cocker Spaniel, Poodle, Pekinese, Gordon Setter, Chow Chow, Golden Retriever, mixed-breed dogs, and Dachshund are the most commonly affected breeds [11,61]. Boxers and German Shepherds appear to be less affected by the disease, as described by Ramos-Vara *et al.* [11].

Dogs with oral malignant melanoma are usually 10.5 to 12 years old, with an average age of 11.4 years [11,54,61]. Males are supposed to be more predisposed to oral malignant melanomas, as verified by Todoroff *et al.* [54] and Vos*et al.* [55]; however,

Ramos-Vara *et al.* [11], in a study of 328 dogs diagnosed with oral melanoma, and Teixeira *et al.*[13] found no such predisposition.

Oral malignant melanoma is a highly locally aggressive disease, with local invasion into bones occurring in 57% of lesions, with metastasis to regional lymph nodes (Figure 4) in 30.3% to 74% of cases, and to the lungs and other distant organs in 14% to 92% of affected dogs [11,61,64].

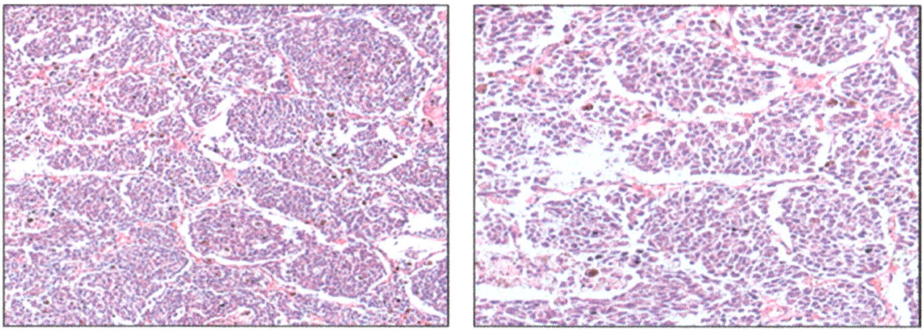

(A) (B)

Figure 4: Photomicrograph of lymph node metastasis from oral melanocytic neoplasm ((**A**), Objective 10x; (**B**), Objective 20x). Hematoxylin and eosin.

Melanoma is one of the few neoplasms in animals for which location is an important prognostic indicator [65]. The statement that all oral melanocytic neoplasms should be considered malignant is commonly found throughout the literature and has become dogma [41].

The prognosis for oral melanoma varies from favorable to unfavorable, with an overall median survival time (MST) of less than 36 months, depending on the intrinsic characteristics of the tumor, and the stage of the disease [61,66,67,68,69].

Historically, many studies confirm that oral and lip melanomas have a poorer prognosis when compared to skin melanomas. The differences concerning the results of different studies of lip melanomas are directly related to the real site of the tumor, that is, either in the skin or in the mucocutaneous junction. In one study, oral melanomas had an MST of 147 days, while the MST of melanoma of the lips and digits were 676 days and 725 days, respectively [18]. Large and poorly or non-pigmented tumors, necrosis, ulceration, high rate of cell proliferation (PCNA expression), and p53 expression are considered poor prognostic factors [29]. Amelanotic melanomas showed a significantly higher amount of mitotic cells when compared to melanotic melanomas [24]. The PCNA (proliferating cell nuclear antigen) in pigmented and non-pigmented melanomas was also assessed. It was demonstrated that cells of all samples stained positive for PCNA, confirming the proliferative activity of this tumor.

The World Health Organization (WHO) staging scheme for dogs with oral melanoma is based on the size of the tumor and the presence of regional and distant metastasis (Table 3) [70]. These staging systems are old and size is not considered a prognostic factor for malignant melanoma [18,28,36], but they are still cited in veterinary practice.

Table 3: TNM classification of tumors in domestic animals, WHO, Geneva, 1980.

Clinical Staging System for Oral Tumor			
Primary Tumor (T)			
Tis	Tumor *in situ*		
T1	Tumor <2 cm in diameter at greatest dimension		
T1a	Without evidence of bone invasion		
T1b	With evidence of bone invasion		
T2	Tumor 2–4 cm in diameter at greatest dimension		
T2a	Without evidence of bone invasion		
T2b	With evidence of bone invasion		
T3	Tumor >4 cm in diameter at greatest dimension		
T3a	Without evidence of bone invasion		
T3b	With evidence of bone invasion		
Regional Lymph Nodes (N)			
N0	No regional lymph node metastasis		
N1	Movable ipsilateral lymph nodes		
N1a	No evidence of lymph mode metastasis		
N1b	Evidence of lymph mode metastasis		
N2	Movable contralateral lymph nodes		
N2a	No evidence of lymph mode metastasis		
N2b	Evidence of lymph mode metastasis		
N3	Fixed lymph nodes		
Metastasis (M)			
M0	No distance metastasis		
M1	Distance metastasis		
Stage Group	**Tumor (T)**	**Nodes (N)**	**Metastasis (M)**
I	T1	N0, N1a, N2a	M0
II	T2	N0, N1a, N2a	M0
III	T3	N0, N1a, N2a	M0
	Any T	N1b	M0
IV	Any T	N2b, N3	M0
	Any T	Any N	M0

Dogs with stage I melanomas have tumors smaller than 2 cm in diameter, while dogs with stage II and III have tumors measuring between 2 to 4 cm, and more than 4 cm, respectively. Dogs with lymph node metastasis are also classified as stage III disease, and dogs with distant metastasis are classified as stage IV disease. Median survival times for dogs with oral melanoma treated with surgery are approximately 17–18 months, 5–6 months, and 3 months for stage I, II, and III disease, respectively [67].

In a study of 70 dogs with oral melanoma, Tuohy *et al.* [71] observed that 11.4% of dogs had mandibular lymph node metastasis and 1.4% of dogs had lung metastasis at the time of diagnosis. After 821 days (mean time of follow-up), 8.6% of mandibular lymph node metastasis, 17.1% of lung metastasis, 5.7% of metastasis to both sites, and 4.2% of metastasis to lung and other locations were observed. Williams *et al.* [64] reported that 70% of canines with melanomas had metastasis when lymphadenomegaly was present, and that 40% had metastasis in the absence of lymphadenomegaly. Harvey *et al.* [72]

observed that dogs with untreated oral melanomas have a median survival time of 65 days.

Gillard *et al.* [19] performed clinical and histopathological analyses of 153 malignant canine melanomas with a four-year follow-up. These samples were histopathological characterization by human classification and showed that most canine tumors are intradermal and homologous to human nevocytoid (72%) type, animal type (16.5%), composite type (6.5%), pleomorphic type (4.5%), and superficial spreading melanoma type (0.5%) [19]. Figure 5shows a representative histology of canine oral malignant melanoma on which local invasion, sparsely pigmented cells, and pleomorphism with variation in shape and cell or nuclear size can be seen.

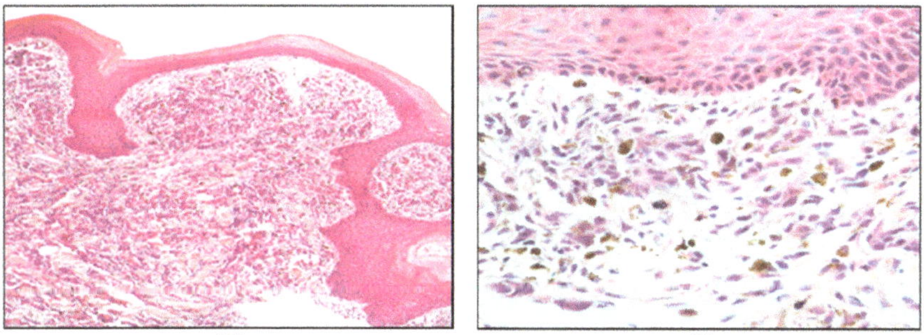

(A) (B)

Figure 5: Photomicrograph of oral melanocytic neoplasm ((**A**), Objective 4 ×; (**B**), Objective 40 ×); Hematoxylin and Eosin.

A recent study of over 382 canine oral melanomas did not find statistically significant differences in survival among different sites or mitotic indices [11].

CANINE OCULAR MELANOMAS

Ocular melanocytic tumors, benign or malignant, may occur in humans and domestic animals. These tumors may affect the eyelids, conjunctiva, orbit, limbo, and uvea [73,74]. Melanomas have different biological behaviors depending on the location in the eye [75]. In general, canine ocular melanomas are less aggressive than oral melanomas. Within the ocular melanoma group, the uveal melanoma is characterized by being more aggressive than the epibulbar melanoma [75].

Eyelid tumors in dogs are usually benign, such as sebaceous adenomas and sebaceous epitheliomas. Among all eyelid tumors, the melanocytic neoplasms account for 20%, and only 8% of these are melanomas [73]. Most, if not all, eyelid skin melanomas are benign [75]. Eyelid melanomas in dogs are usually pedunculated with nodular internal infiltration [73]. They are generally non-aggressive tumors, but occasionally some pigmented melanomas act aggressively and become locally invasive with the development of metastasis [73]. When compared to dogs, melanomas of the eyelid in humans carry a worse prognosis, especially when the tumor is located on the lid margin [76].

Conjunctival melanomas generally affect the nictitating membrane and the bulbar and/or eyelid conjunctiva [77]. Rottweilers and Cockers Spaniels are predisposed [74]. Lesions appear as dark, raised solid masses. Metastasis is rarely seen, but when it occurs it is typically associated with melanomas of the conjunctival eyelid. Complete surgical removal is warranted in early-diagnosed cases [77]. Due to the high risk of local recurrence, enucleation should be considered for invasive tumors [74]. Although conjunctival melanomas in humans are unusual, they have the potential to cause vision impairment and reduce life expectancy, with a mortality rate varying from 18% to 44% [74,78].

Canine and feline limbal melanomas have a benign biological behavior. They appear as raised, well-circumscribed heavily pigmented masses that arise from scleral and subconjunctival connective tissue melanocytes. Most of them develop slowly and are located closely to the superior aspect of the limbus. Labrador Retrievers are genetically predisposed [79].

Among the intraocular melanocytic tumors in the dog, melanocytomas are the most common tumors encountered, representing approximately 80% of the neoplasms. Melanomas account for only 20% of tumors [74]. It is difficult and unreliable to clinically differentiate between melanocytomas and melanomas, since melanocytomas can be locally aggressive and even invade the drainage angle and adjacent tissues [73,80]. Therefore, histopathological analysis is indispensable for a definitive diagnosis [81]. Despite the fact that melanocytomas are benign, when located in the iris, they can spontaneously cause necrosis and pigment dispersion, which may lead to obstruction of drainage and cause glaucoma in dogs and humans [82] (Figure 6).

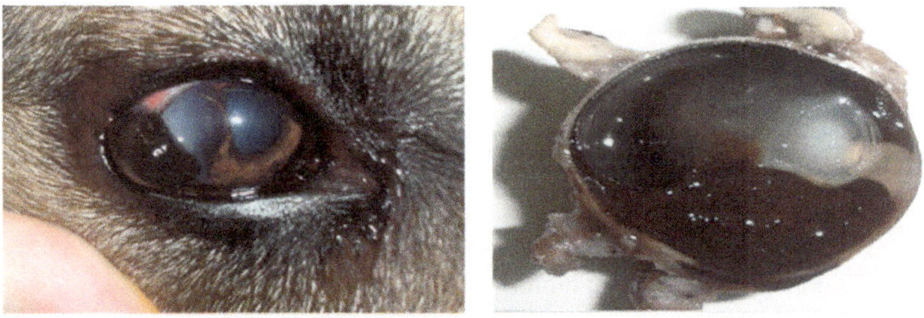

(A) (B)

Figure 6: Photographs showing: blackened mass in the iris with extraocular extension (**A**) and sagittal section of the eyeball revealing melanocytic neoplasia of iris, ciliary body, and choroid (**B**) (*Eduardo Perlmann*).

Melanocytomas most commonly affect the anterior uvea in dogs, but rarely affect the choroid [29]. When located in the uvea, they may cause several changes, such as intraocular hemorrhage, uveitis, and secondary glaucoma. Despite the fact that human intraocular melanocytomas are commonly located at the level of the optical disk or adjacent tissues, this location was never described in dogs [74]. An early diagnosis and rapid surgical treatment increase the chances of a favorable prognosis [83]. Wilcock *et al.* [75] studied 91 canine uveal melanocytic neoplasms, and only three developed metastatic disease. These data emphasize the low metastatic rate of uveal melanoma in dogs. Giuliano *et al.* [84], however, showed that animals affected by uveal melanomas had a lower life expectancy when compared with patients diagnosed with uveal melanocytomas. Tumors located in the uvea most frequently are consistent with primary neoplasia; however, animals presenting with intraocular-pigmented tumors should have a complete diagnostic work-up and physical exam to rule out metastasis [85].

In general, when tumors are only confined to the intraocular space, the recommended treatment is enucleation. Exenteration is indicated when the tumor extends to the extraocular space [83]. Other treatment options include iridectomy or diode laser photocoagulation in small-pigmented tumors of the iris [86]. There is no evidence that chemotherapy is effective in the treatment of ocular melanomas [87], but long-term follow-up evaluation would be needed. Ocular malignant melanoma had significantly shorter survival time than benign melanocytomas [84].

CANINE DIGITAL MELANOMAS

Melanoma is considered the second most common type of cancer of the digits in dogs [22,29,88]. Local invasion is a common feature of digital melanomas and 5%–58% of dogs with this disease have evidence of bone lysis [22,88,89,90]. Tumors of the footpad and interdigital region are less likely to invade into the bone [22,90]. Besides possible local invasion, regional and distant metastasis via lymphatics is frequently noted. It is estimated that 30%–40% of dogs have metastasis at the time of presentation and that even after appropriate local treatment with surgery, subsequent metastasis is frequently seen [22,88].

Due to its aggressive behavior, canine digital melanomas often require digital amputation. The median survival time for dogs without metastasis at the time of diagnosis treated with digital amputation is approximately 12 months, with 42%–57% of dogs surviving one year, and 11%–13% surviving two years [22,88,90,91].

Canine Cutaneous Melanomas

In contrast to digital melanomas, cutaneous melanomas typically have benign behavior in dogs, with the exception of melanomas that develop on the mucocutaneous junctions [18,92]. They account for 0.8%–2% of all canine cutaneous tumors [64] and are more commonly seen in dogs with heavily pigmented skin. Predisposed breeds include Scottish Terrier, Poodle, Golden Retriever, Dachshund, Cocker Spaniel, Miniature Poodle, Chow Chow, and Gordon Setter [93]. Benign skin melanomas are usually solitary, small, pigmented, firm, and freely moveable over deeper structures. Malignant melanomas tend to be fast-growing tumors, and often are ulcerated, and pigmented (grey, brown, or black) [21].

The most common sites for benign cutaneous melanomas are the face (near the eyelids), trunk, and extremities. Malignant melanoma is found most frequently on the head, ventral abdomen, and scrotum. When metastases occur, lymph nodes, followed by lungs, are the main organs involved [29].

Brockley *et al.* [94] studied 63 dogs diagnosed with melanomas at different locations. Surgery was performed in 24 cutaneous melanomas, with 88% of dogs alive a year after treatment.

Most dogs are cured with complete surgical excision, although some characteristics of the tumor, such as a mitotic index of ≥3/10 HPF, the presence of ≥20% of nuclear atypia, a Ki67 index ≥15%, ulceration, lymphatic invasion, and tumors extending beyond dermis, may have a negative influence on prognosis [18,41,92].

TREATMENT MODALITIES FOR CANINE MELANOMAS

Surgery

Surgery is the most common and main treatment option for local management of all melanomas, including oral [69], ocular [74], cutaneous, and digital melanomas [90,92]. Due to its high metastatic potential, systemic therapy should also be considered [61,62].

Tuohy *et al.* [71] studied 70 cases of canine oral malignant melanomas treated with curative intent surgery. Surgical resections were done with wide margins, including 2 to 3 cm of bone margins, and 1 cm of soft tissue margins. Histopathological analysis showed that 72.9% of tumors were completely excised, with 10% of these patients developing local tumor recurrence. In this study, dogs that had surgery as their sole treatment option had a progression-free interval (PFI) longer than 567 days, and an MST of 874 days. In a survey performed by Boston *et al.*[69], among wide-margin surgeries performed, 79.3% (73/92) were completely excised based on histologic evaluation, and the recurrence rate was 8.3% (6/73) in this group. The MST of these dogs was 354 days. Esplin [65] studied 61 dogs diagnosed with well-differentiated oral melanomas that were surgically excised, and reported an MST of 34 months with 3.2% of local recurrence.

Regional lymph node resection has been studied in maxillofacial tumors. The analysis of sentinel lymph nodes provides essential information regarding the clinical stage of disease, and also helps determine the appropriate treatment plan [95,96]. As previously shown, in a survey of 100 dogs with oral malignant melanoma, 53% had cytological or histopathological evidence of mandibular lymph node metastasis, even in normal sized nodes [64]. Therefore, regional lymph node removal is warranted, especially in dogs with oral melanomas.

Radiation Therapy

Radiation therapy is effective for malignant melanomas in dogs and may be useful for the control of local disease and involved regional lymph nodes [97]. Response rates are generally best for smaller tumors rather than for salvage therapy against large tumor burdens late in their clinical progression [98]. Another prognostic factor that appears to affect therapy outcome includes the presence of bone lysis. Proulx *et al.* [97] found that dogs without evidence of radiologic bone destruction experienced longer disease-free intervals and overall survival when compared to dogs with bone invasion.

Although melanoma has traditionally been viewed as a "radio-insensitive" disease, many studies suggest a significant role for radiation therapy in the treatment of melanoma [99]. Optimal fractionation schedules have not yet been established for canine malignant melanoma; however, hypofractionated protocols have been utilized with some success [93]. Overall response rates range from 82% to 94.4%, with the complete and partial resolution of tumors in 51% to 69% and 25% to 31% of cases, respectively [91,92,93,94,95,96,97,98,99,100,101,102]. The reported median time to progression ranges from 3.6 to 7.9 months with a median survival time varying from 5.3 to 11.9 months [97,98,100,101,102,103].

Chemotherapy alone has generally offered little benefit in terms of clinical outcome for the control of local canine melanomas; however, a few published studies have shown that the association of radiation with chemotherapy may potentially slow local progression and/or improve overall survival. Cancedda *et al.* [102] compared the efficacy of radiation therapy (5 × 6 Gy) alone and radiation therapy with post-radiation temozolamide (60 mg/m^2 PO for five consecutive days every 28 days) in dogs with measurable malignant melanoma. Dogs treated with temozolamide had a significantly longer median time to progression (6.8 months) than dogs treated only with radiation (3.6 months). Freeman *et al.* [103] retrospectively looked at dogs with incompletely resected oral melanoma treated with either cisplatin (10–30 mg/m^2 IV) or carboplatin (90 mg/m^2 IV) given once weekly 1 h before receiving radiation therapy (6 × 6 Gy). The reported median survival time was 11.9 months, representing the longest survival time when compared to the survival time previously reported for dogs with incompletely resected oral malignant melanoma [103]. Other studies combining radiation with chemotherapy agents, such as carboplatin, cisplatin, or melphalan, did not have a significant impact on either time to progression or overall survival [97,101,104].

Chemotherapy

Despite treating dogs with appropriate local therapies, such as surgery and/or radiation therapy, the ultimate cause of death, especially in oral melanomas, is metastasis. Therefore, the use of systemic therapies is typically recommended. Many chemotherapy protocols have been published in the veterinary literature with minimal improvement in survival times when compared to local treatment alone.

Many chemotherapy protocols using platinum agents have been studied. Rassnick *et al.* [104] reported an overall response rate of 28% using carboplatin as a single agent (300 to 350mg/m^2/IV/ every 21 days) prior to surgery in dogs with oral (25/27) and cutaneous melanomas (2/27). Boria *et al.* [105] reported an overall response rate of 18% and a MST of 119 days using cisplatin (50 to 55 mg/m^2/IV/ every three weeks) in combination with piroxicam (0.3 mg/kg/PO/24 hs) in oral melanomas.

Brockley *et al.* 2013 [94] evaluated the effect of carboplatin on the survival of 63 canine patients diagnosed with oral, cutaneous, or digital malignant melanomas. In this survey, carboplatin was administered at 300 mg/m^2 IV every 21 days for a total of 4–6 cycles. The addition of carboplatin after local therapy did not lead to a significant increase in survival times, and the anatomic site was significantly associated with survival. The overall median survival time for patients with oral, digital, and cutaneous melanomas were 389 days, 1350 days, with a median follow-up of 776 days, respectively.

In another survey, Dank *et al.* [106] compared the outcome of 17 dogs treated with surgery, adjuvant carboplatin (150 to 300 mg/m²/IV every three weeks), with or without radiation therapy. The MST was 387 days for the group treated with radiotherapy and 440 days for the group without the addition of radiotherapy.

In a comparative study reported by Tuohy *et al.* [71], surgery with or without any adjuvant therapy (carboplatin, cyclophosphamide as a metronomic therapy, radiotherapy, or xenogeneic canine melanoma vaccine) did not improve overall survival time in dogs with oral melanoma. The MST reported was 874 and 396 days for dogs that had surgery or surgery plus adjuvant therapy, respectively. Boston *et al.* [69] treated 151 dogs with oral melanoma and also concluded that there were no benefits in survival times among dogs that had surgery alone (MST of 335 days for 98 dogs) *versus* dogs that had surgery followed by systemic adjuvant therapy (MST of 352 for 53 dogs). Carboplatin, lomustine, dacarbazine, doxorubicin, metronomic chemotherapy, or commercial melanoma vaccine were the adjuvant therapies used in this study. Postoperative radiation therapy was associated with a longer survival time (MST of 1747 days), but was not significant in the multivariate analysis of this study.

Immunotherapy

Many researchers are currently using and developing therapies to activate the immune system of dogs. The immune responses by therapeutic vaccine represent a potential and powerful strategy for the treatment of melanomas [107]. There is wide evidence that the immune system could modulate the progression and metastasis of melanoma.

Many biological agents have the capacity to demonstrate antitumor activation, such as BCG, IFN-alpha, IL-2, and immunization activators, using an anticancer vaccine [108].

Bacillus Calmette–Guérin (BCG) is used intralesionally in melanomas to activate an immune response and induce tumor regression; however, there may be some complications, such as granulomas and hypersensitivity reactions [109].

Corynebacterium parvum is a bacterial substance that has antitumor activity in humans and canines with melanoma. MacEwen *et al.* [67] used *C. parvum* in dogs with stage II and III oral melanomas and compared the outcomes between surgical excision alone and surgery plus *C. parvum* immunotherapy. Animals who received *C. parvum* and surgery had a better prognosis than those with surgery only.

In rodents, dogs, and men, a liposome-encapsulad muramyl tripeptide phosphatidyl ethanolamine (L-MTP-PE), when used *in vivo*, actives monocytes and macrophages, resulting in antitumor activity, which can lead to melanoma metastasis tumor regression or at least stable disease. According to MacEwen *et al.* [108], when L-MTP-PE was used alone or in combination with GM-CSF the antitumor response was minimal, and only prolonged the survival time in dogs with stage I melanoma.

Bianco *et al.* [110], demonstrated that peripheral blood mononuclear cells with apoptotic melanoma cells significantly increased the antitumor immune response, leading to a reduction of the melanoma in three out of five dogs treated intralesionally with FasL-DNA.

Alexander *et al.* [111] used an allogeneic melanoma vaccine in combination with human a glycoprotein 100 (hgp 100), which is a xenogeneic melanoma protein. The vaccine was well tolerated in dogs, and the tumor response rate was 35% for six weeks (including complete response and stable disease).

Hogge *et al.* [112] used an autologous vaccine made of lysate cells transfected with GM-CSF in dogs with soft tissue sarcoma or melanoma. There was a large concentration of inflammatory cells at the site of vaccine administration, different from the ones that received a vaccine placebo only.

A xenogeneic human DNA-encoding tyrosinase protein vaccine (Oncept®) has been developed and used in dogs with stage II and III oral malignant melanoma [113]. This vaccine was generally well tolerated in a study of 111 dogs. No systemic reactions occurred, only local hematomas and pain at the injection site [114]. In another retrospective study, medical records from 45 dogs were reviewed, including 30 dogs with stage II and III disease, treated with the Oncept® vaccine after appropriate achievement of loco-regional cancer control. The review found that dogs that received the vaccine did not achieve a greater progression-free survival, disease-free interval, or median survival time than dogs that did not receive the vaccine [115].

The role of dendritic cells (DCs) as a biological adjuvant against malignant melanoma through the induction of an active immune response in the oncologic patient has been explored. Dendritic cells, as professional antigen-presenting cells with an ability to initiate the immune response, could therefore qualify for vaccination strategies to treat human or canine cancers. Compared with the human clinical trials using DC-based vaccines, reports of testing in dogs are scarce.

For humans, at least 13 clinical trials conducted in the United States have been registered using *ex vivo* autologous DCs [116] and, for dogs, only a few reports have been published to strengthen the rational use of DC vaccination for canine malignant melanoma [117,118]. Both protocols used bone marrow-derived DC of dogs with or without malignant melanoma. Gyorffy *et al.* [117] conducted a study using a few canine melanoma bearers and employed DC transduced with an adenovirus vector encoding a xenoantigen, human melanoma antigen gp100, as a coadjuvant of radiation therapy. One dog had an antigen-specific cytotoxic T lymphocyte (CTL) activity in peripheral blood lymphocytes, with no clinical signs, either locally or systemically, with melanoma recurrence 48 months after initial DC injection. However, another dog, which had a negative CTL activity, relapsed 22 months after vaccination. Tamura *et al.* [118], using an autologous DC pulsed with canine melanoma CMM2 cell lysate, efficiently elicited T cell-mediated immunity against CMM-2 cells *in vivo*, reinforcing the rationale to use DC as a therapeutic vaccine.

Although the immunotherapeutic approach using a DC vaccine to drive tumor-specific immune responses appears to be a promising strategy to control malignant melanoma, there are limitations, such as the cost of vaccine production for veterinary use as well as the very fragmentary designed strategies available.

Outcomes after Treatment

Table 4 describes the reported outcomes for canine oral malignant melanoma treated with different protocols.

Table 4: Outcomes for canine oral malignant melanoma after different therapeutic protocols.

Summary of Treatment Outcome for Canine Oral Malignant Melanoma
Radiation Therapy (RT)
- Response Rate = 82%–94.4% - Local Recurrence = 11%–27% - MST (Median Survival Time) = 5.3–11.9 months
References: Theon *et al.*, 1997 (98); Bateman *et al.*, 1994 (100); Murphy *et al.*, 2005 (101); Cancedda *et al.*, 2014 (102); Proulx *et al.*, 2003 (97); Freeman *et al.*, 2003 (103).
Surgery (SX) with Wide Margins
- Local Recurrence = 3.2%–10% - MST = 11.8–34 months
References: Tuohy *et al.*, 2014 (71); Boston *et al.*, 2014 (69); Esplin *et al.*, 2008 (65).
Chemotherapy (CT) for Macroscopic Disease
- Carboplatin response rate = 28% - Cisplatin + piroxicam response rate = 18%
References: Rassnick *et al.*, 2001 (104); Boria *et al.*, 2004 (105).
Adequate Local Treatment + Systemic Therapy
- SX ± RT + adjuvant carboplatin: MST = 14.6 months - SX ± RT + adjuvant carboplatin, metronomic therapy, or melanoma vaccine: MST = 13.2 months (adjuvant therapy did not improve overall MST) - SX + adjuvant carboplatin, lomustine, dacarbazine, doxorubicin, or melanoma vaccine: MST = 11.7 months (adjuvant therapy did not improve overall MST) - RT + post-RT temozolamide: CT did not improve MST, but was associated with a longer median time to progression when compared to dogs treated with RT alone (6.8 months *versus* 2.6 months) - SX + RT + cisplatin or carboplatin once weekly 1 h before RT: MST = 11.9 months
References: Dank *et al.*, 2012 (106); Tuohy *et al.*, 2014 (71); Boston *et al.*, 2014 (69); Cancedda *et al.*, 2014 (102); Freeman *et al.*, 2003 (103).

Abbreviations: RT = radiotherapy, SX = surgery, CT = chemotherapy, MST = median survival time.

New Perspectives for the Treatment of Canine Melanomas

The aggressive nature of melanomas in canines and humans, with short survival times and minimal clinical outcome benefits after surgery and adjuvant therapy, emphasizes the importance of new studies to find an effective therapy for treatment and prevention of melanomas metastasis.

A canine therapeutic vaccine has been commercially available since 2007. The Merial melanoma vaccine for dogs (Oncept®) consists of DNA encoding the gene for the human melanocyte protein tyrosinase but apparently seems not to cure all melanoma cases. Published studies evaluating the survival times in dogs with melanoma in the mouth undergoing surgery and treatment with the Merial melanoma vaccine report average survival times of 599 days (20 months) or longer [113,114]. These results, though not from randomized studies, are promising and have prompted many veterinary oncologists to recommend the vaccine for patients with stage II and III melanoma despite the lack of FDA-standard clinical trials. The vaccine is well tolerated and has not been reported to be associated with side effects requiring medical intervention. In patients with very large and aggressive melanoma, there may not be sufficient time for an immune response to be mounted against the tyrosinase protein to prevent progression of the melanoma. In fact, 15% of patients treated with the vaccine reportedly die within three months of initiation of treatment, presumably due to the aggressive nature of the melanoma and insufficient time for the vaccine to be effective [119].

Lupeol [120] is among the new therapies under study. Lupeol is a triterpene extracted from various fruits and vegetables that reportedly inhibits melanoma cell proliferation *in vitro* and *in vivo*. A total of 11 dogs bearing buccal melanomas (three, five, and three dogs diagnosed with clinical stage I, II, and III melanoma, respectively) were evaluated. Subcutaneous lupeol (10 mg/kg) was administered postoperatively at various time points. Of the 11 subjects, seven exhibited no local recurrence 180 days postoperatively and no severe adverse effects were observed in any of these cases. Furthermore, no metastases have been detected during the period of the trial.

The current and promising immunotherapy to further augment the options for treatment in malignant melanomas, at least in humans, has been based on checkpoint–blocking antibodies, which can restore anticancer immune responses. Immune checkpoint molecules regulate the immune response avoiding autoimmunity and deleterious effects of an inflammatory response, but when expressed on tumors cells they work as a mechanism of immune evasion. Good examples of immune checkpoint molecules include PD-1 immune checkpoint inhibitor antibody (Pembrolizumab-humanized IgG4; Nivolumab- human IgG4), which was the first drug to gain FDA approval to a phase I trial in patients with BRAF inhibitor-resistant advanced melanoma and BRAFV600 mutation-positive melanoma [121]; and a checkpoint inhibitor (ipilimumab) directed against the cytotoxic T lymphocyte Antigen (CTLA-4). Data from clinical trials has demonstrated the important role this therapeutic approach can play—even with the development of immune-related side effects—since it has been proved a meaningful clinical improvement and an impressive increase in overall survival in melanoma patients [122] when compared to conventional chemotherapy. In the veterinary medicine field, the perspective of this therapy was described by Maekawa *et al.* [123], who demonstrated that an antibovine PD-L1 monoclonal antibody effectively blocked the binding of recombinant PD-1 with PD-L1-expressing tumor cells in a dose-dependent manner, including canine melanoma cells.

Other therapy as future treatment strategy for canine malignant melanoma can be based on oncolytic virotherapy. Basically, the virus infects and kills tumor cells when replication, lysis, and release of viruses occur. Tumor oncolysis by reovirus infection that was related in Ras-transformed cells was studied in six canine malignant melanoma cell lines CMeC1, CMeC2, KMeC, LMeC, CMGD2, and CMGD5. All of them were susceptible to reovirus infection, although Ras activation was not related in these cells, and only one of them (CMGD2) demonstrated more than 50% of cell death [124].

All efforts are geared toward better characterization of malignant melanomas in dogs, for the benefit of these companion animals, and also in an attempt to benefit the treatment of melanoma in humans.

CONCLUSIONS

Melanomas are very aggressive tumors and dogs are considered good models to study this disease. All efforts are geared toward better characterization and control of malignant melanomas in dogs, for the benefit of these companion animals, and also in an attempt to benefit the treatment of human melanomas.

ACKNOWLEDGMENTS

Karen Batschinski is the recipient of a fellowship from Fundação de Amparo a Pesquisa do Estado de São Paulo, FAPESP, Proc. Number 2013/16423-8. The authors are grateful to Jose Guilherme Xavier for supplying photos of canine melanomas.

AUTHOR CONTRIBUTIONS

Adriana Tomoko Nishiya, Claudia Ronca Felizzola, Eduardo Perlmann, Claudia Ronca Felizzola, Priscila Pedra Mendonça, Jéssica Soares Garcia, Tarso Felipe Teixeira, Maria Lucia Zaidan Dagli and Maria Lucia drafted the manuscript, Karen Batschinski, Marcello Vannucci Tedardi and the others revised the manuscript. All authors read and approved the final manuscript.

REFERENCES

1. Sweet, M.; Kirkham, N.; Bendall, M.; Currey, L.; Bythell, J.; Heupel, M. *PLoS ONE* 2012.
2. Starkey, M.P.; Scase, T.J.; Mellersh, C.S.; Murphy, S. Dogs really are man's best friend—Canine genomics has applications in veterinary and human medicine! *Brief. Funct. Genomic. Proteomic.* 2005, *4*, 112–128.
3. Paoloni, M.; Khanna, C. Translation of new cancer treatments from pet dogs to humans. *Nat. Rev. Cancer* 2008,*8*, 147–156.
4. Nowend, K.L.; Starr-Moss, A.N.; Murphy, K.E. The function of dog models in developing gene therapy strategies for human health. *Mamm. Genome* 2011, *22*, 476–485.
5. Khanna, C.; Lindblad-Toh, K.; Vail, D.; London, C.; Bergman, P.; Barber, L.; Breen, M.; Kitchell, B.; McNeil, E.; Modiano, J.F.; *et al.* The dog as a cancer model. *Nat. Biotechnol.* 2006, *24*, 1065–1066.
6. Fowles, J.S.; Denton, C.L.; Gustafson, D.L. Comparative analysis of MAPK and PI3K/AKT pathway activation and inhibition in human and canine melanoma. *Vet. Comp. Oncol.* 2015, *13*, 288–304.

7. Haass, N.K.; Smalley, K.S.; Herlyn, M. The role of altered cell–cell communication in melanoma progression. *J. Mol. Histol.* 2004, *35*, 309–318.

8. Marcus, D.M.; Marcus, P.M.; Prabhu, R.S.; Owonikoko, T.K.; Lawson, D.H.; Switchenko, J.; Beither, J. Rising incidence of mucosal melanoma of the head and neck in the United States. *J. Skin Cancer* 2012, 231693.

9. Gavriel, H.; McArthur, G.; Sizeland, A.; Henderson, M. Review: Mucosal melanoma of the head and neck.*Melanoma Res.* 2011, *21*, 257–266.

10. Meleti, M.; Leemans, C.R.; De Bree, R.; Vescovi, P.; Sesenna, E.; van der Waal, I. Head and neck mucosal melanoma: Experience with 42 patients, with emphasis on the role of postoperative radiotherapy. *Head Neck*2008, *30*, 1543–1551.

11. Ramos-Vara, J.A.; Beissenherz, M.E.; Miller, M.A.; Johnson, G.C.; Pace, L.W.; Fard, A.; Kottler, S.J. Retrospective study of 338 canine oral melanomas with clinical, histologic, and immunohistochemical review of 129 cases.*Vet. Pathol.* 2000, *37*, 597–608.

12. Kimura, K.C.; Garate, A.P.; Dagli, M.L.Z. Retrospective study of neoplasms in domestic animals: A survey between 1993 and 2002 of the service of animal pathology, department of pathology, school of veterinary medicine and animal science, University of Sao Paulo, Southeast Brazil. *Braz. J. Vet. Pathol.* 2012, *5*, 60–69.

13. Teixeira, T.F.; Silva, T.C.; Cogliati, B.; Nagamine, N.K.; Dagli, M.L.Z. Retrospective study of melanocytic neoplasms in dogs and cats. *Braz. J. Vet. Pathol.* 2010, *3*, 100–104.

14. Omholt, K.; Grafström, E.; Kanter-Lewensohn, L.; Hansson, J.; Ragnarsson-Olding, B.K. KIT pathway alterations in mucosal melanomas of the vulva and other sites. *Clin. Cancer Res.* 2011, *17*, 3933–3942.

15. Zanoni, M.T.; Medicina, D.; Lombardi, D.; Ungari, M.; Balzarini, P.; Rossini, C.; Pellegrini, W.; Battaglia, P.; Capella, C.; Castelnuovo, P.; *et al.* Sinonasal mucosal melanoma: Molecular profile and therapeutic implications from a series of 32 cases. *Head Neck* 2013, *35*, 1066–1077.

16. Lyu, J.; Wu, Y.; Li, C.; Wang, R.; Song, H.; Ren, G.; Guo, W. Mutation scanning of BRAF, NRAS, KIT, and GNAQ/GNA11 in oral mucosal melanoma: A study of 57 cases. *J. Oral Pathol. Med.* 2015.

17. Curtin, J.A.; Fridlyand, J.; Kageshita, T.; Patel, H.N.; Busam, K.J.; Kutzner, H.; Cho, K.H.; Aiba, S.; Bröcker, E.B.; LeBoit, P.E.; *et al.* Distinct sets of genetic alterations in melanoma. *N. Engl. J. Med.* 2005, *353*, 2135–2147.

18. Spangler, W.L.; Kass, P.H. The histologic and epidemiologic bases for prognostic consideration in canine melanocytic neoplasia. *Vet. Pathol.* 2006, *43*, 136–149.

19. Gillard, M.; Cadieu, E.; De Brito, C.; Abadie, J.; Vergier, B.; Devauchelle, P.; Degorce, F.; Dreano, S.; Primot, A.; Dorso, L.; *et al.* Naturally occurring melanomas in dogs as models for non-UV pathways of human melanomas. *Pigment Cell Melanoma Res.* 2014, *27*, 90–102.

20. Priester, W.A. Skin tumors in domesticated animals. Data from 12 United States and Canadian Colleges of Veterinary Medicine. *J. Natl. Cancer Insit.* 1973, *50*, 457–466.
21. Goldschmidt, M.H. Pigmented lesions of the skin. *Clin. Dermatol.* 1994, *12*, 507–514.
22. Marino, D.J.; Matthiesen, D.T.; Stefanacci, J.D.; Moroff, S.D. Evaluation of dogs with digit masses: 117 cases (1981–1991). *J. Am. Vet. Med. Assoc.* 1995, *207*, 726–728.
23. Miller, W.H.; Griffin, I.; Campbell, K.L. *Muller and Kirk's Small Animal Dermatology*, 7th ed.; Elsevier Mosby: St. Louis, MO, USA, 2013; pp. 774–843.
24. Teixeira, T.F.; Gentile, L.B.; Silva, T.C.; Mennecier, G.; Chaible, L.M.; Cogliati, B.; Roman, M.A.; Gioso, M.A.; Dagli, M.L.Z. Cell proliferation and expression of connexins differ in melanotic and amelanotic canine oral melanomas. *Vet. Res. Commun.* 2014, *38*, 29–38.
25. Tedardi, M.V.; Biondi, L.R.; Kimura, K.C.; Pedra Mendonça, P.; Grandi, F.; Latorre, A.M.; Dagli, M.L.Z. Comparative oncology in Sao Paulo, Brazil—What to learn from cancer registry. *Source J. Vet. Sci.* 2014, *1*, 1–8.
26. Tedardi, M.V.; Veneziano, D.B.; Kimura, K.C.; Pedra Mendonça, P.; Biondi, L.R.; Grandi, F.; Latorre, A.M.; Dagli, M.L.Z. Sao Paulo animal cancer registry, the first in Latin America. *Vet. Comp. Oncol.* 2015, *13*, 154–155.
27. Haass, N.K.; Ripperger, D.; Wladykowski, E.; Dawson, P.; Gimotty, P.A.; Blome, C.; Fischer, F.; Schmage, P.; Moll, I.; Brandner, J.M. Melanoma progression exhibits a significant impact on connexin expression patterns in the epidermal tumor microenvironment. *Histochem. Cell Biol.* 2010, *133*, 113–124.
28. Modiano, J.F.; Ritt, M.G.; Wojcieszyn, J. The molecular basis of canine melanoma: Pathogenesis and trends in diagnosis and therapy. *J. Vet. Intern. Med.* 1999, *13*, 163–174.
29. Smith, H.; Goldschmidt, H.; Mcmanus, P.M. A Comparative review of melanocytic neoplasms. *Vet. Pathol.* 2002,*39*, 651–678.
30. Dzutsev, A.; Goldszmid, R.S.; Viaud, S.; Zivtogel, L.; Trinchieri, G. The role of the microbiota in inflammation, carcinogenesis, and cancer therapy. *Eur. J. Immunol.* 2015, *45*, 17–31.
31. Goldschmidt, M.H.; Hendrick, M.J. Tumors of the skin and soft tissues. In *Tumors in Domestic Animals*, 4th ed.; Meuten, D.J., Ed.; Iowa State Press: Ames, IA, USA, 2002; pp. 78–82.
32. Scott, D.W.; Miller, W.H., Jr.; Griffin, C.E. *Muller & Kirk's Small Animal Dermatology*, 6th ed.; Elsevier Saunders: Philadelphia, PA, USA, 2001; pp. 1–70.
33. Li, G.; Herlyn, M. Dynamics of intercellular communication during melanoma development. *Mol. Med. Today*2000, *6*, 163–169.
34. Chin, L. The genetics of malignant melanoma: Lessons from mouse and man. *Nat. Rev. Cancer* 2003, *3*, 559–570.

35. Gaggioli, C.; Sahai, E. Melanoma invasion—Current knowledge and future directions. *Pigment Cell Res.* 2007,*20*, 161–172.

36. Head, K.W.; Else, R.W.; Dubielzig, R.R. Tumors of the Alimentary Tract. In *Tumors in Domestic Animals*, 4th ed.; Meuten, D.J., Ed.; Iowa State Press: Ames, IA, USA, 2002; pp. 426–430.

37. Tajima, S.; Ura-Ishiko, A.; Hayashi, A. Melanogenesis, biosynthetic phenotype of fibronectin and collagen, and migrating activity in cloned B16 mouse melanoma cells. *J. Dermatol. Sci.* 1996, *12*, 24–30.

38. Simonetti, O.; Lucarini, G.; Brancorsini, D.; Nita, P.; Bernardini, M.L.; Biagini, G.; Offidani, A. Immunohistochemical expression of vascular endothelial growth factor, matrix metalloproteinase 2 and matrix metalloproteinase 9 in cutaneous melanocytic lesions. *Cancer* 2002, *95*, 602–624.

39. Nakhleh, R.E.; Wick, M.R.; Rocamora, A.; Swanson, P.E.; Dehner, L.P. Morphologic diversity in malignant melanomas. *Am. J. Clin. Pathol.* 1990, *93*, 731–740.

40. Chénier, S.; Doré, M. Oral Malignant Melanoma with Osteoid Formation in a Dog. *Vet. Pathol.* 1999, *36*, 74–76.

41. Smedley, R.C.; Spangler, W.L.; Esplin, D.G.; Kitchell, B.E.; Bergman, P.J.; Ho, H.Y.; Bergin, I.L.; Kiupel, M. Prognostic markers for canine melanocytic neoplasms: A comparative review of the literature and goals for future investigation. *Vet. Pathol.* 2011, *48*, 54–72.

42. Sandusky, G.E.; Carlton, W.W.; Wightman, K.A. Diagnostic immunohistochemistry of canine round cell tumors. *Vet. Pathol.* 1987, *24*, 495–499.

43. Silva, A.P.; Silva, R.G.; Cogliati, B.; Dias, A.S.M.; Le Bas, A.E.; Hernandez-Blazquez, F.J. Bleaching of melanin in the epidermis of South American fur seal and its application on enzyme immunohistochemistry. *Pesqui. Vet. Bras.* 2011, *31*, 267–270.

44. Fisher, D.E.; Kwong, L.N.; Chin, L. Melanoma. In *DeVita VT, Hellman and Rosenberg's Cancer Principles & Practice of Oncology*, 8th ed.; De Vita, V.T., Jr., Lawrence, T.S., Rosenberg, S.A., Eds.; Lippincott Williams & Wilkins: Philadelphia, PA, USA, 2008; pp. 1889–1951.

45. Shelly, S.; Chien, M.B.; Yip, B.; Kent, M.S.; Theon, A.P.; McCallan, J.L.; London, C.A. Exon 15 BRAF mutations are uncommon in canine oral malignant melanomas. *Mamm. Genome* 2004, *16*, 211–217.

46. Chu, P.Y.; Pan, S.L.; Liu, C.H.; Lee, J.; Yeh, L.S.; Liao, A.T. KIT gene exon 11 mutations in canine malignant melanoma. *Vet. J.* 2013, *196*, 226–230.

47. Curtin, J.A.; Busam, K.; Pinkel, D.; Bastian, B.C. Somatic activation of KIT in distinct subtypes of melanoma. *J. Clin. Oncol.* 2006, *24*, 4340–4346.

48. Maldonado, J.L.; Fridlyand, J.; Patel, H.; Jain, A.N.; Busam, K.; Kageshita, T.; Ono, T.; Albertson, D.G.; Pinkel, D.; Bastian, B.C. Determinants of BRAF mutations in primary melanomas. *J. Natl. Cancer Inst.* 2003, *95*, 1878–1890.

49. Murakami, A.; Mori, T.; Sakai, H.; Murakami, M.; Yanai, T.; Hoshino, Y.; Maruo, K. Analysis of KIT expression and KIT exon 11 mutations in canine oral malignant melanomas. *Vet. Comp. Oncol.* 2011, *9*, 219–224.

50. Zebary, A.; Jangard, M.; Omholt, K.; Ragnarsson-Olding, B.; Hansson, J. KIT, NRAS and BRAF mutations in sinonasal melanoma. *Br. J. Cancer* 2013, *109*, 559–564.

51. Goel, V.K.; Lazar, A.J.; Warneke, C.L.; Redston, M.S.; Haluska, F.G. Examination of mutations in BRAF, NRAS, and PTEN in primary cutaneous melanoma. *J. Investig. Dermatol.* 2006, *126*, 154–160.

52. Mochizuki, H.; Kennedy, K.; Shapiro, S.G.; Breen, M. BRAF Mutations in Canine Cancers. *PLoS ONE* 2015.

53. Bergman, P.J. Canine Oral Melanoma. *Clin. Tech. Small Anim. Pract.* 2007, *22*, 55–60.

54. Todoroff, R.J.; Brodey, R.S. Oral and pharyngeal neoplasia in the dog: A retrospective survey of 361 cases. *J. Am. Vet. Med. Assoc.* 1979, *175*, 567–571.

55. Vos, J.H.; Gaag, I.V.D. Canine and feline oral-pharyngeal tumours. *J. Vet. Med.* 1987, *34*, 420–427.

56. Guerra, J.L.; Dagli, M.L.; Godoy, L.F.; Birman, E.G. A retrospective study of oral neoplasms in dogs: A survey from 1941 to 1986. *Rev. Fac. Med. Vet. Zootec. Univ. S. Paulo* 1989, *26*, 207–212.

57. Stopiglia, A.J.; Felizzola, C.R.; Dagli, M.L.Z.; Xavier, J.G.; Guerra, J.L.; Birman, E. Estudo clínico e anátomo-patológico das formações neoplásicas e não neoplásicas da cavidade bucal de cães. *Comun. Cient. Fac. Med. Vet. Zootec. USP* 1992, *16*, 33–39.

58. Ghirelli, C.D.O. In Biblioteca Digital USP. Available online: http://www.teses.usp.br/teses/disponiveis/10/10137/tde-22072008-090727/pt-br.php (assecced on 15 November 2015).

59. Requicha, J.F.M.F. Repositório Universidade de Trás-os-Montes e Alto Douro. Available online: https://repositorio.utad.pt/bitstream/10348/711/1/MsC_jfmfrequicha.pdf (accessed on 15 November 2015).

60. Bronden, L.B.; Eriksen, T.; Kristensen, A.T. Oral malignant melanomas and other head and neck neoplasms in Danish dogs-data from the Danish Veterinary Cancer Registry. *Acta Vet. Scand.* 2009, *51*, 1–6.

61. Liptak, J.M.; Withrow, S.J. Cancer of gastrointestinal tract. In *Small Animal Clinical Oncology*, 5th ed.; Withrow, S.J., Vail, D.M., Page, R.L., Eds.; Elsevier Saunders: St. Louis, MO, USA, 2013; pp. 381–395.

62. McEntee, M.C. Clinical behavior of nonodontogenic tumors. In *Oral and Maxillofacial Surgery in Dogs and Cats*; Verstraete, F.J.M., Lommer, M.J., Eds.; Elsevier Saunders: Pennsylvania, PA, USA, 2012; pp. 387–402.

63. Dennis, M.; Ehrhart, N.; Duncan, C.; Barnes, A.; Ehrhart, E. Frequency of and risk factors associated with lingual lesions in dogs: 1196 cases (1995–2004). *J. Am. Vet. Med. Assoc.* 2006, *228*, 1533–1537.

64. Williams, L.E.; Packer, R.A. Association between lymph node size and metastasis in dogs with oral malignant melanoma: 100 cases (1987–2001). *J. Am. Vet. Med. Assoc.* 2003, *222*, 1234–1236.

65. Esplin, D.G. Survival of dogs following surgical excision of histologically well-differentiated melanocytic neoplasms of the mucous membranes of the lips and oral cavity. *Vet. Pathol.* 2008, *45*, 889–896.

66. White, R.A.S.; Jefferies, A.R.; Freedman, L.S. Clinical staging for oropharyngeal malignancies in the dog. *J. Small Anim. Pract.* 1985, *26*, 581–594.

67. MacEwen, E.G.; Patnaik, A.K.; Harvey, H.J.; Hayes, A.A.; Matus, R. Canine oral melanoma: Comparison of surgery *versus* surgery plus Corynebacterium parvum. *Cancer Investig.* 1986, *4*, 397–402.

68. Hahn, K.A.; Denicola, D.B.; Richardson, R.C.; Hahn, E.A. Canine oral malignant melanoma: Prognostic utility of an alternative staging system. *J. Small Anim. Pract.* 1994, *35*, 251–256.

69. Boston, S.E.; Lu, X.; Culp, W.T.N.; Montinaro, V.; Romanelli, G.; Dudley, R.M.; Liptak, J.M.; Mestrinho, L.A.; Buracco, P. Efficacy of systemic adjuvant therapies administered to dogs after excision of oral malignant melanomas: 151 cases (2001–2012). *J. Am. Vet. Med. Assoc.* 2014, *245*, 401–407.

70. Owen, L.N. *TNM Classification of Tumours in Domestic Animals*; World Health Organization: Geneve, Switzerland, 1980.

71. Tuohy, J.L.; Selmic, L.E.; Worley, D.R.; Ehrhart, N.P.; Withrow, S.J. Outcome following curative-intent surgery for oral melanoma in dogs: 70 cases (1998–2011). *J. Am. Vet. Med. Assoc.* 2014, *245*, 1266–1273.

72. Harvey, H.J.; MacEwen, E.G.; Braun, D.; Patnaik, A.K.; Withrow, S.J.; Jongeward, S. Prognostic criteria for dogs with oral melanoma. *J. Am. Vet. Med. Assoc.* 1981, *178*, 580–582.

73. Mould, J.R.B.; Petersen-Jones, S.M.; Peruccio, C.; Ratto, A.; Sassani, J.W.; Harbour, J.W. Uveal melanocytic tumors. In *Ocular Tumors in Animals and Humans*; Peiffer, R.L., Jr., Simons, K.B., Eds.; Iowa State Press: Ames, IA, USA, 2002; pp. 225–282.

74. Dubielzig, R.R.; Ketring, K.L.; Mclellan, G.J.; Albert, D.M. *Veterinary Ocular Pathology: A Comparative Review*; W.B. Saunders: Philadelphia, PA, USA, 2010; p. 472.

75. Wilcock, B.P.; Peiffer, J.R. Morphology and behavior of primary ocular melanomas in 91 dogs. *Vet. Pathol.* 1986,*23*, 418–424.

76. Garner, A.; Koornneef, L.; Levene, A.; Collin, J.R. Malignant melanoma of the eyelid skin: Histopathology and behaviour. *Br. J. Ophthalmol.* 1985, *69*, 180–186.

77. Conceição, L.F.; Ribeiro, A.P.; Piso, D.Y.T.; Laus, J.L. Considerations about ocular neoplasia of dogs and cats.*Cienc. Rural* 2010, *40*, 2235–2242.

78. Lim, L.A.; Madigan, M.C.; Conway, R.M. Conjunctival melanoma: A review of conceptual and treatment advances. *Clin. Ophthalmol.* 2013, *7*, 521–531.

79. Donaldson, D.; Sansom, J.; Scase, T.; Adams, V.; Mellersh, C. Canine Limbal melanoma: 30 cases (1992–2004). Part 1. Signalment, clinical and histological features and pedigree analysis. *Vet. Ophthalmol.* 2006, *9*, 115–119.

80. Perlmann, E.; Barros, P.S.M.; Fernandez, L.; Di Cesare, S.; Bakalian, S.; Burnier, M.N., Jr. Histopathological evaluation of pigmented intraocular tumors in dogs. *Investig. Ophthalmol. Vis. Sci.* 2010, *5*, 5159.

81. Esson, D.; Fahrer, C.; Zarfoss, M.K.; Dubielzig, R.R. Suspected uveal metastasis of a nail bed melanoma in a dog. *Vet. Ophthalmol.* 2007, *10*, 262–266.

82. Fineman,M.S.;Eagle,R.C.;Shields,J.A.;Shields,C.L.;Potter,P.Melanocytomalytic glaucoma in eyes with necrotic iris melanocytoma. *Ophthalmology* 1998, *105*, 492–496.

83. Ryan, A.M.; Diters, R.W. Clinical and pathologic features of canine ocular melanomas. *J. Am. Med. Assoc.* 1984,*184*, 60–67.

84. Giuliano, E.A.; Chappell, R.; Fischer, B.; Dubielzig, R.R. A matched observational study of canine survival with primary intraocular melanocytic neoplasia. *Vet. Ophthalmol.* 1999, *2*, 185–190.

85. Konrade, K.A.; Hoffman, A.; Schubert, C.S.; Dubielzig, R.R. A histologic series of secondary uveal melanomas in eleven dogs. In Proceedings of the 40th Annual Meeting of the American College of Veterinary Ophthalmologist, Chicago, IL, USA, 4–7 November 2009.

86. Willis, A.M.; Wilkie, D.A. Ocular oncology. *Clin. Tech. Small Anim. Pract.* 2001, *16*, 77–85.

87. Cazalot, G.; Raymond-Letron, I.; Regnier, A. Choroidal melanoma presented as glaucoma in a dog: Case report and review of the literature. *Rev. Med. Vet.* 2008, *159*, 74–78.

88. Henry, C.J.; Brewer, W.G.; Whitley, E.M.; Tyler, J.W.; Ogilvie, G.K.; Norris, A.; Fox, L.E.; Morrison, W.B.; Hammer, A.; Vail, D.M.; *et al.* Canine digital tumors: Veterinary cooperative oncology group retrospective study of 64 dogs. *J. Vet. Intern. Med.* 2005, *19*, 720–724.

89. Aronsohn, M.G.; Carpenter, J.L. Distal extremity melanocytic nevi an malignant melanomas in dogs. *J. Am. Anim. Hosp. Assoc.* 1990, *26*, 605–612.

90. Wobeser, B.K.; Kidney, B.A.; Powers, B.E.; Withrow, S.J.; Mayer, M.N.; Spinato, M.T.; Allen, A.L. Diagnosis and clinical outcomes associated with surgically amputated canine digit submitted to multiple veterinary diagnostic laboratories. *Vet. Pathol.* 2007, *44*, 355–361.

91. Manley, C.A.M.; Leibman, N.F.; Wolchok, J.D.; Riviere, I.C.M.; Bartido, S.; Craft, D.M.; Bergman, P.J. Xenogeneic Murine Tyrosinase DNA Vaccine for Malignant Melanoma of the Digit of Dogs. *J. Vet. Intern. Med.*2011, *25*, 94–99.

92. Bostock, D.E. Prognosis after surgical excision of canine melanoma. *Vet. Pathol.* 1979, *16*, 32–40.

93. Bergman, P.J.; Kent, M.S.; Farese, J.P. Melanoma. In *Small Animal Clinical Oncology*, 5th ed.; Withrow, S.J., Vail, D.M., Page, R.L., Eds.; Elsevier Saunders: St. Louis, MO, USA, 2013; pp. 321–334.

94. Brockley, L.K.; Cooper, M.A.; Bennett, P.F. Malignant melanoma in 63 dogs (2001–2011): The effect of carboplatin chemotherapy on survival chemotherapy on survival. *N. Z. Vet. J.* 2013, *61*, 25–31.

95. Smith, M.M. Surgical approach for lymph node staging of oral and maxillofacial neoplasms in dogs. *J. Am. Anim. Hosp. Assoc.* 1995, *31*, 514–518.

96. Herring, E.S.; Smith, M.M.; Robertson, J.L. Lymph node staging of oral and maxillofacial neoplasms in 31 dogs and cats. *J. Vet. Dent.* 2002, *19*, 122–126.

97. Proulx, D.R.; Ruslander, D.M.; Dodge, R.K.; Hauck, M.L.; Williams, L.E.; Horn, B.; Price, G.S.; Thrall, D.E. A retrospective analysis of 140 dogs with oral melanoma treated with external beam radiation. *Vet. Radiol. Ultrasound.* 2003, *44*, 352–359.

98. Théon, A.P.; Rodriguez, C.; Madewell, B.R. Analysis of prognostic factors and patterns of failure in dogs with malignant oral tumors treated with megavoltage irradiation. *J. Am. Vet. Med. Assoc.* 1997, *210*, 778–784.

99. Khan, N.; Mohammad, K.K.; Almasan, A.; Singh, A.D.; Macklis, R. The evolving role of radiation therapy in the management of malignant melanoma. *Int. J. Radiat. Oncol. Biol. Phys.* 2011, *80*, 645–654.

100. Bateman, K.E.; Catton, P.A.; Pennock, P.W.; Kruth, S.A. 0-7-21 radiation therapy for the treatment of canine oral melanoma. *J. Vet. Intern. Med.* 1994, *8*, 267–272.

101. Murphy, S.; Hayes, A.M.; Blackwood, L.; Maglennon, G.; Pattinson, H.; Sparkes, A.H. Oral malignant melanoma: The effect of coarse fractionation alone or with adjuvant carboplatin therapy. *Vet. Comp. Oncol.*2005, *3*, 222–229.

102. Cancedda, S.; Bley, C.R.; Aresu, L.; Dacasto, M.; Leone, V.F.; Pizzoni, S.; Gracis, M.; Marconato, L. Efficacy and side effects of radiation therapy in comparison with radiation therapy and temozolomide in the treatment of measurable canine malignant melanoma. *Vet. Comp. Oncol.* 2014.

103. Freeman, K.P.; Hahn, K.A.; Harris, F.D.; King, G.K. Treatment of dogs with oral melanoma by hypofractionated radiation therapy and platinum-based chemotherapy (1987–1997). *J. Vet. Intern. Med.* 2003, *17*, 96–101.

104. Rassnick, K.M.; Ruslender, D.M.; Cotter, S.M.; Al-Sarraf, R.; Bruyette, D.S.; Gamblin, R.M.; Meleo, K.A.; Moore, A.S. Use of carboplatin for treatment of dogs with malignant melanoma: 27 cases (1989–2000). *J. Am. Vet. Med. Assoc.* 2001, *218*, 1444–1448.

105. Boria, P.A.; Murry, D.J.; Bennett, P.F.; Glickman, N.W.; Snyder, P.W.; Merkel, B.L.; Schlittler, D.L.; Mutsaers, A.J.; Thomas, R.M.; Knapp, D.W. Evaluation of cisplatin combined with piroxicam for the treatment of oral malignant melanoma and oral squamous cell carcinoma in dogs. *J. Am. Vet. Med. Assoc.* 2004, *224*, 388–394.

106. Dank, G.; Rassnick, K.M.; Sokolovsky, Y.; Garrett, L.D.; Post, G.S.; Kitchell, B.E.; Sellon, R.K.; Kleiter, M.; Northrup, N.; Segev, G. Use of adjuvant carboplatin for treatment of dogs with oral malignant melanoma following surgical excision. *Vet. Comp. Oncol.* 2014, *12*, 78–84.

107. Bergman, P.J.; Mcknight, J.; Novosad, A.; Charney, S.; Farrelly, J.; Craft, D.; Wulderk, M.; Jeffers, Y.; Sadelain, M.; Hohenhaus, A.E.; *et al.* Long-term survival of dogs with advanced malignant melanoma after DNA vaccination with xenogeneic human tyrosinase: A phase I trial. *Clin. Cancer Res.* 2003, *9*, 1284–1290.

108. MacEwen, E.G.; Kurzman, I.D.; Vail, D.M.; Dubielzig, R.R.; Everlith, K.; Madewell, B.R.; Rodriguez, C.O., Jr.; Phillips, B.; Zwahlen, C.H.; Obradovich, J.; *et al.* Adjuvant therapy for melanoma in dogs: Results of randomized clinical trials using surgery, liposome-encapsulated muramyl triptide, and granulocyte macrophage colony-stimulang factor. *Clin. Cancer Res.* 1999, *5*, 4249–4258.

109. Moff, S.L.; Corey, G.R.; Gottfredsson, M. Distant cutaneous granulomas after bacille Calmette-Guérin immunotherapy for malignant melanoma: Case for direct infection. *Clin. Infect. Dis.* 1999, *29*, 1569–1570.

110. Bianco, S.R.; Sun, J.; Fosmire, S.P.; Hance, K.; Padilla, M.L.; Ritt, M.G.; Getzy, D.M.; Duke, R.C.; Withrow, S.J.; Lana, S.; *et al.* Enhancing anti melanoma immune responses through apoptosis. *Cancer Gene Ther.* 2003, *10*, 726–736.

111. Alexander, A.N.; Huelsmeyr, M.K.; Mitzey, A.; Dubielzig, R.R.; Kurzman, I.D.; MacEwen, E.G.; Vail, D.M. Development of an allogenic whole-cell tumor vaccine expressing xenogenic gp100 and implementation in phase II clinical trial in canine patients with malignant melanoma. *Cancer Immunol. Immunother.* 2006, *55*, 433–442.

112. Hogge, G.S.; Burkholder, J.K.; Culp, J.; Albertini, M.R.; Dubielzig, R.R.; Keller, E.T.; Yang, N.S.; MacEwen, E.G. Development of human granulocyte-macrophage colony-stimulating factor- transfected tumor cell vaccines for treatment of spontaneous canine cancer. *Hum. Gene Ther.* 1998, *9*, 1851–1861.

113. Bergman, P.J.; Wolchok, J.D. Of mice and men (and dogs): Development of a xenogeneic DNA vaccine for canine oral malignant melanoma. *Cancer Ther.* 2008, *6*, 817–826.

114. Grosenbaugh, D.A.; Leard, A.T.; Bergman, P.J.; Klein, M.K.; Meleo, K.; Susaneck, S.; Hess, P.R.; Jankowski, M.K.; Jones, P.D.; Leibman, N.; *et al.* Safety and efficacy of a xenogeneic DNA vaccine encoding for human tyrosinase as adjunctive treatment for oral malignant melanoma in dogs following surgical excision of the primary tumor. *Am. J. Vet. Res.* 2011, *72*, 1631–1638.

115. Ottnod, J.M.; Smedley, R.C.; Walshaw, R.; Hauptman, J.G.; Kiupel, M.; Obradovich, J.E. A retrospective analysis of the efficacy of Oncept vaccine for the adjunct treatment of canine oral malignant melanoma. *Vet. Comp. Oncol.* 2013, *11*, 219–229.

116. Rotte, A.; Bhandaru, M.; Zhou, Y.; Mcelwee, K.J. Immunotherapy of melanoma: Present options and future promises. *Cancer Metastasis Rev.* 2015, *34*, 115–128.

117. Gyorffy, S.; Rodriguez-Lecompte, J.C.; Woods, J.P.; Foley, R.; Kruth, S.; Liaw, P.C.; Gauldie, J. Bone marrow-derived dendritic cell vaccination of dogs with naturally occurring melanoma by using human gp100 antigen.*J. Vet. Intern. Med.* 2005, *19*, 56–63.

118. Tamura, K.; Yamada, M.; Isotani, M.; Arai, H.; Yagihara, H.; Ono, K.; Washizu, T.; Bonkobara, M. Induction of dendritic cell-mediated immune responses against canine malignant melanoma cells. *Vet. J.* 2008, *175*, 126–129.

119. Elmslie, R. VRCC Veterinary Speciality & Emergency Hospital. Available online: http://www.vetcancerspecialists.com/blog/2013/1/31/the-controversy-surrounding-the-melanoma-vaccine-for-dogs/ (accesse on 15 November 2015).

120. Yokoe, I.; Azuma, K.; Hata, K.; Mukaiyama, T.; Goto, T.; Tsuka, T.; Imagawa, T.; Itoh, N.; Murahata, Y.; Osaki, T.; *et al.* Clinical systemic lupeol administration for canine oral malignant melanoma. *Mol. Clin. Oncol.* 2015, *3*, 89–92.

121. Robert, C.; Ribas, A.; Wolchok, J.D.; Hodi, F.S.; Hamid, O.; Kefford, R.; Weber, J.S.; Joshua, A.M.; Hwu, W.J.; Gangadhar, T.C.; *et al.* Anti-programmed-death-receptor-1 treatment with pembrolizumab in ipilimumab-refractory advanced melanoma: A randomised dose-comparison cohort of a phase 1 trial. *Lancet* 2014, *384*, 1109–1117.

122. Schadendorf, D.; Hodi, F.S.; Robert, C.; Weber, J.S.; Margolin, K.; Hamid, O.; Patt, D.; Chen, T.T.; Berman, D.M.; Wolchok, J.D. Pooled analysis of long-term survival data from phase II and phase III trials of ipilimumab in unresectable or metastatic melanoma. *J. Clin. Oncol.* 2015, *33*, 1889–1894.

123. Maekawa, N.; Konnai, S.; Ikebuchi, R.; Okagawa, T.; Adachi, M.; Takagi, S.; Kagawa, Y.; Nakajima, C.; Suzuki, Y.; Murata, S.; *et al.* Expression of PD-L1 on canine tumor cells and enhancement of IFN-c production from tumor infiltrating cells by PD-L1 blockade. *PLoS ONE* 2014.

124. Igase, M.; Hwang, C.C.; Coffey, M.; Okuda, M.; Noguchi, S.; Mizuno, T. The oncolytic effects of reovirus in canine solid tumor cell lines. *J. Vet. Med. Sci.* 2015, *77*, 541–548.

8

CHAPTER

THERAPEUTIC INNOVATIONS: TYROSINE KINASE INHIBITORS IN CANCER

Nikolaos Dervisis and Shawna Klahn

Virginia Maryland College of Veterinary Medicine, 245 Duck Pond Dr., Blacksburg, VA 24061, USA

ABSTRACT

Conventional cytotoxic chemotherapy involving DNA-interacting agents and indiscriminate cell death is no longer the future of cancer management. While chemotherapy is not likely to completely disappear from the armamentarium; the use of targeted therapies in combination with conventional treatment is becoming the standard of care in human medicine. Tyrosine kinases are pivotal points of functional cellular pathways and have been implicated in malignancy, inflammatory, and immune-mediated diseases. Pharmaceutical interventions targeting aberrant tyrosine kinase signaling has exploded and is the second most important area of drug development. The "Valley of Death" between drug discovery and approval threatens to blunt the enormous strides in cancer management seen thus far. Kinase inhibitors, as targeted small molecules, hold promise in the treatment and diagnosis of cancer. However, there are still many unanswered questions regarding the use of kinase inhibitors in the interpretation and management of cancer. Comparative oncology has the potential to address restrictions and limitations in the advancement in kinase inhibitor therapy.

INTRODUCTION

Kinases are among the first oncogenes identified. Initial understanding of oncogene function originates from experiments utilizing retroviruses expressing oncogenic kinases. Murine, feline, and avian retroviruses were the first to demonstrate integration into the host genome, thereby transducing genes harbored at the insertion site. Src kinase is transduced within the avian genome by the Rous sarcoma virus and is the driving

Citation: Nikolaos Dervisis and Shawna Klahn, Therapeutic Innovations: Tyrosine Kinase Inhibitors in Cancer, doi:10.3390/vetsci3010004

force behind Rous sarcoma. Similarly, Raf kinase is transduced by the same retrovirus. Activation of genes encoding kinases contribute to oncogenic transformation of the infected cell. An array of over 500 kinases have since been identified using animal tissue culture models and genetic methodologies [1,2]. Their role in tumorigenesis, tumor progression, and metastasis has been expanding, along with pharmacological attempts to therapeutically intervene the aberrant functions.

DIGITAL AGE IN CELLULAR BIOLOGY

Kinases catalyze the transfer of the gamma-phosphate group of ATP onto a substrate. Kinases mediate nearly all signal transductions, thereby regulating multiple cellular activities such as proliferation, survival, apoptosis, metabolism, transcription, differentiation [3,4]. Accumulating pharmacological and pathological evidence demonstrate that kinases are promising drug targets for the treatment of numerous diseases, such as cancer, inflammatory diseases, central nervous system disorders, cardiovascular diseases, and diabetes [5]. The catalytic activity depends on the phosphorylation status of specific amino-acid residues. Conformational and other changes induced by phosphorylation events result in dramatic shifts in the kinase catalytic activity, manifesting as a binary switch in functional behavior of the enzyme [6,7,8].

Kinases are located at key positions within the cell. Intercellular communication and the extracellular environment are monitored through signal receptors, while intracellular communication is conducted through secondary signaling molecules and at specific functional checkpoints. Individual subcircuits representing relative simplified functions, such as cellular growth and energy metabolism, have multiple interconnections and crosstalk, forming a functional signaling network that is characterized by higher-level complexity [9]. Kinases have an important role in the amplification and termination of signals, facilitating communication between integral parts of the cell, and between cells. Thus, kinases can be thought as the molecular receptors, amplifiers and transducers of extra and intracellular signals, facilitating the cell's response to the challenges of life.

A consequence of this complex and intricate signaling network is that kinases exhibit pleiotropy and locus heterogeneity. Mutations within the same gene may result in several phenotypes, while the same disease phenotype can sometimes result from mutations in different kinase genes. For example, gain-of-function mutations in the region of the immunoglobulin domain of fibroblast growth factor receptor 1 (FGFR1) result in Pfeiffer syndrome and osteoglophonic dysplasia, whereas loss-of-function mutations throughout the protein cause hypogonadotrophic hypogonadism [10,11].

DISEASE AS A KINASE DYSFUNCTION

Despite the enormous amount of research and rapid developments during the past decades, cancer continues to be a worldwide killer. In the USA, cancer accounts for 23% of the total deaths, and is the second most common cause of death after heart disease. It is expected to surpass heart disease as the leading cause of death in the next few years [12,13]. The intense research in the molecular biology of cancer resulted in an explosion of candidate genes that drive oncogenesis. Nearly simultaneous with the discovery of cancer-associated genes, strategies to repair them were explored. Early attempts focusing on gene replacement therapies were not translated into clinical use due to technological, ethical, and biological barriers. Efforts were soon turned towards pharmacologic methods of blocking specific aberrant oncogenic signaling.

Mutations in protein kinases are overrepresented approximately four-fold compared with a random selection of genes, and reportedly the most frequently mutated family of genes contributing to neoplastic diseases [14,15]. Protein kinases may act as tumor suppressors or proto-oncogenes in normal, healthy cells. Aberrations in protein kinase function can lead to tumorigenesis through numerous mechanisms, including the activation of proliferative pathways, genomic instability, reduction of the DNA damage response, deactivation of apoptotic pathways and/or the promotion of angiogenesis and cellular motility [15]. Gain-of-function mutations typically increase constitutive kinase activity, leading to unrestrained cellular signaling, while loss of-function mutations can lead to a loss in cell signaling. The combined signal aberrations can have a profound effect on the cell, leading to oncogenesis, tumor growth and metastasis.

KINASES AS AN ATTRACTIVE DRUG TARGET

Protein kinases are considered to be the second most important group of drug targets after G-protein-coupled receptors [16,17]. Aberrant kinase activity is implicated in a large variety of diseases, particularly those involving inflammatory or proliferative responses, such as cancer, rheumatoid arthritis, cardiovascular and neurological disorders, asthma and psoriasis. Directly or indirectly, hundreds of human diseases have been connected to protein kinase dysfunction. The ability to modulate kinase activity therefore represents an attractive therapeutic strategy for the treatment of human illnesses [18].

Kinase activity is typically regulated by interconverting between two structural conformations via phosphorylation of key amino acid residues, shifting the balance between active and inactive. These two states are characterized by movements in conformationally mobile loops that border or block the ATP binding site of the kinase. For this reason, the dissociation constant for ATP may be significantly higher for the inactive conformation than for the active conformation. This kinase activation model provides the framework for drugs designed to interact with specific kinase domains. A large number of kinase inhibitors selectively target the inactive conformation, whereas other compounds bind to both conformations with similar affinity [19,20,21]. Inhibitors that bind to the inactive conformation likely face weaker competition with cellular ATP. The potential result is enhanced activity *in vivo*, acting primarily to shift equilibria between conformational states to prevent kinase activation, indirectly inhibiting activity [22].

The modulation of kinase activity can be achieved through either direct or indirect strategies (Figure 1). Imatinib (Gleevec; Novartis) is the prototype of direct protein-tyrosine kinase inhibitors that inhibits the BCR-ABL phosphorylation activity through blocking ATP binding. Imatinib has been approved for the treatment of patients with BCR-ABL positive chronic myeloid leukemia (CML) and patients with Kit (CD117)-

positive gastrointestinal stromal tumors. BCR-ABL is the constitutively active tyrosine kinase in CML and in certain forms of acute lymphoblastic leukemia. Imatinib also inhibits the kinase activity of platelet derived growth factor receptor, stem-cell factor receptor and c-kit. Indirect kinase inhibition involves disruption of protein-protein interactions. Cetuximab (Erbitux; ImClone/Bristol-Myers Squibb) is a monoclonal antibody that selectively binds to the extracellular domain of human epidermal growth factor receptor (EGFR), and competitively inhibits binding of epidermal growth factor (EGF) to its receptor tyrosine kinase. Bevacizumab (Avastin; Genentech) is the first anti-angiogenesis cancer drug approved by the FDA. Bevacizumab binds to human vascular endothelial growth factor A (VEGF-A), and prevents it from binding to its receptor tyrosine kinases, Flt-1/VEGFR1 and KDR/VEGRF2. Inhibition of VEGF signaling interferes with tumor blood vessel development, a process that is crucial for tumor growth and metastasis [23].

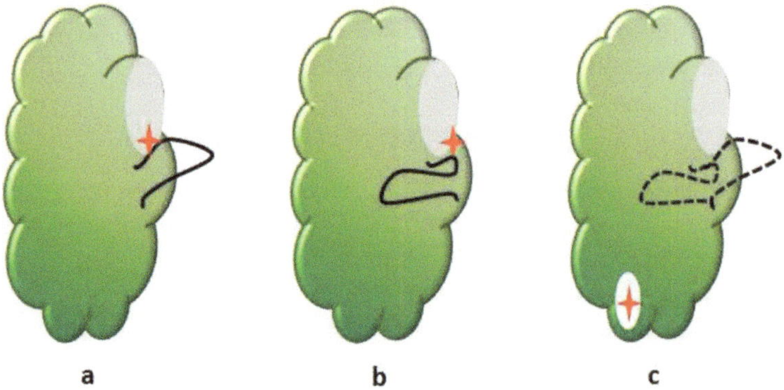

Figure 1: The activation loop of the protein kinase domain regulates access to the ATP binding site. The conformation of a conserved Asp-Phe-Gly (DFG) motif within the activation loop is used to categorize the binding mode of inhibitors. The common types of kinase—kinase inhibitor interactions include: (**a**) Type I inhibitors (**red** star) bind the ATP binding site (grey) of the protein kinase domain (green). The aspartate side chain in the conserved DFG motif at the beginning of the activation loop (black) faces into the active site; (**b**) Type II inhibitors bind a flipped conformation of the DFG motif in which the aspartate side chain faces outwards; (**c**) Allosteric ligands bind to binding pockets (white) that do not overlap with the active site of the kinase. The DFG motif conformation is not important. These binding pockets can be adjacent to the active site or distant from the active site.

Compounds that bind to protein kinases outside of the ATP-binding pocket may possess advantages over ATP-competitive counterparts. Drugs can be administered at concentrations closer to their biochemical inhibition constant, as inhibition is not affected by fluctuations in the cellular concentration of ATP. There is a potential for greater selectivity as residues outside the ATP binding pocket tend to be less conserved. In certain cases, noncompetitive inhibitors can be substrate selective, inhibiting the activity of a kinase against only a subset of its targets. Rapamycin, the first noncompetitive kinase inhibitor to be identified, is a cyclic macrolide that inhibits the protein kinase mammalian target of rapamycin (mTOR) [24]. MEK1 inhibitor PD098059, the first synthetic noncompetitive kinase inhibitor to be described, acts by binding to inactive MEK1 and preventing its phosphorylation by the upstream kinase Raf [25,26]. Several such inhibitors, termed allosteric, have been described, targeting kinases such as Akt, and inhibitor of nuclear factor kappa-B kinase (IKK-2) [27,28].

The target regions for most kinase inhibitors are intracellular. As small molecules, kinase inhibitors enter the cell by diffusion down the concentration gradient that exists across the membrane. The rate at which this process occurs, and the rate of active efflux, are important determinantsof the intracellular bioavailability of a kinase. How quickly the intracellular inhibitor concentration reaches a steady state and the relative concentrations of inhibitor inside and outside the cell at steady state rely on the relative lipophilicity *vs.* hydrophilicity characteristics of the drug. The rate that it permeates the cellular membrane and non-specific binding to proteins and may affect the route of administration and dosing schedule [29,30]. Expression of drug efflux pump transporters has been shown to reduce the steady-state intracellular drug concentration, although most mammalian cells in culture appear to have less efflux activity for kinase inhibitors compared to chemotherapeutics such as doxorubicin.

HITTING THE TARGET

The transition from cytotoxic chemotherapy to molecularly targeted cancer drug discovery and development has resulted in an increasing number of successful therapies that have impacted the lives of a large number of cancer patients. The BCR-ABL inhibitor imatinib is generally regarded as a trailblazer drug that most impressively validated the concept of designing a small molecule therapeutic. Imatinib is designed to treat a defined patient population with chronic myeloid leukemia in which the malignancy is driven by the BCR-ABL translocation. The improvement in survival has been dramatic [31]. These successes were followed by a number of other small molecule drugs inhibiting critical cancer targets, essentially changing the anti-neoplastic armamentarium of modern Oncology. There has been an explosion of approved kinase inhibitors, with nearly 20 drugs approved by the FDA in a four-year period (Table 1). Veterinary Oncology has been slowly following the fast pace of human Oncology, and there are currently three kinase inhibitors approved by FDA, and a number of small molecular inhibitors under various stages of development (Table 2). The clinical success of such targeted therapeutics depends to a large degree to the availability of predictive markers. The specific histopathologic diagnosis may not be of such importance, as the presence of markers associated with specific genetic aberrations (mutations, internal tandem duplications, gene amplifications) [32,33,34,35]. For example, the anaplastic lymphoma kinase (ALK) was first implicated in the pathogenesis of an aggressive type of non-Hodgkin's lymphoma [36]. Rearrangements of the ALK gene were subsequently discovered to be are present in 3% to 5% of non-small-cell lung cancers (NSCLC) [37]. These genetic lesions define a distinct subgroup of NSCLC that typically occurs in younger patients who have never smoked or have a history of light smoking [38]. Knowing the presence of these rearrangements can guide the treatment protocol selection, alter the prognosis, and essentially result in a truly personalized approach in cancer therapy [29,35].

Table 1: Approved tyrosine kinase inhibitors in human medicine, 2011–2015 [a].

Drug	Target	Year Approved	Indication
Vandetanib (Caprelsa®)	Flt1, Flt4, KDR, EGFR, Ret	2011	MTC
Crizotinib (Xalkori®)	ALK, MET, EML4-ALK fusion protein	2011	NSCLC
Ruxolitinib (Jakafi®/Jakavi®)	JAK1, JAK2	2011	Myelofibrosis
Vemurafenib (Zelboraf®)	BRAF	2011	Melanoma
Bosutinib (Bosulif®)	BCR/ABL1	2012	CML
Axitinib (Inlyta®)	Flt1, Flt4, KDR, Kit, PDGF-Rα/β	2012	RCC
Cabozantinib (Cometriq®)	KDR, Mek	2012	MTC
Regorafinib (Stivarga®)	KDR, TEK	2012	CC, GIST
Ponatinib (Iclusig®)	BCR/ABL1	2012	CML, ALL
Dabrafenib (Tafinlar®)	BRAF	2013	Melanoma
Trametinib (Mekinist®)	MEK1, MEK2	2013	Melanoma
Afatinib (Gilotrif®)	ERBB2, EGFR	2013	NSCLC
Ibrutinib (Imbruvica®)	BTK	2013	MCL, CLL
Tofacitinib (Xeljanz®)	JAK3	2013	Rheumatoid arthritis
Idelalisib (Zydelig®)	PI3-K	2014	CLL
			Follicular B-cell NHL
Ceritinib (Zykadia®)	ALK	2014	ALK⁺ NSCLC
Lenvatinib (Lenvima®)	VEGFR2 and VEGFR3	2015	Radioactive iodine-refractory DTC
Palbociclib (Ibrance®)	CDK4 and CDK6	2015	Breast carcinoma

[a] Abbreviations: ALL, acute lymphoblastic leukemia; CC, colorectal cancer; CML, chronic myelogenous leukemia; DTC, differentiated thyroid cancer; GIST, gastrointestinal stromal tumor; MCL, mantle cell lymphoma; MTC, medullary thyroid carcinoma; NHL, Non-Hodgkin's lymphoma; NSCLC, non-small-cell lung carcinoma; RCC, renal cell carcinoma.

Table 2: Approved tyrosine kinase inhibitors in veterinary medicine, all drugs.

Drug	Targets	Year Approved	Indication
Toceranib (Palladia®)	VEGF-R2 PDGF-Rα Kit Flt-3 *RET* *JAK family*	2009	Patnaik grade 2 or 3, recurrent, cutaneous mast cell tumors with or without regional lymph node involvement in dogs
Masitinib (Kinavet-CA1®)	Kit PDGF-Rα/β Lyn FGF-R3	2010 [a]	Nonresectable grade 2 and 3 cutaneous mast cell tumors in dogs that have not previously received radiotherapy and/or chemotherapy except corticosteroids
Oclacitinib (Apoquel®)	JAK1 JAK 2	2013	Control of pruritus associated with allergic dermatitis and control of atopic dermatitis in dogs at least 12 mos of age

[a] Conditional approval by the FDA expired in December 2015 and the drug is not commercially available in the US. The drug can only be obtained through the FDA's personal import mechanism.

MISSING THE POINT

The high specificity of the kinase inhibitors appears to be their Achilles heel. As many of the kinase inhibitors exert their tumoricidal effects primarily by inhibiting a specific kinase, there is a strong selective pressure for cells to acquire resistance through mutations in the kinase gene that abrogate drug binding. Additional non-mutation kinase inhibitor resistance mechanisms have been documented, including target amplification and upregulation of alternative kinase pathways such as hepatocyte growth factor receptor in the acquisition of resistance to EGFR kinase inhibitors in lung cancer [30,39,40]. The rapid proliferation of cancer cells and the acquisition of mutations conferring drug resistance has become a recurring theme in the clinic. To date the most extensive clinical and laboratory characterization of resistance-causing mutations has been performed for BCR–ABL in the context of imatinib and second-generation inhibitors. Furthermore, it has been shown in specific hematological tumors that quiescent stem cells are refractory to tyrosine kinase inhibitors, and these cell populations may be instrumentally involved in resistance mechanisms [41].

Inhibitor resistance conferred by mutations at the gatekeeper residue appears to be the common theme for a variety of kinases. The gatekeeper residue term refers to the amino acid side chain at the position that determines the relative accessibility of the hydrophobic pocket located near the ATP/drug binding site. Access to this pocket is important to many kinase inhibitors because hydrophobic interactions in this site are crucial for the binding affinity of the drug. Several strategies are being investigated to overcome kinase inhibitor resistance mutants. A first approach was to develop inhibitors that can tolerate diverse amino acids at the gatekeeper position [42,43]. A second approach is to target the kinase with inhibitors that bind at alternative binding sites [44]. A third approach involves targeting other molecules that may be required for signal transduction in the specific kinase pathway [45]. These approaches have been demonstrated to work in cell culture, and rodent models and clinical trials are currently underway.

UNANSWERED QUESTIONS

Considerable progress made with the new molecularly targeted therapies. Significant advances have occurred in the treatment of diseases in which few treatment options are available, such NSCLC and melanoma. However, for many patients the therapeutic options are still limited, and the process of bringing a new drug to patients is frustratingly slow with very high failure rates [46,47]. The point of failure between basic research and new drug approval has often referred to as the "Valley of Death" [48,49].

The current model of targeted drug development is severely flawed. The inefficiency of translating seemingly important discoveries from the lab to the clinic can be demonstrated by a simple comparison between the research publications on kinase function and the drug approvals. Multiple obstacles within the current framework severely restrict the timely exploration of combinatorial kinase inhibitor therapies. Regulatory, patent secrets, and risk-averse corporate cultures need to be quickly remedied in order to be prepared, as cancer is becoming the leading cause of death in both humans and veterinary patients.

Scientific questions potentially affecting patient clinical management and treatment options include:

- *When to treat with kinase inhibitors?*
- What is the biologically sound way to combine kinase inhibitors with cytotoxic chemotherapy?
- *How to combine multiple kinase inhibitors in a treatment protocol*
- *How to determine efficacy when tumor size is not an appropriate measure*
- *How to manage treatment failure? Switch to different kinase inhibitors, or add different kinase inhibitors to the current therapy?*

The canine cancer patient can help in answering some of these questions. Spontaneous cancers in pet dogs offer a unique and largely unexploited translational research opportunity for cancer imaging, device and drug development. Dogs suffer from spontaneous malignancies at similar rates and types as humans. Limitations with rodent models stem from development from inbred strains of mice kept in controlled environments. Companion animals, like humans, are genetically diverse and are exposed to many of the same environmental influences. Furthermore, purebred dogs represent unique gene pools, with genetic predisposition to cancers segregating within specific breeds. This provides the opportunity to study complex phenotypes in a relatively simplified genetic background, allowing the identification of critical genetic events that drive malignant behavior.

Dogs suffering from cancer have been successfully used in elegantly designed studies, providing useful and translatable pharmacokinetic/pharmacodynamic data [50,51,52,53,54,55]. Data from canine clinical trials have informed on the scheduling and dosing of small molecular inhibitors in human cancer patients [56]. The availability of the canine genome and growth of high throughput genomic technologies and informatics has enabled comparative oncology to describe canine cancer biology and define potential therapeutic targets in many of the same ways as human cancers [57,58]. Canine cancer patients offer an unparalleled resource for targeting the tumor stroma and tumor/host immune interactions, due to the presence of syngeneic host-tumor relationship and a competent immune function [50].

Using spontaneous pet dog oncology modeling does not require up-front treatment with specific cancer treatment regimens. Thus, novel therapeutic agents can be offered through clinical trials at any stage in cancer presentation. The disease progression times in pet dogs is compressed, allowing for evaluation of a variety of pharmacodynamics intervention outcomes and providing longitudinal endpoints of cancer response through serial sampling. Randomized controlled trials can be conducted in the newly-diagnosed, adjuvant, or metastatic settings, evaluating the utility of drug combinations and drug selection algorithms across a range of tumor and genetic background scenarios [51].

Finally, the infrastructure and resources to realize the potential of the canine cancer patient as an additional tool in conquering cancer exists. The National Cancer Institute's Comparative Oncology Trials Consortium (NCI-COTC;http://ccr.cancer.gov/resources/cop/COTC.asp) brings together study sponsors with academic veterinary oncology centers in North America to support multicenter clinical trials of investigational therapeutics [59]. High-quality biologic samples (tumor, normal, biologic fluids) from dogs with various malignancies are available via the Pfizer-Canine Comparative

Oncology and Genomics Consortium (CCOGC) biospecimen repository (www.ccogc.net) [60]. As a direct result of such mechanisms drugable target identification and signaling pathway similarities have been identified between canine and human cancer patients [61,62,63,64,65].

FUTURE DIRECTIONS

The use of pet dogs in translational medicine may be the "bridge" to the Death Valley [66]. Translational medicine is the process of applying knowledge gained from basic biomedical research to clinical practice. It involves bridging new research findings, scientific discoveries and new techniques to approaches in the prevention, diagnosis or treatment of diseases. The ultimate outcome is the patient's health. The paradigm shift is that scientific discoveries should not only be celebrated in basic laboratories and research institutes, or published (and archived) in prestigious medical journals—they need to make their way to hospitals, clinics, and into patients' lives to be real successes. Translational medicine involves a longer-term strategy for research that is beyond the immediate outcomes of a research project [67].

A major hurdle in therapeutic development is the translation of efficacy determined during the drug discovery phase into efficacy in the clinic. There are often discrepancies between drug efficacy, demonstrated in the current preclinical experimental models, and final efficacy, or lack thereof, in patients. Tissue culture and various rodent models have been and are used as potential predictive models for response in human cancers. It remains to be decided which model is most predictive, however, it is clear that none can reliably predict significant clinical efficacy.

CONCLUDING REMARKS

Veterinary cancer patients can provide the solution for some of the current limitations faced in targeted therapies. Several of the features that define human cancer, including long periods of latency, the complex biology of cancer recurrence and metastasis, the stromal interactions, and outcomes to novel therapies are frequently not adequately represented in murine cancer [68]. Dogs develop cancer and are diagnosed, staged, and treated in an almost identical manner to human cancer patients. Canine tumors develop in a complex genetic background, in the backdrop of intact immune system, and are exposed to the same environmental carcinogens as their human counterparts. Many dogs are essentially family members. Their owners are motivated to treat their pets, and as advocates for their pet, they actively seek participation in Clinical Trials. With the continuous improvement of the canine genomic annotation, dogs with cancer may represent an excellent opportunity for bridging the Valley of Death. One of the payoffs for human cancer patients is reduced exposure to ineffective clinical trials. The partnership under One Medicine of basic science researchers, veterinary and human oncologists, and pharmaceutical industry, has significant potential to advance drug discovery and approval. Ultimately, this ideal could result in improved cancer management, regardless of species.

AUTHOR CONTRIBUTIONS

Nikolaos Dervisis and Shawna Klahn equally contributed to the writing, revisions and editing of the paper. They are both veterinary oncologists with extensive experience in cancer chemotherapy.

REFERENCES

1. Zhang, J.; Yang, P.L.; Gray, N.S. Targeting cancer with small molecule kinase inhibitors. *Nat. Rev. Cancer* 2009,*9*, 28–39.
2. Tsatsanis, C.; Spandidos, D.A. Oncogenic kinase signaling in human neoplasms. *Ann. N. Y. Acad. Sci.* 2004,*1028*, 168–175.
3. Johnson, L.N.; Lewis, R.J. Structural basis for control by phosphorylation. *Chem. Rev.* 2001, *101*, 2209–2242.
4. Adams, J.A. Kinetic and catalytic mechanisms of protein kinases. *Chem. Rev.* 2001, *101*, 2271–2290.
5. Rask-Andersen, M.; Zhang, J.; Fabbro, D.; Schioth, H.B. Advances in kinase targeting: Current clinical use and clinical trials. *Trends Pharmacol. Sci.* 2014, *35*, 604–620.
6. Burnett, G.; Kennedy, E.P. The enzymatic phosphorylation of proteins. *J. Biol. Chem.* 1954, *211*, 969–980.
7. Cohen, P. The origins of protein phosphorylation. *Nat. Cell Biol.* 2002, *4*, 127–130.
8. UniProt, C. Uniprot: A hub for protein information. *Nucleic Acids Res.* 2015, *43*, 204–212.
9. Hanahan, D.; Weinberg, R.A. Hallmarks of cancer: The next generation. *Cell* 2011, *144*, 646–674.
10. Muenke, M.; Schell, U.; Hehr, A.; Robin, N.H.; Losken, H.W.; Schinzel, A.; Pulleyn, L.J.; Rutland, P.; Reardon, W.; Malcolm, S.; *et al.* A common mutation in the fibroblast growth factor receptor 1 gene in Pfeiffer syndrome.*Nat. Genet.* 1994, *8*, 269–274.
11. Pitteloud, N.; Acierno, J.S., Jr.; Meysing, A.; Eliseenkova, A.V.; Ma, J.; Ibrahimi, O.A.; Metzger, D.L.; Hayes, F.J.; Dwyer, A.A.; Hughes, V.A.; *et al.* Mutations in fibroblast growth factor receptor 1 cause both kallmann syndrome and normosmic idiopathic hypogonadotropic hypogonadism. *Proc. Natl. Acad. Sci. USA* 2006, *103*, 6281–6286.
12. CDC. Leading Causes of Death. Available online: http://www.cdc.gov/nchs/fastats/leading-causes-of-death.htm(accessed on 19 January 2016).
13. Siegel, R.L.; Miller, K.D.; Jemal, A. Cancer statistics, 2015. *CA Cancer J. Clin.* 2015, *65*, 5–29.
14. Futreal, P.A.; Coin, L.; Marshall, M.; Down, T.; Hubbard, T.; Wooster, R.; Rahman, N.; Stratton, M.R. A census of human cancer genes. *Nat. Rev. Cancer* 2004, *4*, 177–183.

15. Lahiry, P.; Torkamani, A.; Schork, N.J.; Hegele, R.A. Kinase mutations in human disease: Interpreting genotype-phenotype relationships. *Nat. Rev. Genet.* 2010, *11*, 60–74.

16. Vlahovic, G.; Crawford, J. Activation of tyrosine kinases in cancer. *Oncologist* 2003, *8*, 531–538.

17. Cohen, P. Protein kinases—The major drug targets of the twenty-first century? *Nat. Rev. Drug Discov.* 2002, *1*, 309–315.

18. Melnikova, I.; Golden, J. Targeting protein kinases. *Nat. Rev. Drug Discov.* 2004, *3*, 993–994.

19. Schindler, T.; Bornmann, W.; Pellicena, P.; Miller, W.T.; Clarkson, B.; Kuriyan, J. Structural mechanism for STI-571 inhibition of abelson tyrosine kinase. *Science* 2000, *289*, 1938–1942.

20. Wan, P.T.; Garnett, M.J.; Roe, S.M.; Lee, S.; Niculescu-Duvaz, D.; Good, V.M.; Jones, C.M.; Marshall, C.J.; Springer, C.J.; Barford, D.; *et al.* Mechanism of activation of the RAF-ERK signaling pathway by oncogenic mutations of β-RAF. *Cell* 2004, *116*, 855–867.

21. Frantz, B.; Klatt, T.; Pang, M.; Parsons, J.; Rolando, A.; Williams, H.; Tocci, M.J.; O'Keefe, S.J.; O'Neill, E.A. The activation state of p38 mitogen-activated protein kinase determines the efficiency of ATP competition for pyridinylimidazole inhibitor binding. *Biochemistry* 1998, *37*, 13846–13853.

22. Knight, Z.A.; Shokat, K.M. Features of selective kinase inhibitors. *Chem. Biol.* 2005, *12*, 621–637.

23. Ferrara, N.; Hillan, K.J.; Novotny, W. Bevacizumab (avastin), a humanized anti-VEGF monoclonal antibody for cancer therapy. *Biochem. Biophys. Res. Commun.* 2005, *333*, 328–335.

24. Benjamin, D.; Colombi, M.; Moroni, C.; Hall, M.N. Rapamycin passes the torch: A new generation of mTOR inhibitors. *Nat. Rev. Drug Discov.* 2011, *10*, 868–880.

25. Alessi, D.R.; Cuenda, A.; Cohen, P.; Dudley, D.T.; Saltiel, A.R. PD 098059 is a specific inhibitor of the activation of mitogen-activated protein kinase kinase *in vitro* and *in vivo*. *J. Biol. Chem.* 1995, *270*, 27489–27494.

26. Dudley, D.T.; Pang, L.; Decker, S.J.; Bridges, A.J.; Saltiel, A.R. A synthetic inhibitor of the mitogen-activated protein kinase cascade. *Proc. Natl. Acad. Sci. USA* 1995, *92*, 7686–7689.

27. Lindsley, C.W.; Zhao, Z.; Leister, W.H.; Robinson, R.G.; Barnett, S.F.; Defeo-Jones, D.; Jones, R.E.; Hartman, G.D.; Huff, J.R.; Huber, H.E.; *et al.* Allosteric AKT (PKB) inhibitors: Discovery and SAR of isozyme selective inhibitors. *Bioorg. Med. Chem. Lett.* 2005, *15*, 761–764.

28. Yang, J.; Amiri, K.I.; Burke, J.R.; Schmid, J.A.; Richmond, A. Bms-345541 targets inhibitor of κβ kinase and induces apoptosis in melanoma: Involvement of nuclear factor κβ and mitochondria pathways. *Clin. Cancer Res.* 2006, *12*, 950–960.

29. Shaw, A.T.; Kim, D.W.; Nakagawa, K.; Seto, T.; Crino, L.; Ahn, M.J.; de Pas, T.; Besse, B.; Solomon, B.J.; Blackhall, F.; *et al.* Crizotinib versus chemotherapy in advanced alk-positive lung cancer. *N. Engl. J. Med.* 2013,*368*, 2385–2394.

30. le Coutre, P.; Tassi, E.; Varella-Garcia, M.; Barni, R.; Mologni, L.; Cabrita, G.; Marchesi, E.; Supino, R.; Gambacorti-Passerini, C. Induction of resistance to the abelson inhibitor sti571 in human leukemic cells through gene amplification. *Blood* 2000, *95*, 1758–1766.

31. Druker, B.J.; Guilhot, F.; O'Brien, S.G.; Gathmann, I.; Kantarjian, H.; Gattermann, N.; Deininger, M.W.; Silver, R.T.; Goldman, J.M.; Stone, R.M.; *et al.* Five-year follow-up of patients receiving imatinib for chronic myeloid leukemia. *N. Engl. J. Med.* 2006, *355*, 2408–2417.

32. Yang, J.C.; Sequist, L.V.; Geater, S.L.; Tsai, C.M.; Mok, T.S.; Schuler, M.; Yamamoto, N.; Yu, C.J.; Ou, S.H.; Zhou, C.; *et al.* Clinical activity of afatinib in patients with advanced non-small-cell lung cancer harbouring uncommon EGFR mutations: A combined post-hoc analysis of LUX-Lung 2, LUX-Lung 3, And LUX-Lung 6.*Lancet Oncol.* 2015, *16*, 830–838.

33. Lorenzen, S.; Riera Knorrenschild, J.; Haag, G.M.; Pohl, M.; Thuss-Patience, P.; Bassermann, F.; Helbig, U.; Weissinger, F.; Schnoy, E.; Becker, K.; *et al.* Lapatinib *versus* lapatinib plus capecitabine as second-line treatment in human epidermal growth factor receptor 2-amplified metastatic gastro-oesophageal cancer: A randomised phase II trial of the arbeitsgemeinschaft internistische onkologie. *Eur. J. Cancer* 2015, *51*, 569–576.

34. London, C.A.; Malpas, P.B.; Wood-Follis, S.L.; Boucher, J.F.; Rusk, A.W.; Rosenberg, M.P.; Henry, C.J.; Mitchener, K.L.; Klein, M.K.; Hintermeister, J.G.; *et al.* Multi-center, placebo-controlled, double-blind, randomized study of oral toceranib phosphate (SU11654), a receptor tyrosine kinase inhibitor, for the treatment of dogs with recurrent (either local or distant) mast cell tumor following surgical excision. *Clin. Cancer Res.* 2009, *15*, 3856–3865.

35. Solomon, B.J.; Mok, T.; Kim, D.W.; Wu, Y.L.; Nakagawa, K.; Mekhail, T.; Felip, E.; Cappuzzo, F.; Paolini, J.; Usari, T.; *et al.* First-line crizotinib *versus* chemotherapy in ALK-positive lung cancer. *N. Engl. J. Med.* 2014, *371*, 2167–2177.

36. Duyster, J.; Bai, R.Y.; Morris, S.W. Translocations involving anaplastic lymphoma kinase (ALK). *Oncogene* 2001,*20*, 5623–5637.

37. Rikova, K.; Guo, A.; Zeng, Q.; Possemato, A.; Yu, J.; Haack, H.; Nardone, J.; Lee, K.; Reeves, C.; Li, Y.; *et al.* Global survey of phosphotyrosine signaling identifies oncogenic kinases in lung cancer. *Cell* 2007, *131*, 1190–1203.

38. Blackhall, F.H.; Peters, S.; Bubendorf, L.; Dafni, U.; Kerr, K.M.; Hager, H.; Soltermann, A.; O'Byrne, K.J.; Dooms, C.; Sejda, A.; *et al.* Prevalence and clinical outcomes for patients with ALK-positive resected stage I to III adenocarcinoma: Results from the european thoracic oncology platform lungscape project. *J. Clin. Oncol.*2014, *32*, 2780–2787.

39. Engelman, J.A.; Zejnullahu, K.; Mitsudomi, T.; Song, Y.; Hyland, C.; Park, J.O.; Lindeman, N.; Gale, C.M.; Zhao, X.; Christensen, J.; *et al.* Met

amplification leads to gefitinib resistance in lung cancer by activating ERBB3 signaling. *Science* 2007, *316*, 1039–1043.

40. Cui, J.J. Targeting receptor tyrosine kinase met in cancer: Small molecule inhibitors and clinical progress. *J. Med. Chem.* 2014, *57*, 4427–4453.
41. Copland, M.; Hamilton, A.; Elrick, L.J.; Baird, J.W.; Allan, E.K.; Jordanides, N.; Barow, M.; Mountford, J.C.; Holyoake, T.L. Dasatinib (BMS-354825) targets an earlier progenitor population than imatinib in primary cml but does not eliminate the quiescent fraction. *Blood* 2006, *107*, 4532–4539.
42. Weisberg, E.; Manley, P.W.; Breitenstein, W.; Bruggen, J.; Cowan-Jacob, S.W.; Ray, A.; Huntly, B.; Fabbro, D.; Fendrich, G.; Hall-Meyers, E.; *et al.* Characterization of AMN107, a selective inhibitor of native and mutant BCR-ABL. *Cancer Cell* 2005, *7*, 129–141.
43. Shah, N.P.; Lee, F.Y.; Luo, R.; Jiang, Y.; Donker, M.; Akin, C. Dasatinib (BMS-354825) inhibits kitd816v, an imatinib-resistant activating mutation that triggers neoplastic growth in most patients with systemic mastocytosis. *Blood* 2006, *108*, 286–291.
44. Gumireddy, K.; Reddy, M.V.; Cosenza, S.C.; Boominathan, R.; Baker, S.J.; Papathi, N.; Jiang, J.; Holland, J.; Reddy, E.P. ON01910, a non-ATP-competitive small molecule inhibitor of Plk1, is a potent anticancer agent.*Cancer Cell* 2005, *7*, 275–286.
45. Copland, M.; Pellicano, F.; Richmond, L.; Allan, E.K.; Hamilton, A.; Lee, F.Y.; Weinmann, R.; Holyoake, T.L. BMS-214662 potently induces apoptosis of chronic myeloid leukemia stem and progenitor cells and synergizes with tyrosine kinase inhibitors. *Blood* 2008, *111*, 2843–2853.
46. Yap, T.A.; Workman, P. Exploiting the cancer genome: Strategies for the discovery and clinical development of targeted molecular therapeutics. *Annu. Rev. Pharmacol. Toxicol.* 2012, *52*, 549–573.
47. DiMasi, J.A.; Grabowski, H.G. Economics of new oncology drug development. *J. Clin. Oncol.* 2007, *25*, 209–216.
48. Adams, D.J. The valley of death in anticancer drug development: A reassessment. *Trends Pharmacol. Sci.* 2012,*33*, 173–180.
49. Wong, T.Y. How to bridge the "valley of death" between a research discovery and clinical application? *Ann. Acad. Med. Singap.* 2014, *43*, 422–424.
50. Paoloni, M.; Mazcko, C.; Selting, K.; Lana, S.; Barber, L.; Phillips, J.; Skorupski, K.; Vail, D.; Wilson, H.; Biller, B.; *et al.* Defining the pharmacodynamic profile and therapeutic index of NHS-IL12 immunocytokine in dogs with malignant melanoma. *PLoS ONE* 2015.
51. Paoloni, M.; Webb, C.; Mazcko, C.; Cherba, D.; Hendricks, W.; Lana, S.; Ehrhart, E.J.; Charles, B.; Fehling, H.; Kumar, L.; *et al.* Prospective molecular profiling of canine cancers provides a clinically relevant comparative model for evaluating personalized medicine (PMed) trials. *PLoS ONE* 2014.

52. Paoloni, M.; Lana, S.; Thamm, D.; Mazcko, C.; Withrow, S. The creation of the comparative oncology trials consortium pharmacodynamic core: Infrastructure for a virtual laboratory. *Vet. J.* 2010, *185*, 88–89.

53. Paoloni, M.C.; Mazcko, C.; Fox, E.; Fan, T.; Lana, S.; Kisseberth, W.; Vail, D.M.; Nuckolls, K.; Osborne, T.; Yalkowsy, S.; *et al.* Rapamycin pharmacokinetic and pharmacodynamic relationships in osteosarcoma: A comparative oncology study in dogs. *PLoS ONE* 2010.

54. Gordon, I.; Paoloni, M.; Mazcko, C.; Khanna, C. The comparative oncology trials consortium: Using spontaneously occurring cancers in dogs to inform the cancer drug development pathway. *PLoS Med.* 2009.

55. Paoloni, M.C.; Tandle, A.; Mazcko, C.; Hanna, E.; Kachala, S.; Leblanc, A.; Newman, S.; Vail, D.; Henry, C.; Thamm, D.; *et al.* Launching a novel preclinical infrastructure: Comparative oncology trials consortium directed therapeutic targeting of TNFα to cancer vasculature. *PLoS ONE* 2009, *4*, e4972.

56. London, C.A.; Bernabe, L.F.; Barnard, S.; Kisseberth, W.C.; Borgatti, A.; Henson, M.; Wilson, H.; Jensen, K.; Ito, D.; Modiano, J.F.; *et al.* Preclinical evaluation of the novel, orally bioavailable selective inhibitor of nuclear export (SINE) KPT-335 in spontaneous canine cancer: Results of a phase I study. *PLoS ONE* 2014.

57. Lindblad-Toh, K.; Wade, C.M.; Mikkelsen, T.S.; Karlsson, E.K.; Jaffe, D.B.; Kamal, M.; Clamp, M.; Chang, J.L.; Kulbokas, E.J., 3rd; Zody, M.C.; *et al.* Genome sequence, comparative analysis and haplotype structure of the domestic dog. *Nature* 2005, *438*, 803–819.

58. Hoeppner, M.P.; Lundquist, A.; Pirun, M.; Meadows, J.R.; Zamani, N.; Johnson, J.; Sundstrom, G.; Cook, A.; FitzGerald, M.G.; Swofford, R.; *et al.* An improved canine genome and a comprehensive catalogue of coding genes and non-coding transcripts. *PLoS ONE* 2014.

59. LeBlanc, A.K.; Mazcko, C.N.; Khanna, C. Defining the value of a comparative approach to cancer drug development. *Clin. Cancer Res.* 2015.

60. Webster, J.D.; Simpson, E.R.; Michalowski, A.M.; Hoover, S.B.; Simpson, R.M. Quantifying histological features of cancer biospecimens for biobanking quality assurance using automated morphometric pattern recognition image analysis algorithms. *J. Biomol. Tech.* 2011, *22*, 108–118.

61. Simpson, R.M.; Bastian, B.C.; Michael, H.T.; Webster, J.D.; Prasad, M.L.; Conway, C.M.; Prieto, V.M.; Gary, J.M.; Goldschmidt, M.H.; Esplin, D.G.; *et al.* Sporadic naturally occurring melanoma in dogs as a preclinical model for human melanoma. *Pigment Cell Melanoma Res.* 2014, *27*, 37–47.

62. Bushell, K.R.; Kim, Y.; Chan, F.C.; Ben-Neriah, S.; Jenks, A.; Alcaide, M.; Fornika, D.; Grande, B.M.; Arthur, S.; Gascoyne, R.D.; *et al.* Genetic inactivation of TRAF3 in canine and human B-cell lymphoma. *Blood* 2015, *125*, 999–1005.

63. Elvers, I.; Turner-Maier, J.; Swofford, R.; Koltookian, M.; Johnson, J.; Stewart, C.; Zhang, C.Z.; Schumacher, S.E.; Beroukhim, R.; Rosenberg, M.; *et al.* Exome sequencing of lymphomas from three dog breeds reveals somatic mutation patterns reflecting genetic background. *Genome Res.* 2015, *25*, 1634–1645.

64. Mochizuki, H.; Kennedy, K.; Shapiro, S.G.; Breen, M. BRAF mutations in canine cancers. *PLoS ONE* 2015.

65. Decker, B.; Parker, H.G.; Dhawan, D.; Kwon, E.M.; Karlins, E.; Davis, B.W.; Ramos-Vara, J.A.; Bonney, P.L.; McNiel, E.A.; Knapp, D.W.; *et al.* Homologous mutation to human BRAF V600E is common in naturally occurring canine bladder cancer—Evidence for a relevant model system and urine-based diagnostic test. *Mol. Cancer Res.* 2015, *13*, 993–1002.

66. Butler, D. Translational research: Crossing the valley of death. *Nature* 2008, *453*, 840–842.

67. Jiang, F.; Zhang, J.; Wang, X.; Shen, X. Important steps to improve translation from medical research to health policy. *J. Transl. Med.* 2013.

68. Ranieri, G.; Gadaleta, C.D.; Patruno, R.; Zizzo, N.; Daidone, M.G.; Hansson, M.G.; Paradiso, A.; Ribatti, D. A model of study for human cancer: Spontaneous occurring tumors in dogs. Biological features and translation for new anticancer therapies. *Crit. Rev. Oncol. Hematol.* 2013, *88*, 187–197.

9

CHAPTER

UNDERSTANDING THE OSTEOSARCOMA PATHOBIOLOGY: A COMPARATIVE ONCOLOGY APPROACH

Jyotika Varshney [1,2], Milcah C. Scott [1,3,4], David A. Largaespada [1,5], and Subbaya Subramanian [1,2]

[1]Masonic Cancer Center, University of Minnesota, Minneapolis, MN 55455, USA

[2]Department of Surgery, University of Minnesota Medical School, Moos Tower, 11-212420 Delaware Street, S.E.; MMC 195, Minneapolis, MN 55455, USA

[3]Animal Cancer Care and Research Program, University of Minnesota, St. Paul, MN 55455, USA

[4]Department of Veterinary Clinical Sciences, College of Veterinary Medicine, University of Minnesota, St. Paul, MN 55108, USA

[5]Department of Pediatrics, University of Minnesota, Minneapolis, MN 55455, USA

ABSTRACT

Osteosarcoma is an aggressive primary bone tumor in humans and is among the most common cancer afflicting dogs. Despite surgical advancements and intensification of chemo- and targeted therapies, the survival outcome for osteosarcoma patients is, as of yet, suboptimal. The presence of metastatic disease at diagnosis or its recurrence after initial therapy is a major factor for the poor outcomes. It is thought that most human and canine patients have at least microscopic metastatic lesions at diagnosis. Osteosarcoma in dogs occurs naturally with greater frequency and shares many biological and clinical similarities with osteosarcoma in humans. From a genetic perspective, osteosarcoma in both humans and dogs is characterized by complex karyotypes with highly variable structural and numerical chromosomal aberrations. Similar molecular abnormalities have been observed in human and canine osteosarcoma. For instance, loss of *TP53* and *RB* regulated pathways are common. While there are several oncogenes that are commonly amplified in both humans and dogs, such as *MYC* and *RAS*, no commonly activated proto-oncogene has been identified that could form the basis for targeted therapies. It remains

Citation: Varshney, J.; Scott, M.C.; Largaespada, D.A.; Subramanian, S.Understanding the Osteosarcoma Pathobiology: A Comparative Oncology Approach. Vet. Sci. 2016, 3,3

possible that recurrent aberrant gene expression changes due to gene amplification or epigenetic alterations could be uncovered and these could be used for developing new, targeted therapies. However, the remarkably high genomic complexity of osteosarcoma has precluded their definitive identification. Several advantageous murine models of osteosarcoma have been generated. These include spontaneous and genetically engineered mouse models, including a model based on forward genetics and transposon mutagenesis allowing new genes and genetic pathways to be implicated in osteosarcoma development. The proposition of this review is that careful comparative genomic studies between human, canine and mouse models of osteosarcoma may help identify commonly affected and targetable pathways for alternative therapies for osteosarcoma patients. Translational research may be found through a path that begins in mouse models, and then moves through canine patients, and then human patients.

INTRODUCTION

Osteosarcoma is an aggressive primary bone tumor most prevalent in human patients. It mostly occurs during adolescence, with a second peak at middle age (older than 40) [1,2]. The tumor is characterized by increased production of osteoid (abnormal bone matrix) and by exceptionally complex karyotypes [3,4]. While the target cell for malignant transformation in the formation of osteosarcoma is not known with certainty, it is thought to be a mesenchymal stem cell (MSC) or a cell committed to the osteoblast lineage [5]. Evidence from mouse models indicates that any of several cell stages could serve as target cells for osteosarcoma development [6]. There are three common histologic types of osteosarcoma: osteoblastic, where tumor cells produce large amounts of tumor osteoid; chondroblastic, where tumor cells produce chondroid (cartilage) in addition to some amount of tumor osteoid; and fibroblastic, where tumor cells are predominantly fibroblasts and can produce both collagen and tumor osteoid [7]. The disease is highly metastatic, with distant spread mostly to lungs and other sites in bone, but osteosarcoma can also metastasize to lymph nodes and intra-abdominal organs [8,9]. The metastatic pattern (lungs, bones, lymph nodes) is similar for dogs and humans [10]. Osteosarcoma may present with macroscopic metastatic disease or metastatic disease can occur after therapy. In either case, prognosis is significantly worse once metastasis has been detected [11,12].

In canine patients, osteosarcoma is a disease primarily of adult dogs; the median age at diagnosis is approximately eight years, with a small peak of incidence in young animals (younger than 3 years) [10,13]. This differs from the situation in human patients where the peak age of incidence is in adolescence. Nevertheless, the natural history of the disease is similar in canine and human osteosarcoma patients [14]. Moreover, we have observed that genome wide expression profiles of canine osteosarcoma are indistinguishable from human pediatric osteosarcoma and more like human osteosarcoma than any other human cancer [14,15]. In dogs, there is generally a strong breed preference in the risk for cancer, such as osteosarcoma [16,17]. Many large breed dogs have an increased risk for osteosarcoma compared to other breeds [4,18,19]. The genetic determinants of osteosarcoma susceptibility in dogs are not fully elucidated, and it is possible that these factors will also be important in human osteosarcoma susceptibility. The development of treatment strategies in dogs and people has proven mutually beneficial for both species [20]. In fact, current treatment options are similar in both species.

Osteosarcoma is treated using surgery, radiation and chemotherapy. Surgical techniques have greatly improved with time, and in many cases limb salvage is feasible with low rates of local recurrence in humans [21]. Combination chemotherapies are vital for effective treatment of osteosarcoma [22]. However, despite decades of effort, nothing better than the most often used combination of three chemotherapeutic agents (*i.e.*, methotrexate, doxorubicin and cisplatin) has been found [22].The adjuvant chemotherapy is generally administered prior to surgery and, according to many studies, the extent of necrosis observed in the primary tumor after surgical removal is correlated with the outcome. [21]. The goal of the adjuvant chemotherapy is to eliminate the micrometastases that are thought to be present in >80% of all patients at the time of diagnosis, thus preventing relapse [1]. New research is underway to define specific molecular targets that could be utilized to treat this disease, but their elucidation has been proven difficult. It is possible that osteosarcoma may also be treated using recently developed immunotherapies, such as immune checkpoint blockade or chimeric antigen receptor-engineered T cells [21].

Osteosarcoma is characterized by aneuploidy and extensive genetic instability [23]. Due to this extreme genetic instability, common causes of osteosarcoma development have largely been limited to implicating loss of *RB* and*TP53* regulated cellular activities and upregulation of *MYC* transcriptional activity reviewed by Morrow *et al.* [24]. Beyond these, few alterations are common or well accepted as osteosarcoma drivers. Gene amplification and protein overexpression of the *RUNX2* transcription factor, which is a regulator of bone renewal, has been proposed to drive osteosarcoma [25]. Conflicting data on activation of beta-catenin dependent transcription in osteosarcoma has been reported [26]. In addition, TGF-β signaling has been proposed to promote the acquisition of metastatic disease [27]. Notable, expression of Ezrin at high levels has been found in metastatic human and canine osteosarcoma and functionally validated in model systems as a driver of osteosarcoma metastasis [28]. Recently, a large scale Sleeping Beauty (SB) transposon-based forward genetic screen was carried out for osteosarcoma in mice [29]. From this screen, a large number of new candidate osteosarcoma proto-oncogene and tumor suppressors were reported. These included the candidate oncogenes *SEMA4D* and *SEMA6D*, which were partially functionally validated as well as tumor suppressors like *NF1*, *NF2* and *PTEN* [29]. Beyond protein encoding genes, several micro RNAs (miRNAs) and miRNA clusters have been suggested as drivers or suppressors of osteosarcoma development and progression [30]. What remains unclear is which common oncogenic drivers for osteosarcoma should be targeted and how they would be targeted. Unlike the case for other malignancies, osteosarcoma is genetically heterogeneous and common molecular targets may not be present.

Osteosarcoma is much more common in dogs than in people (greater than 15 times) and can be experimentally induced in mice via transgenesis. Perceivably, the opportunity to study osteosarcoma in three different species may make it possible to identify core genes and pathways, whose alterations are central to the osteosarcoma phenotype and that would make good targets for therapy. In the past, the main challenges were the development of improved surgical techniques for limb salvage, prevention of local recurrence and the identification of effective combination chemotherapies. Currently, a major pressing need is the development of new therapies to prevent the outgrowth of metastatic disease and to treat it once it has occurred. It is possible that germline or somatic mutations or tumor gene expression signatures identified through multi-species approaches could help predict which patients will respond well to current treatment regimes and which need to be referred for more intensive therapy or follow-up screening. However, much remains to be learned about what allows microscopic osteosarcoma lesions to resist chemotherapy and to suddenly break tumor dormancy and form a macroscopic mass. Until these questions are answered, we are not fully capable to help many human and canine osteosarcoma patients.

This review is an attempt to address many of the unanswered questions pertaining to osteosarcoma by focusing on recently acquired knowledge from a multi-species approach.

HUMAN OSTEOSARCOMA

Osteosarcoma in human patients is a rare tumor with a peak incidence in the second decade of life. The incidence is roughly 25 cases per 10 million per year in the United States [31]. A second wave of osteosarcoma is diagnosed in individuals between 70 and 80 years of age, often in association with Paget's disease. Paget's disease is an abnormality of bone homeostasis in which excessive bone reabsorption and reformation occur. Genetic and viral origins of Paget's disease have been suggested. While osteosarcoma is a rare manifestation of the disease, risk for osteosarcoma is increased. Osteosarcoma can occur in nearly any part of the skeleton, but commonly affects one of the long bones. As it occurs during a period of intense bone growth, there may be an association between this growth and sensitivity to osteoblast transformation [31]. Indeed, children with osteosarcoma are on average tall for their age [32]. Genetic studies also have suggested an association between the inheritance of certain forms of growth control genes and risk for osteosarcoma [33]. Other risk factors for human osteosarcoma include prior radiation therapy, male gender, and possibly African ancestry [34,35]. A genome-wide association study (GWAS) revealed possible risk alleles in the glutamate receptor, metaotropic 4 (*GRM4*) gene and a gene desert at chromosome 2p25.2 [36]. A recent GWAS also identified a potential high-risk allele for osteosarcoma metastasis at presentation within the transcriptional activator *NFIB* [37], a gene that was also identified as a potential tumor/metastasis suppressor in a transposon-based genetic screen in mice [29].

Some rare inherited cancer predisposition syndromes increase the risk for osteosarcoma. These rare cancers include Li-Fraumeni syndrome, hereditary retinoblastoma and Rothman-Thompson syndrome caused by germline mutations in *TP53, RB1*, and *RECQL4*, respectively [38]. Certain other cancer predisposition syndromes also seem to increase the risk of osteosarcoma development including

Neurofibromatosis Type 1 syndrome, Werner's syndrome and Diamond-Blackfan anemia [24]. Patients with hereditary multiple osteochondromas, due to inheritance of mutations in the*EXT1* or *EXT2* genes, are predisposed to development of osteosarcoma also [24].

Human osteosarcoma is typically diagnosed due to swelling and pain often in the limbs. This can cause a limp if the involved limb is a leg or immobility of a joint. Pain may be constant or associated with exertion. In rare cases osteosarcoma will trigger a bone fracture. Diagnosis is made following a complete medical exam and imaging studies. Often an X-ray is done, followed by positron emission tomography or a bone scan. As osteosarcoma can often metastasize to the lungs, lung X-rays are utilized. A definitive diagnosis requires a biopsy. Staging of osteosarcoma is controversial. Most believe that all osteosarcoma should be considered high grade and treated as such although low grade osteosarcoma seems to be a distinct entity [38]. The only commonly accepted staging is localized *versus* metastatic disease.

Human osteosarcoma is commonly treated using surgery and chemotherapy [38]. Chemotherapy for roughly ten weeks that precedes surgery and the extent of necrosis in the surgically removed primary tumor has been suggested to be associated with long term risk for disease recurrence [38]. Chemotherapy is also given after surgery for a period of up to a year. Usually two or three chemotherapeutic agents are given for osteosarcoma treatment. Common combinations include high-dose methotrexate, doxorubicin and cisplatin (sometimes with ifosfamide); doxorubicin and cisplatin; ifosfamide and etoposide; ifosfamide, cisplatin (or carboplatin) and epirubicin [38]. Radiation therapy is used in some cases for non-resectable tumors [38].

The prognosis of human osteosarcoma is affected largely by the presence or absence of metastases. The 5-year survival rate for localized osteosarcoma is estimated to be between 50% and 60%. For metastatic disease the 5-year survival rate is 15% to 30% [39]. There is a better prognosis if metastatic osteosarcoma is present only in the lungs and is all metastatic lesions can be removed surgically [39]. That said, there is a dire need to develop therapies that can be used to treat patients who present with extensive metastatic disease or who recur with metastatic disease. At present, palliative care is often used in such cases or referral for clinical trials [38].

CANINE OSTEOSARCOMA

Canine osteosarcoma accounts for 80%–90% of canine primary bone tumors [40]. Dogs often present with a history of lameness or in some cases with a pathologic fracture of the affected bone. Diagnosis is based on clinical signs, imaging and biopsy. The metaphyseal region of long bones is the most common primary site with front limbs affected twice as often as rear limbs and the distal radius and proximal humerus being the two most common locations [41,42].

It is believed that external factors such as chemical carcinogens, ionization radiation, metallic implants to fix fractures and precedent skeletal disorders such as osteomyelitis and microscopic fractures can lead to canine osteosarcoma [10]. There are implications of genetic factors such as *TP53* and RB1 aberrations, as well as certain viruses and growth factor alterations [43]. Osteosarcoma can affect any breed of dog, but it is more commonly found in the larger breeds. Some breeds, such as the Scottish Deerhound, Great Dane, St. Bernard and Greyhound, are at high risk for developing primary bone tumors suggesting a genetic predilection [40]. In fact, the CDKN2A locus has been recently linked to osteosarcoma risk in dogs, and the risk allele is fixed in certain breeds like Rottweilers and Irish Wolfhounds [4].

Without treatment, the estimated survival for a dog with osteosarcoma is less than 3 months. On the other hand, survival times of approximately 1 year (or about 10% of a dog's lifetime) are achievable for 20%–50% of dogs with osteosarcoma treated using the current standard of care, and a small percentage of dogs can survive up to 5–6 years after diagnosis [44]. Standard of care for dogs is surgery (amputation of limb sparing surgery) with adjuvant chemotherapy [45]. The choice of chemotherapy drugs does not seem to influence survival, thus, toxicity, quality of life and cost tend to be the factors that guide treatment decisions [44]. Chemotherapy is only recommended when the primary tumor is removed and as of current, the drug of choice is carboplatin.

Many well-controlled studies show that a clinical response for osteosarcoma is only achievable with accepted standard of care. In very rare cases, dogs with osteosarcoma that receive palliative care may have prolonged (>1 year) survival, even in face of metastatic disease. Anecdotal benefits reported from herbal or "alternative" treatments, have not been reproducible, and no alternative therapies have been shown to have efficacy or provide consistent clinical benefit in controlled trials.

Metastatic bone cancer is the common cause of death or euthanasia, in 90% of dogs by 1 year [46]. Reducing the primary tumor's ability to metastasize and enhancing the antitumor activity of chemotherapy drugs and yet having minimal negative side effects is still a challenge for veterinary practitioners [10]. Treatment options for canine patients with metastases include pulmonary metastasectomy, but treatment for metastatic disease is only recommended if the primary tumor remains in complete remission [47]. The median survival after pulmonary metastasectomy can be up to 6 months; but without standard surgical procedure, survival outcome is usually less than 2 months [46].

MOUSE MODELS OF OSTEOSARCOMA

The number of genetically engineered or other mouse models of osteosarcoma are fairly restricted. However, these have been useful for studies on the cell of origin for osteosarcoma development and gaining insight into new genes and pathways that influence osteosarcoma initiation, progression and the process of metastasis. Most of the reported models utilize Cre/LoxP mediated deletion of *Trp53* and/or *Rb1* (reviewed in [48]). A few other models have been created by transgenic overexpression of various oncogenes including *Fos* and SV40 large T antigen [49], or co-deletion of one copy of *Twist* and mutation of *Apc* [50]. Osteosarcoma can be induced with high efficiency in mice by osteoblast lineage specific deletion of the *Trp53* gene, although the latency and penetrance is greatly enhanced by co-deletion of both copies of the *Rb1* gene [51].These data are consistent with the centrality of *TP53* and *RB1* loss of function alterations in human osteosarcoma [23]. Mouse osteosarcoma induced by deletion of *Trp53* is genomically unstable, as is seen in human osteosarcoma [52].

Others have created mouse cell lines from spontaneously occurring osteosarcoma. In cases in which these osteosarcoma were induced on a uniform strain background, the osteosarcoma cells can be grown in syngeneic hosts by intravenous, subcutaneous, or orthotopic injections into the tibia (reviewed in [53]). Examples include the K12 and K7M2 derivative that is highly metastatic, and the Dunn along with its metastatic derivative LM8. These cell lines have been useful for testing the role of various components of the immune system on primary osteosarcoma tumor growth and osteosarcoma metastasis [54]. Such cell lines have also been used to create matched pairs of poorly and highly metastatic cell lines for study [53]. These have been useful for developing candidate genes and pathways that may regulate the process of metastasis, such as high-level expression of ezrin [28].

Quist *et al.* reported that osteosarcoma could be induced in mice via homozygous Cre/LoxP-mediated deletion of*Trp53* and *Rb1* in undifferentiated mesenchyme, pre-osteoblasts or infrequently cycling mature osteoblasts [6]. These data suggest that a variety of cell types could be targets for osteosarcoma development. This plasticity may also be the basis for the ready acquisition of new osteosarcoma phenotypes in patients, including chemo/radiotherapy resistance and the ability to readily colonize the lung.

From osteosarcoma mouse models, we have learned that osteosarcoma cells have a predilection to metastatic colonization of the lung, but, interestedly, have observed a metastatic potential spectrum across various cell lines. Intriguingly, in mouse models of Li-Fraumeni, the rate of lung metastasis is influenced by the nature of the p53 mutant allele used and when in the lifetime of the mouse Cre is used to induce mutation of the p53 gene [51]. The rate of spontaneous development of osteosarcoma and the frequency of lung metastasis is higher in mice heterozygous for the *Trp53*^{R272H} allele than in mice heterozygous for the carry *Trp53*^{R270H} allele [55].

Recently, a new mouse model of osteosarcoma was developed which utilizes the *Sleeping Beauty* (SB) transposon mutagenesis system [29]. In this project, a SB transposon vector designed to activate proto-oncogenes or inactivate tumor suppressor genes by insertional mutagenesis, was mobilized specifically in *Osx1*+ cells using a tissue-specific mutagenesis approach. Mutagenesis by SB was able to induce osteosarcoma in otherwise wild type mice or accelerate osteosarcoma in mice with tissue-specific induction of the *Trp53*^{R270H} allele. Transposon insertion mutations in specific regions of the genome are found recurrently in SB induced tumors and these regions are called "common insertion sites" or CIS [29]. CIS result from selection for insertions that occur within or near a cancer gene in the right position and the right orientation so as to give the cell a selective advantage and drive the development of a tumor. Thus, the identification of genes at or near CIS defines new candidate drivers of cancer development.

CONSERVED DRIVERS OF OSTEOSARCOMA

Genomic Alterations

It has been reported that genomic alterations are necessary for development of osteosarcoma in mouse models (*TP53*) and are accepted as being commonly shared in humans and dogs [13,29,56].

Highly chaotic karyotypes encompass a key feature that characterizes some mouse models used for osteosarcoma studies, and naturally occurring osteosarcoma in dogs, as well as in human patients. The average human osteosarcoma harbors roughly 30 coding alterations [23,57] while in dog osteosarcoma and mouse models, this figure is not known with certainty. Many of the candidate genes implicated in the pathogenesis and progression of osteosarcoma in people have also been characterized in the canine disease. Notable examples of these genes are *PTEN*(phosphatase and tensin homolog), *RB1* (retinoblastoma), and *TP53* (tumor protein 53), and *MET* (mesenchymal-epithelial transition factor).

Genetic alterations of the retinoblastoma susceptibility (*RB1*) gene have been implicated in the development and progression of osteosarcoma. In people, almost 70% of osteosarcomas have at least one *RB1* gene alteration and the percentage is similar in dog osteosarcomas [13]. We recently reported that an aberrant RB-E2F1 regulatory pathway is predictive of biological behavior [58]. Since our work, another group has reported that RB1 alterations may serve as a prognostic marker for the management of osteosarcoma patients [59].

Approximately 50% of human osteosarcomas have been reported to have somatic *TP53* deletions or point mutations detected using exon sequencing strategies [23]. However, a recent study that used whole genome sequencing of human osteosarcomas suggests that nearly all osteosarcoma tumors have p53 pathways lesions, which in many cases are translocations that break in the first intron of *TP53* gene [57]. Thus, it would appear that p53 pathway loss might be a requirement for osteosarcoma development in people. Clearly, germline *TP53* mutations, which cause Li-Fraumeni syndrome, predispose to osteosarcoma. However, it is unclear whether *TP53* mutations act as initiating mutations or progression mutations in sporadic osteosarcoma. In any case, p53 pathway alterations are common in genetically engineered mouse models as well as spontaneous canine and human osteosarcoma. Therefore, mouse models could be used to develop therapies that exploit p53 pathway alterations in patient osteosarcoma.

In humans and dogs, several oncogenes have been identified as possibly playing a role in osteosarcoma including*MET*, *FOS*, *IGF1R* (Insulin-Like Growth Factor 1 Receptor), *PVT1/MYC*, *RUNX2*, and *HER2*. Some of these changes involve copy number alterations. Consistent genome and chromosome copy number changes have been reported in canine and human osteosarcoma [17]. For instance, a high copy number gain of the *RUNX2* locus has been reported in both human and dog osteosarcoma [56].

Some of these genes, or the pathways they regulate, including the *PVT1/MYC* locus, *MET* signaling, and *IGF1R*have been implicated in genetically engineered mouse models of osteosarcoma [29,52].

Recurrent point mutations have been observed in osteosarcoma, but there are few beyond *RB1* and *TP53* that reach statistical significance. This is in part because too few samples have been sequenced. However, point mutations or deletions of several tumor suppressor genes, likely to be drivers of osteosarcomagenesis, were observed in a recent report of human osteosarcoma including *NF1*, *NF2* and *PTEN*, all of which were also recovered in a transposon-based screen for osteosarcoma in mice [29]. Overlap exists between other reported candidate human osteosarcoma genes after genome-wide copy number and whole exome sequencing were done [23], and also after transposon based screening in a mouse model including activation of *PI3KCA*, and *AKT1*, and inactivation of *ARID1A* [29].

Deregulation of Micrornas in Canine and Human Osteosarcoma

microRNAs (miRNAs) are small non coding RNAs that regulate more than 60% of the genome post transcriptionally. Several studies have identified deregulated miRNAs in osteosarcoma [60,61,62,63,64,65,66]. One of the earliest studies reported four differentially expressed miRNAs in a handful of osteosarcoma samples compared to controls [67]. Since these initial studies, additional research has shown that miRNA deregulation is potentially central to osteosarcoma development and progression [68]. Indeed, our group generated a Sarcoma MicroRNA Expression Database (S-MED) that represents 22 different sarcoma types, including osteosarcoma [69]. Through S-MED we found that osteosarcoma clustered separately from all other sarcoma types indicating the presence of potentially biologically important miRNAs. One of the unique miRNA signatures we found revealed the significant downregulation of around 50 miRNAs in the human 14q32 locus compared to the controls [65]. Most importantly, we have also shown a comparable decrease in expression of orthologous 14q32 miRNAs in canine osteosarcoma samples [65]. Interestingly we did not observe any copy number changes at the 14q32 locus, suggesting epigenetic changes at the locus. We confirmed that subset of these 50 miRNAs (miR-382, miR-369-5p, miR-544 and miR-134) could target the 3′ UTR of cMYC transcript. Additionally, overexpression of these miRNAs in osteosarcoma cells decreased the cMYC levels and induced apoptosis [65,70]. Also cMYC has been shown to transactivate a commonly known miRNA cluster, miR-17-92 [71]. We showed that restoration of the 14q32 miRNAs not only did decrease the cMYC levels but also significantly reduced the levels of mir-17-92 [70].

It was observed in other studies that miR-135b, -150, -370, -542-5p, -652, and -654 were highly expressed compared to osteoblasts [72,73,74]. Many of them play crucial roles in bone differentiation and key signaling pathways (miR-206 and -286) [75]. Additionally, miRNAs target *TP53*, which is an important tumor suppressor gene, was mutated in more than 60% osteosarcoma tumors [76]. One of the key miRNAs in the *TP53* pathway is miR-34, which is significantly downregulated in many osteosarcoma tumors that affects the cell cycle and proliferation [77,78,79].

The role of miRNAs in canine osteosarcoma remains to be fully elucidated. Since the discovery of miRNAs, there have been few studies that show a correlation between deregulation of miRNAs and canine osteosarcoma. A recent study investigated the role of miR-196a and its target Annexin V in human (143B, MG63) and canine (DAN) osteosarcoma cell lines to identify potential targets for new therapeutic agents in both the species [80]. They observed that miR-196a is downregulated in many of the canine osteosarcoma tumors compared to the normal bone, which is in contradiction with some earlier studies [66,81]. Further studies need to be performed on a larger cohort to establish that miR-196a is a potential therapeutic target and can impact multiple downstream targets in canine osteosarcoma.

A study led by Fenger *et al.*, sought to characterize miRNA expression in canine primary tumors among the major large breeds (greyhounds, rottweilers, golden retrievers and some mixed breeds) [43,82]. Using Nanominer software, they determined 189 miRNAs that were differentially expressed. Of these, miR-494 was highly expressed in all the breeds compared to normal canine osteoblasts.

As mentioned earlier, our group was among the first groups to observe a significant downregulation of around 50 miRNAs in the human 14q32 chromosomal region, which was highly conserved in the dog genome. Out of the 50 miRNAs, 2 miRNAs, miR-134 and mir-544, shared 100% conservation with the canine genome and mapped to the predicted synteny in canine osteosarcoma [14]. We have comprised a table of key miRNAs that play an important role in survival outcome and chemoresponse that can potentially lead to osteosarcoma diagnosis, subtyping and therapeutics in human and canine osteosarcoma (Table 1).

Table 1: miRNAs as potential markers for survival outcome and/ or chemosensitivity

Table 1. miRNAs as potential markers for survival outcome and/ or chemosensitivity.

miRNAs Deregulated in OS	Expression Levels Compared to the Controls	Overall Function	References
miR-382	Down-regulated	Poor survival outcome and metastasis marker	[70,83]
miR-154	Down-regulated	Poor survival outcome	[70]
miR-33a	Up-regulated	Chemoresistance	[84]
miR-34c	Down-regulated	Chemoresistance	[85]

Epigenetic Changes in Osteosarcoma

Most forms of human cancer have changes in the epigenome compared to the normal cellular counterparts from which they are derived. Indeed, changes to the epigenome seem to be a ubiquitous feature of cancer. Epigenetic changes are revealed in alterations to the pattern of DNA methylation, histone modifications and nucleosome remodeling (reviewed in [24]). Osteosarcoma, like other forms of human cancer, seems to have many such epigenome changes compared to normal osteoblasts, the presumptive target cell for transformation. Several studies have analyzed the epigenome in a genome-wide manner, albeit with low numbers of cases [86,87]. These studies confirm that specific methylation events are heterogeneous among different cases of human osteosarcoma and that these differences may help explain differences in the clinical behavior of different osteosarcomas. These genome wide studies in human osteosarcoma have been restricted to the study of DNA methylation. Work on other chromatin modification remains to be done. The study of genome wide epigenetic changes has not been undertaken on a large scale in genetically engineered mouse models or canine osteosarcoma samples.

Many studies in osteosarcoma have focused on methylation of specific genes or gene regions. These studies suggest that certain genes and genetic pathways are subject to control by DNA methylation and attendant modifications to the histone code. Among these are alterations to the RB and p53 pathways. While these specific genes are not frequent targets of methylation based gene silencing, genes in these pathways have been reported as targets for pathogenic methylation. Specifically the *CDKN2A* locus, encoding the cyclin dependent kinase inhibitor $p16^{INK4a}$ and the Mdm2 inhibitor $p14^{Arf}$, has been reported [88,89]. Several genes that are targets of p53, or modulate p53 activity, have been shown to be methylated and silenced in osteosarcoma cell lines or xenograft tumors including *CDKN1A,HIC1* and *GADD45* [90,91,92]. Many other tumor suppressor genes are silenced by promoter hypermethylation in osteosarcoma cell lines including *RASSF1A*, *TIMP3*, DAPK1 and others (review in Morrow and Khanna, Critical Reviews in Oncogenesis, 2015). Methylation and silencing of tumor suppressive miRNA genes has also been observed as specific events in human osteosarcoma cell lines and primary tumors. Promoter hypomethyation, and probable overexpression, of oncogenes is less well studied in osteosarcoma, but several reports have been made suggesting such a mechanism, notably for the metastasis promoting gene *IRX1* and the growth factor gene *IGF2* [93,94]. Several candidate osteosarcoma oncogenes found in a transposon-based forward genetic screen in mice are also hypomethylated and overexpressed in human osteosarcoma compared to normal osteoblasts, including *SEMA4D,RAF1* and *PAK1* [29]. Some of these epigenetic changes, including aberrant repression and activation, are associated with loss of imprinting control at specific loci in osteosarcoma cells [95,96,97].

Genome wide studies of epigenetic alterations in human osteosarcoma need to incorporate many more samples before we learn to what extent they may explain molecular subtypes and clinical behavior of different cases. No such studies have been reported for canine osteosarcomas or mouse models either. When they are, they will allow cross-species comparisons that could help reveal the most meaningful alterations. Despite these limitations, it is apparent that osteosarcoma development is accompanied by changes to the epigenome that drive progression and confer specific cancer phenotypes. Published data does suggest that epigenome targeted therapies, including histone deacetylase inhibitors and DNA demethylating agents, can alter gene expression and inhibit osteosarcoma growth and/or metastasis [93,98]. Indeed, one study suggests that osteosarcoma cell lines can be reprogrammed using induced pluripotency genes and that the accompanying epigenetic changes reduce tumorigenic potential [99]. Taken together, these data suggest that modification of osteosarcoma epigenomes will be a useful therapeutic approach.

ADVANTAGES OF A MULTI-SPECIES, COMPARATIVE OSTEOSARCOMA STUDY APPROACH

Using comparative genetic studies in multiple organisms, it is possible to understand more about the inherited and somatically acquired genetic alterations that are informative of osteosarcoma risk and clinical behavior, especially metastasis. It is reasonable that genetic alterations that are present in human, dog, and mouse osteosarcomas represent the most likely true drivers of osteosarcoma progression, based on the concept of convergent evolution. Singly, mouse models offer opportunities to discover new genes and pathways important in disease initiation and progression. Dogs bring many other advantages to the table. Notably, since they show remarkable intra-breed homogeneity, which, together with noticeable interbreed heterogeneity, the dog offers distinctive opportunities to understand the genetics underlying osteosarcoma. Taken all together, an interspecies approach offers a possibly broader view and understanding of osteosarcoma since, for example, what is found to be altered at the genetic level in one species may be epigenetically silenced altered in another, but would be hard to pick out based on changes to gene expression alone.

Findings from mouse models and naturally occurring osteosarcoma in dogs need to be translated into therapeutic approaches in a clinically relevant model. Advantages of clinical trials in dogs are numerous and include that there are many more cases of canine osteosarcoma than human osteosarcoma [100,101]. In addition, disease progression in dogs, even with standard of care, is rapid so that assessments of improvement can be made in comparatively short periods of time [102].

It has been shown that histological response is not a good predictor (St. Jude, CTOS 20th Annual Meeting) in human osteosarcoma patients, and so there is an urgent need for informative biomarkers. The 14q32 locus is a new and promising marker, which was discovered by our group through a comparative species approach [65].

CONCLUSIONS

In more than 70% of osteosarcoma patients, current standard-of-care therapies ultimately fail to prevent relapse and metastasis. This dismal outcome has not improved over the past three decades, indicating a desperate need for novel drugs and treatment strategies. As osteosarcoma is genetically heterogeneous, successful therapies will need to target conserved pathobiology. In this review, we discussed the presence of multiple conserved signaling mechanisms as well as some of the approaches for understanding osteosarcoma pathobiology. Recent studies highlight the role of microRNAs in regulation of these conserved signaling pathways. In addition, we have just begun to understand the roles of the regulatory small RNAs and long-noncoding RNAs (lncRNAs). Further, intricacy in gene regulations does not end with identification of regulatory RNAs and its interacting partners. Molecular intricacy is also heavily dependent on our understanding of the implications of other layers of gene regulation such as role for competing endogenous RNAs along with pseudogenes, circular RNAs and lncRNAs. Acquiring such breadth and depth of knowledge is critical for developing therapies that will prevent bypass mechanisms of resistance to therapies. Moreover, cell non-autonomous functions of secreted factors such as exosomes are currently being investigated. In addition, emerging concepts of immune regulation by cancer and recent advancements in immunotherapy hold promise for treating and better outcomes in osteosarcoma.

ACKNOWLEDGMENTS

We thank Jaime Modiano and Aaron Sarver for helpful discussions and Anne Sarver for assisting in manuscript preparation. Due to the space restrictions we could not cite many other significant contributions made by numerous researchers and laboratories in this potentially important and rapidly progressing field. Subbaya Subramanian and

David A. Largaespada are supported by research grants funded by American Cancer Society Grant (RSG 13-381-01-RMC), the Sobiech osteosarcoma fund, Children's cancer research funds, the Wyckoff Rein in Sarcoma Foundation.

AUTHOR CONTRIBUTIONS

Jyotika Varshney and Subbaya Subramanian developed the concept for the review. Milcah C. Scott and David A. Largaespada provided input in the canine osteosarcoma and epigenetics of osteosarcoma.

REFERENCES

1. Moore, D.D.; Luu, H.H. Osteosarcoma. *Cancer Treat Res.* 2014, *162*, 65–92.
2. Ottaviani, G.; Jaffe, N. The epidemiology of osteosarcoma. *Cancer Treat Res.* 2009, *152*, 3–13.
3. Letson, G.D.; Muro-Cacho, C.A. Genetic and molecular abnormalities in tumors of the bone and soft tissues.*Cancer Control* 2001, *8*, 239–251.
4. Karlsson, E.K.; Sigurdsson, S.; Ivansson, E.; Thomas, R.; Elvers, I.; Wright, J.; Howald, C.; Tonomura, N.; Perloski, M.; Swofford, R.; *et al.* Genome-wide analyses implicate 33 loci in heritable dog osteosarcoma, including regulatory variants near CDKN2A/B. *Genome Biol.* 2013, *14*, R132.
5. Mutsaers, A.J.; Walkley, C.R. Cells of origin in osteosarcoma: Mesenchymal stem cells or osteoblast committed cells? *Bone* 2014, *62*, 56–63.
6. Quist, T.; Jin, H.; Zhu, J.F.; Smith-Fry, K.; Capecchi, M.R.; Jones, K.B. The impact of osteoblastic differentiation on osteosarcomagenesis in the mouse. *Oncogene* 2015, *34*, 4278–4284.
7. Yoshida, H.; Adachi, H.; Hamada, Y.; Aki, T.; Yumoto, T.; Morimoto, K.; Orido, T. Osteosarcoma. Ultrastructural and immunohistochemical studies on alkaline phosphatase-positive tumor cells constituting a variety of histologic types. *Acta Pathol. Jpn.* 1988, *38*, 325–338.
8. Dirik, Y.; Cinar, A.; Yumrukcal, F.; Eralp, L. Popliteal lymph node metastasis of tibial osteoblastic osteosarcoma. *Int. J. Surg. Case Rep.* 2014, *5*, 840–844.
9. Jeffree, G.M.; Price, C.H.; Sissons, H.A. The metastatic patterns of osteosarcoma. *Brit. J. Cancer* 1975, *32*, 87–107.
10. Morello, E.; Martano, M.; Buracco, P. Biology, diagnosis and treatment of canine appendicular osteosarcoma: Similarities and differences with human osteosarcoma. *Vet. J.* 2011, *189*, 268–277.
11. Gill, J.; Ahluwalia, M.K.; Geller, D.; Gorlick, R. New targets and approaches in osteosarcoma. *Pharmacol. Ther.*2013, *137*, 89–99.
12. Jaffe, N. Osteosarcoma: Review of the past, impact on the future. The American experience. *Cancer Treat Res.*2009, *152*, 239–262.
13. Modiano, J.F.; Breen, M.; Lana, S.E.; Ehrhart, N.; Fosmire, S.P.; Thomas, R.; Jubala, C.M.; Lamerato-Kozicki, A.R.; Ehrhart, E.J.; Schaack, J.; *et al.* Naturally

occurring translational models for development of cancer therapy. *Gene Ther. Mol. Biol.* 2006, *10*, 31–40.

14. Scott, M.C.; Sarver, A.L.; Gavin, K.J.; Thayanithy, V.; Getzy, D.M.; Newman, R.A.; Cutter, G.R.; Lindblad-Toh, K.; Kisseberth, W.C.; Hunter, L.E.; *et al.* Molecular subtypes of osteosarcoma identified by reducing tumor heterogeneity through an interspecies comparative approach. *Bone* 2011, *49*, 356–367.
15. Paoloni, M.; Davis, S.; Lana, S.; Withrow, S.; Sangiorgi, L.; Picci, P.; Hewitt, S.; Triche, T.; Meltzer, P.; Khanna, C. Canine tumor cross-species genomics uncovers targets linked to osteosarcoma progression. *BMC Genom.*2009, *10*, 625.
16. Schiffman, J.D.; Breen, M. Comparative oncology: What dogs and other species can teach us about humans with cancer. *Philos. Trans. R. Soc. Lond. B Biol. Sci.* 2015, *370*.
17. Thomas, R.; Wang, H.J.; Tsai, P.C.; Langford, C.F.; Fosmire, S.P.; Jubala, C.M.; Getzy, D.M.; Cutter, G.R.; Modiano, J.F.; Breen, M. Influence of genetic background on tumor karyotypes: Evidence for breed-associated cytogenetic aberrations in canine appendicular osteosarcoma. *Chromosome Res.* 2009, *17*, 365–377.
18. McNeill, C.J.; Overley, B.; Shofer, F.S.; Kent, M.S.; Clifford, C.A.; Samluk, M.; Haney, S.; van Winkle, T.J.; Sorenmo, K.U. Characterization of the biological behaviour of appendicular osteosarcoma in Rottweilers and a comparison with other breeds: A review of 258 dogs. *Vet. Comp. Oncol.* 2007, *5*, 90–98.
19. Dobson, J.M. Breed-predispositions to cancer in pedigree dogs. *ISRN Vet. Sci.* 2013, *2013*, 941275.
20. Paoloni, M.; Khanna, C. Translation of new cancer treatments from pet dogs to humans. *Nat. Rev. Cancer* 2008,*8*, 147–156.
21. Isakoff, M.S.; Bielack, S.S.; Meltzer, P.; Gorlick, R. Osteosarcoma: Current treatment and a collaborative pathway to success. *J. Clin. Oncol.* 2015, *33*, 3029–3035.
22. Ferrari, S.; Serra, M. An update on chemotherapy for osteosarcoma. *Expert Opin. Pharmacother.* 2015, *16*, 2727–2736.
23. Perry, J.A.; Kiezun, A.; Tonzi, P.; van Allen, E.M.; Carter, S.L.; Baca, S.C.; Cowley, G.S.; Bhatt, A.S.; Rheinbay, E.; Pedamallu, C.S.; *et al.* Complementary genomic approaches highlight the PI3K/mTOR pathway as a common vulnerability in osteosarcoma. *Proc. Natl. Acad. Sci. USA* 2014, *111*, 5564–5573.
24. Morrow, J.J.; Khanna, C. Osteosarcoma genetics and epigenetics: Emerging biology and candidate therapies.*Crit. Rev. Oncog.* 2015, *20*, 173–197.
25. Li, N.; Luo, D.; Hu, X.; Luo, W.; Lei, G.; Wang, Q.; Zhu, T.; Gu, J.; Lu, Y.; Zheng, Q. RUNX2 and osteosarcoma.*Anticancer Agents Med. Chem.* 2015, *15*, 881–887.
26. Tian, J.; He, H.; Lei, G. Wnt/beta-catenin pathway in bone cancers. *Tumour Biol.* 2014, *35*, 9439–9445.
27. Lamora, A.; Talbot, J.; Bougras, G.; Amiaud, J.; Leduc, M.; Chesneau, J.; Taurelle, J.; Stresing, V.; Le Deley, M.C.; Heymann, M.F.; *et al.* Overexpression

of smad7 blocks primary tumor growth and lung metastasis development in osteosarcoma. *Clin. Cancer Res.* 2014, *20*, 5097–5112.

28. Khanna, C.; Wan, X.; Bose, S.; Cassaday, R.; Olomu, O.; Mendoza, A.; Yeung, C.; Gorlick, R.; Hewitt, S.M.; Helman, L.J. The membrane-cytoskeleton linker ezrin is necessary for osteosarcoma metastasis. *Nat. Med.* 2004,*10*, 182–186.
29. Moriarity, B.S.; Otto, G.M.; Rahrmann, E.P.; Rathe, S.K.; Wolf, N.K.; Weg, M.T.; Manlove, L.A.; LaRue, R.S.; Temiz, N.A. A Sleeping Beauty forward genetic screen identifies new genes and pathways driving osteosarcoma development and metastasis. 2015, *47*, 615–624.
30. Chang, L.; Shrestha, S.; LaChaud, G.; Scott, M.A.; James, A.W. Review of microRNA in osteosarcoma and chondrosarcoma. *Med. Oncol.* 2015, *32*, 613.
31. Geller, D.S.; Gorlick, R. Osteosarcoma: A review of diagnosis, management, and treatment strategies. *Clin. Adv. Hematol. Oncol.* 2010, *8*, 705–718.
32. Mirabello, L.; Pfeiffer, R.; Murphy, G.; Daw, N.C.; Patino-Garcia, A.; Troisi, R.J.; Hoover, R.N.; Douglass, C.; Schuz, J.; Craft, A.W.; *et al.* Height at diagnosis and birth-weight as risk factors for osteosarcoma. *Cancer Causes Control* 2011, *22*, 899–908.
33. Savage, S.A.; Woodson, K.; Walk, E.; Modi, W.; Liao, J., Douglass, C.; Hoover, R.N.; Chanock, S.J. Analysis of genes critical for growth regulation identifies Insulin-like Growth Factor 2 Receptor variations with possible functional significance as risk factors for osteosarcoma. *Cancer Epidemiol. Biomark. Prev.* 2007, *16*, 1667–1674.
34. Miller, R.W. Contrasting epidemiology of childhood osteosarcoma, Ewing's tumor, and rhabdomyosarcoma.*Natl. Cancer Inst. Monogr.* 1981, *56*, 9–15.
35. Jawad, M.U.; Cheung, M.C.; Min, E.S.; Schneiderbauer, M.M.; Koniaris, L.G.; Scully, S.P. Ewing sarcoma demonstrates racial disparities in incidence-related and sex-related differences in outcome: An analysis of 1631 cases from the SEER database, 1973–2005. *Cancer* 2009, *115*, 3526–3536.
36. Savage, S.A.; Mirabello, L.; Wang, Z.; Gastier-Foster, J.M.; Gorlick, R.; Khanna, C.; Flanagan, A.M.; Tirabosco, R.; Andrulis, I.L.; Wunder, J.S.; *et al.* Genome-wide association study identifies two susceptibility loci for osteosarcoma. *Nat. Genet.* 2013, *45*, 799–803.
37. Mirabello, L.; Koster, R.; Moriarity, B.S.; Spector, L.G.; Meltzer, P.S.; Gary, J.; Machiela, M.J.; Pankratz, N.; Panagiotou, O.A.; Largaespada, D.; *et al.* A Genome-wide scan identifies variants in NFIB associated with metastasis in patients with osteosarcoma. *Cancer Discov.* 2015, *5*, 920–931.
38. Gorlick, R.; Khanna, C. Osteosarcoma. *J. Bone Miner. Res.* 2010, *25*, 683–691.
39. Hameed, M.; Dorfman, H. Primary malignant bone tumors—Recent developments. *Semin. Diagn. Pathol.* 2011,*28*, 86–101.
40. Anfinsen, K.P.; Grotmol, T.; Bruland, O.S.; Jonasdottir, T.J. Breed-specific incidence rates of canine primary bone tumors—A population based survey of dogs in Norway. *Can. J. Vet. Res.* 2011, *75*, 209–215.

41. Liptak, J.M.; Dernell, W.S.; Straw, R.C.; Rizzo, S.A.; Lafferty, M.H.; Withrow, S.J. Proximal radial and distal humeral osteosarcoma in 12 dogs. *J. Am. Anim. Hosp. Assoc.* 2004, *40*, 461–467.

42. Boerman, I.; Selvarajah, G.T.; Nielen, M.; Kirpensteijn, J. Prognostic factors in canine appendicular osteosarcoma—A meta-analysis. *BMC Vet. Res.* 2012, *8*, 56–56.

43. Fenger, J.M.; London, C.A.; Kisseberth, W.C. Canine osteosarcoma: A naturally occurring disease to inform pediatric oncology. *ILAR J.* 2014, *55*, 69–85.

44. Szewczyk, M.; Lechowski, R.; Zabielska, K. What do we know about canine osteosarcoma treatment? Review.*Vet. Res. Commun.* 2015, *39*, 61–67.

45. Berg, J. Canine osteosarcoma: Amputation and chemotherapy. *Vet. Clin. N. Am. Small Anim. Pract.* 1996, *26*, 111–121.

46. Straw, R.C.; Withrow, S.J.; Powers, B.E. Management of canine appendicular osteosarcoma. *Vet. Clin. North Am. Small Anim. Pract.* 1990, *20*, 1141–1161.

47. Gilson, S.D. Principles of surgery for cancer palliation and treatment of metastases. *Clin. Tech. Small Anim. Pract.* 1998, *13*, 65–69.

48. Guijarro, M.V.; Ghivizzani, S.C.; Gibbs, C.P. Animal models in osteosarcoma. *Front. Oncol.* 2014, *4*, 189.

49. Ruther, U.; Komitowski, D.; Schubert, F.R.; Wagner, E.F. c-fos expression induces bone tumors in transgenic mice. *Oncogene* 1989, *4*, 861–865.

50. Entz-Werle, N.; Choquet, P.; Neuville, A.; Kuchler-Bopp, S.; Clauss, F.; Danse, J.M.; Simo-Noumbissie, P.; Guerin, E.; Gaub, M.P.; Freund, J.N.; *et al.* Targeted apc;twist double-mutant mice: A new model of spontaneous osteosarcoma that mimics the human disease. *Transl. Oncol.* 2010, *3*, 344–353.

51. Walkley, C.R.; Qudsi, R.; Sankaran, V.G.; Perry, J.A.; Gostissa, M.; Roth, S.I.; Rodda, S.J.; Snay, E.; Dunning, P.; Fahey, F.H.; *et al.* Conditional mouse osteosarcoma, dependent on p53 loss and potentiated by loss of Rb, mimics the human disease. *Genes Dev* 2008, *22*, 1662–1676.

52. Rao, P.H.; Zhao, S.; Zhao, Y.J.; Yu, A.; Rainusso, N.; Trucco, M.; Allen-Rhoades, W.; Satterfield, L.; Fuja, D.; Borra, V.J.; *et al.* Coamplification of Myc/Pvt1 and homozygous deletion of Nlrp1 locus are frequent genetics changes in mouse osteosarcoma. *Genes Chromosomes Cancer* 2015, *54*, 796–808.

53. Mohseny, A.B.; Hogendoorn, P.C.; Cleton-Jansen, A.M. Osteosarcoma models: From cell lines to zebrafish.*Sarcoma* 2012, *2012*, 417271.

54. Merchant, M.S.; Melchionda, F.; Sinha, M.; Khanna, C.; Helman, L.; Mackall, C.L. Immune reconstitution prevents metastatic recurrence of murine osteosarcoma. *Cancer Immunol. Immunother.* 2007, *56*, 1037–1046.

55. Olive, K.P.; Tuveson, D.A.; Ruhe, Z.C.; Yin, B.; Willis, N.A.; Bronson, R.T.; Crowley, D.; Jacks, T. Mutant p53 gain of function in two mouse models of Li-Fraumeni syndrome. *Cell* 2004, *119*, 847–860.

56. Angstadt, A.Y.; Thayanithy, V.; Subramanian, S.; Modiano, J.F.; Breen, M. A genome-wide approach to comparative oncology: High-resolution

oligonucleotide aCGH of canine and human osteosarcoma pinpoints shared microaberrations. *Cancer Genet.* 2012, *205*, 572–587.

57. Chen, X.; Bahrami, A.; Pappo, A.; Easton, J.; Dalton, J.; Hedlund, E.; Ellison, D.; Shurtleff, S.; Wu, G.; Wei, L.; *et al.* Recurrent somatic structural variations contribute to tumorigenesis in pediatric osteosarcoma. *Cell Rep.*2014, *7*, 104–112.

58. Scott, M.C.; Sarver, A.L.; Tomiyasu, H.; Cornax, I.; van Etten, J.; Varshney, J.; O'Sullivan, M.G.; Subramanian, S.; Modiano, J.F. Aberrant RB-E2F transcriptional regulation defines molecular phenotypes of osteosarcoma. *J. Biol. Chem.* 2015.

59. Ren, W.; Gu, G. Prognostic implications of RB1 tumour suppressor gene alterations in the clinical outcome of human osteosarcoma: A meta-analysis. *Eur. J. Cancer Care* 2015.

60. Sampson, V.B.; Yoo, S.; Kumar, A.; Vetter, N.S.; Kolb, E.A. MicroRNAs and potential targets in osteosarcoma: Review. *Front. Pediatr.* 2015, *3*, 69.

61. Zhang, J.; Yan, Y.G.; Wang, C.; Zhang, S.J.; Yu, X.H.; Wang, W.J. MicroRNAs in osteosarcoma. *Clin. Chim. Acta*2015, *444*, 9–17.

62. Miao, J.; Wu, S.; Peng, Z.; Tania, M.; and Zhang, C. MicroRNAs in osteosarcoma: Diagnostic and therapeutic aspects. *Tumour Biol.* 2013, *34*, 2093–2098.

63. Zhou, G.; Shi, X.; Zhang, J.; Wu, S.; Zhao, J. MicroRNAs in osteosarcoma: From biological players to clinical contributors, a review. *J. Int. Med. Res.* 2013, *41*, 1–12.

64. Li, Y.; Zhang, J.; Zhang, L.; Si, M.; Yin, H.; Li, J. Diallyl trisulfide inhibits proliferation, invasion and angiogenesis of osteosarcoma cells by switching on suppressor microRNAs and inactivating of Notch-1 signaling. *Carcinogenesis* 2013, *34*, 1601–1610.

65. Sarver, A.L.; Thayanithy, V.; Scott, M.C.; Cleton-Jansen, A.M.; Hogendoorn, P.C.; Modiano, J.F.; Subramanian, S. MicroRNAs at the human 14q32 locus have prognostic significance in osteosarcoma. *Orphanet J. Rare Dis.*2013, *8*, 7.

66. Namlos, H.M.; Meza-Zepeda, L.A.; Baroy, T.; Ostensen, I.H.; Kresse, S.H.; Kuijjer, M.L.; Serra, M.; Burger, H.; Cleton-Jansen, A.M.; Myklebost, O. Modulation of the osteosarcoma expression phenotype by microRNAs.*PloS ONE* 2012, *7*, e48086.

67. Lulla, R.R.; Costa, F.F.; Bischof, J.M.; Chou, P.M.; de, F.B.M.; Vanin, E.F.; Soares, M.B. Identification of differentially expressed MicroRNAs in osteosarcoma. *Sarcoma* 2011, *2011*, 732690.

68. Varshney, J.; Subramanian, S. MicroRNAs as potential target in human bone and soft tissue sarcoma therapeutics. *Front. Mol. Biosci.* 2015, *2*, 31.

69. Sarver, A.L.; Phalak, R.; Thayanithy, V.; Subramanian, S. S-MED: Sarcoma microRNA expression database. *Lab. Investig. J. Tech. Methods Pathol.* 2010, *90*, 753–761.

70. Thayanithy, V.; Sarver, A.L.; Kartha, R.V.; Li, L.; Angstadt, A.Y.; Breen, M.; Steer, C.J.; Modiano, J.F.; Subramanian, S. Perturbation of 14q32 miRNAs-cMYC gene network in osteosarcoma. *Bone* 2012, *50*, 171–181.
71. Li, Y.; Choi, P.S.; Casey, S.C.; Dill, D.L.; Felsher, D.W. MYC through miR-17–92 suppresses specific target genes to maintain survival, autonomous proliferation, and a neoplastic state. *Cancer Cell* 2014, *26*, 262–272.
72. Schaap-Oziemlak, A.M.; Raymakers, R.A.; Bergevoet, S.M.; Gilissen, C.; Jansen, B.J.; Adema, G.J.; Kogler, G.; le Sage, C.; Agami, R.; van der Reijden, B.A.; *et al.* MicroRNA hsa-miR-135b regulates mineralization in osteogenic differentiation of human unrestricted somatic stem cells. *Stem. Cells Dev.* 2010, *19*, 877–885.
73. Wei, J.Q.; Chen, H.; Zheng, X.F.; Zhang, B.X.; Wang, Y.; Tang, P.F.; She, F.; Song, Q.; Li, T.S. Hsa-miR-654–5p regulates osteogenic differentiation of human bone marrow mesenchymal stem cells by repressing bone morphogenetic protein 2. *J. Southern Med. Univ.* 2012, *32*, 291–295.
74. Fang, S.; Deng, Y.; Gu, P.; Fan, X. MicroRNAs regulate bone development and regeneration. *Int. J. Mol. Sci.*2015, *16*, 8227–8253.
75. Inose, H.; Ochi, H.; Kimura, A.; Fujita, K.; Xu, R.; Sato, S.; Iwasaki, M.; Sunamura, S.; Takeuchi, Y.; Fukumoto, S.; *et al.* A microRNA regulatory mechanism of osteoblast differentiation. *Proc. Natl. Acad. Sci. USA* 2009, *106*, 20794–20799.
76. Feng, Z.; Zhang, C.; Wu, R.; Hu, W. Tumor suppressor p53 meets microRNAs. *J. Mol. Cell Biol.* 2011, *3*, 44–50.
77. Wang, Y.; Jia, L.S.; Yuan, W.; Wu, Z.; Wang, H.B.; Xu, T.; Sun, J.C.; Cheng, K.F.; Shi, J.G. Low miR-34a and miR-192 are associated with unfavorable prognosis in patients suffering from osteosarcoma. *Am. J. Transl. Res.* 2015,*7*, 111–119.
78. Zhao, H.; Ma, B.; Wang, Y.; Han, T.; Zheng, L.; Sun, C.; Liu, T.; Zhang, Y.; Qiu, X.; Fan, Q. miR-34a inhibits the metastasis of osteosarcoma cells by repressing the expression of CD44. *Oncol. Rep.* 2013, *29*, 1027–1036.
79. He, C.; Xiong, J.; Xu, X.; Lu, W.; Liu, L.; Xiao, D.; Wang, D. Functional elucidation of MiR-34 in osteosarcoma cells and primary tumor samples. *Biochem. Biophys. Res. Commun.* 2009, *388*, 35–40.
80. Pazzaglia, L.; Leonardi, L.; Conti, A.; Novello, C.; Quattrini, I.; Montanini, L.; Roperto, F.; del Piero, F.; di Guardo, G.; Piro, F.; *et al.* miR-196a expression in human and canine osteosarcomas: A comparative study. *Res. Vet. Sci.* 2015, *99*, 112–119.
81. Zhang, W.; Zhang, C.; Chen, H.; Li, L.; Tu, Y.; Liu, C.; Shi, S.; Zen, K.; Liu, Z. Evaluation of microRNAs miR-196a, miR-30a-5P, and miR-490 as biomarkers of disease activity among patients with FSGS. *Clin. J. Am. Soc. Nephrol.* 2014, *9*, 1545–1552.
82. Gardner, H.L.; Fenger, J.M.; London, C.A. Dogs as a model for cancer. *Annu. Rev. Anim. Biosci.* 2015. in print.

83. Xu, M.; Jin, H.; Xu, C.X.; Sun, B.; Song, Z.G.; Bi, W.Z.; Wang, Y. miR-382 inhibits osteosarcoma metastasis and relapse by targeting Y box-binding protein 1. *Mol. Ther.* 2015, *23*, 89–98.

84. Zhou, Y.; Huang, Z.; Wu, S.; Zang, X.; Liu, M.; Shi, J. miR-33a is up-regulated in chemoresistant osteosarcoma and promotes osteosarcoma cell resistance to cisplatin by down-regulating TWIST. *J. Exp. Clin. Cancer Res.*2014, *33*, 12.

85. Xu, M.; Jin, H.; Xu, C.X.; Bi, W.Z.; Wang, Y. MiR-34c inhibits osteosarcoma metastasis and chemoresistance.*Med. Oncol.* 2014, *31*, 972.

86. Rosenblum, J.M.; Wijetunga, N.A.; Fazzari, M.J.; Krailo, M.; Barkauskas, D.A.; Gorlick, R.; Greally, J.M. Predictive properties of DNA methylation patterns in primary tumor samples for osteosarcoma relapse status.*Epigenetics* 2015, *10*, 31–39.

87. Kresse, S.H.; Rydbeck, H.; Skarn, M.; Namlos, H.M.; Barragan-Polania, A.H.; Cleton-Jansen, A.M.; Serra, M.; Liestol, K.; Hogendoorn, P.C.; Hovig, E.; *et al.* Integrative analysis reveals relationships of genetic and epigenetic alterations in osteosarcoma. *PLoS ONE* 2012, *7*, e48262.

88. Oh, J.H.; Kim, H.S.; Kim, H.H.; Kim, W.H.; Lee, S.H. Aberrant methylation of p14ARF gene correlates with poor survival in osteosarcoma. *Clin. Orthop. Relat. Res.* 2006, *442*, 216–222.

89. Park, Y.B.; Park, M.J.; Kimura, K.; Shimizu, K.; Lee, S.H.; Yokota, J. Alterations in the INK4a/ARF locus and their effects on the growth of human osteosarcoma cell lines. *Cancer Genet. Cytogenet.* 2002, *133*, 105–111.

90. Al-Romaih, K.; Sadikovic, B.; Yoshimoto, M.; Wang, Y.; Zielenska, M.; Squire, J.A. Decitabine-induced demethylation of 5′ CpG island in GADD45A leads to apoptosis in osteosarcoma cells. *Neoplasia* 2008, *10*, 471–480.

91. Badal, V.; Menendez, S.; Coomber, D.; Lane, D.P. Regulation of the p14ARF promoter by DNA methylation.*Cell Cycle* 2008, *7*, 112–119.

92. Chen, W.; Cooper, T.K.; Zahnow, C.A.; Overholtzer, M.; Zhao, Z.; Ladanyi, M.; Karp, J.E.; Gokgoz, N.; Wunder, J.S.; Andrulis, I.L.; *et al.* Epigenetic and genetic loss of Hic1 function accentuates the role of p53 in tumorigenesis. *Cancer Cell* 2004, *6*, 387–398.

93. Lu, J.; Song, G.; Tang, Q.; Zou, C.; Han, F.; Zhao, Z.; Yong, B.; Yin, J.; Xu, H.; Xie, X.; *et al.* IRX1 hypomethylation promotes osteosarcoma metastasis via induction of CXCL14/NF-kappaB signaling. *J. Clin. Investig.* 2015, *125*, 1839–1856.

94. Li, Y.; Meng, G.; Huang, L.; Guo, Q.N. Hypomethylation of the P3 promoter is associated with up-regulation of IGF2 expression in human osteosarcoma. *Hum. Pathol.* 2009, *40*, 1441–1447.

95. Ulaner, G.A.; Vu, T.H.; Li, T.; Hu, J.F.; Yao, X.M.; Yang, Y.; Gorlick, R.; Meyers, P.; Healey, J.; Ladanyi, M.; *et al.* Loss of imprinting of IGF2 and H19 in osteosarcoma is accompanied by reciprocal methylation changes of a CTCF-binding site. *Hum. Mol. Genet.* 2003, *12*, 535–549.

96. Li, Y.; Meng, G.; Guo, Q.N. Changes in genomic imprinting and gene expression associated with transformation in a model of human osteosarcoma. *Exp. Mol. Pathol.* 2008, *84*, 234–239.

97. Lee, D.F.; Su, J.; Kim, H.S.; Chang, B.; Papatsenko, D.; Zhao, R.; Yuan, Y.; Gingold, J.; Xia, W.; Darr, H.; *et al.* Modeling familial cancer with induced pluripotent stem cells. *Cell* 2015, *161*, 240–254.

98. Thayanithy, V.; Park, C.; Sarver, A.L.; Kartha, R.V.; Korpela, D.M.; Graef, A.J.; Steer, C.J.; Modiano, J.F.; Subramanian, S. Combinatorial treatment of DNA and chromatin-modifying drugs cause cell death in human and canine osteosarcoma cell lines. *PLoS ONE* 2012, *7*, e43720.

99. Zhang, X.; Cruz, F.D.; Terry, M.; Remotti, F.; Matushansky, I. Terminal differentiation and loss of tumorigenicity of human cancers via pluripotency-based reprogramming. *Oncogene* 2013, *32*, 2249–2260.

100. Maniscalco, L. Canine osteosarcoma: Understanding its variability to improve treatment. *Vet. J.* 2015, *203*, 135–136.

101. Rodriguez, C.O., Jr. Using canine osteosarcoma as a model to assess efficacy of novel therapies: Can old dogs teach us new tricks? *Adv. Exp. Med. Biol.* 2014, *804*, 237–256.

102. Modiano, J.F.; Bellgrau, D.; Cutter, G.R.; Lana, S.E.; Ehrhart, N.P.; Ehrhart, E.; Wilke, V.L.; Charles, J.B.; Munson, S.; Scott, M.C.; *et al.* Inflammation, apoptosis, and necrosis induced by neoadjuvant fas ligand gene therapy improves survival of dogs with spontaneous bone cancer. *Mol. Ther.* 2012, *20*, 2234–2243.

10
CHAPTER

CATS, CANCER AND COMPARATIVE ONCOLOGY

Claire M. Cannon

University of Tennessee College of Veterinary Medicine, 2407 River Drive, Knoxville, TN 37996, USA

ABSTRACT

Naturally occurring tumors in dogs are well established models for several human cancers. Domestic cats share many of the benefits of dogs as a model (spontaneous cancers developing in an immunocompetent animal sharing the same environment as humans, shorter lifespan allowing more rapid trial completion and data collection, lack of standard of care for many cancers allowing evaluation of therapies in treatment-naïve populations), but have not been utilized to the same degree in the One Medicine approach to cancer. There are both challenges and opportunities in feline compared to canine models. This review will discuss three specific tumor types where cats may offer insights into human cancers. Feline oral squamous cell carcinoma is common, shares both clinical and molecular features with human head and neck cancer and is an attractive model for evaluating new therapies. Feline mammary tumors are usually malignant and aggressive, with the 'triple-negative' phenotype being more common than in humans, offering an enriched population in which to examine potential targets and treatments. Finally, although there is not an exact corollary in humans, feline injection site sarcoma may be a model for inflammation-driven tumorigenesis, offering opportunities for studying variations in individual susceptibility as well as preventative and therapeutic strategies.

INTRODUCTION

'Cats are not small dogs' is an oft-quoted phrase in veterinary medicine. Nowhere is this more true than in comparative oncology, and it is both the advantage and disadvantage of the cat as a model.

Citation: Claire M. Cannon, Cats, Cancer and Comparative Oncology, Vet. Sci. 2015, 2(3), 111-126; doi:10.3390/vetsci2030111

Although domestic cats have been used as models for various non-neoplastic diseases and are of particular value for investigation of inherited ophthalmic diseases and type 2 diabetes [1,2], to date the dog has been the focus in comparative oncology [3,4]. This may be due, in part, to the fact that the complete feline genome has only very recently become available [5], whereas the canine genome has been available since 2005 [6]. The resources are now available to begin to fully investigate naturally-occurring cancers in cats as models for human diseases beyond the clinical and histological similarities. Greater coverage of the feline genome and development of a feline microarray chip similar to those developed for humans and dogs, allowing genome-wide assessments, would assist in fully investigating cats as cancer models.

Cancer is common in domestic cats, though likely somewhat less common than in dogs [7,8]. Like dogs, cats with cancer have clear benefits over laboratory models of human cancers (*i.e.*, induced tumors or xenografted human cell lines in rodents). Cats and dogs experience the same environmental risk factors as humans and are immunocompetent, more accurately reflecting the complex interplay of genetics and environmental risk factors as well as the role of the immune system and tumor microenvironment. There is greater homology between dogs and humans for key cancer-related genes than there is between rodents and humans [9], and there is also significant homology between cats and humans for specific genes [10,11,12]. Comparative genomics in feline cancers are reviewed in detail elsewhere in this issue [13]. The shorter lifespan and more rapid progression of cancers in animals allows more rapid trial completion and data collection, potentially identifying therapies that are more likely to succeed in human trials. There is a lack of standard of care for many cancers in animals and new therapies are more likely to be evaluated in treatment-naïve patients, which may give better determination of toxicity and efficacy. The cat may be superior to the dog as a model for some specific tumors, e.g., oral squamous cell carcinoma (SCC) and aggressive mammary tumors, due to the increased frequency in this species. Sarcoma formation secondary to inflammation (at injection sites or following trauma), while rarely reported in dogs, is well-recognized in cats, and may offer insights into inflammation-driven tumorigenesis in general. Published feline cell lines for these tumor types are included in Table 1.

When considering potential benefits of the cat as a model, there are some species-specific challenges to be considered. Although 2012 data suggest that there are more cats than dogs owned as pets in the United States, they are less likely to be seen by veterinarians, either at primary care or referral hospitals [14,15,16,17,18]. This effect is more pronounced in cats greater than 9 years of age [17], meaning that cats at highest risk of cancer are least likely to be seen for routine veterinary care. Cat owners are more likely to perceive their pet being stressed by veterinary visits than dog owners [17]. In the specific situation of clinical trials, a recent survey found that most cat owners were unsure about whether they would consider enrolling their cat in a hypothetical trial, though 71% of owners who had previously participated in a clinical trial would consider participating again. Important factors in owners' decisions included the recommendation of their primary veterinarian, the number of visits, and the risk of discomfort to their cat [19]. Although there are barriers to clinical trials in cats, there are opportunities at every level to improve recruitment including education of the public about the importance of routine veterinary care and the existence of clinical trials, of primary care veterinarians about clinical trial opportunities and of both primary care and specialist veterinarians about 'feline-friendly' or low-stress handling techniques.

One of the strengths of the dog in comparative oncology is the relatively genetically homogenous breeds (compared to humans) with breed predispositions to different cancers, simplifying identification of genetic signatures related to cancer predisposition (for example, DNA repair deficiency in Golden Retrievers associated with higher risk of lymphoma) [20]. Dogs have undergone major selection pressure by humans for hundreds, if not thousands, of years, resulting in genetically distinct groups. Most cat breeds developed within the past century and there are fewer genetically distinct breeds than in dogs [21,22]. The fact that there are very few specific breed predispositions reported for cancer in cats may reflect this, although Siamese cats are over-represented in cats with cancer in general, and specifically with mammary gland and intestinal neoplasia [23,24,25]. The recently available feline genome may allow identification of genetic signatures of cancer risk in Siamese compared to other cats.

In terms of using cats as pre-clinical models for assessment of new drugs, thorough consideration needs to be given to drug metabolism and pharmacokinetics in this species before determination of applicability in people can be made. Cats are known to have reduced overall hepatic glucuronidation capacity compared to dogs and humans, though this seems to be drug-specific [26,27]. Consideration of metabolic pathways prior to clinical trials of potential new drugs in cats is recommended. Examples of chemotherapeutic drugs with differing toxicities in dogs and cats include cisplatin (fatal pulmonary edema in cats) [28], 5-fluorouracil (fatal neurotoxicity in cats, which is not due to reduced DPD function) [29], CCNU (lower apparent risk of hepatotoxicity in cats) [30], doxorubicin (nephrotoxic in cats, cardiotoxic in dogs) [31] and ifosfamide (higher maximum tolerated dose in cats) [31].

Despite the potential challenges, investigating cancer in cats is likely to add to the field of comparative oncology and complement the use of the canine model, especially in some specific instances.

FELINE ORAL SQUAMOUS CELL CARCINOMA

Squamous cell carcinoma represents 70–80% of all oral tumors in domestic cats. Increased risk has been associated with exposure to environmental tobacco smoke, flea collars and feeding canned food [32], although specific risk factors are not identified in most patients. Tobacco use, along with alcohol, is a major risk factor in human head and neck cancer (HHNC), most of which are SCC affecting the oral/oropharyngeal cavity [33,34]. Papillomavirus infection plays a role in a significant proportion of HHNC, and is associated with less aggressive disease and better outcome [34]. Although papillomavirus may play a role in feline cutaneous SCC and has been isolated from oral papillomas in cats, it has not been demonstrated to be involved in the vast majority of feline oral SCC [35,36,37,38]. In humans, it seems that many oral/oropharyngeal SCC arise from pre-existing disorders such as leukoplakia and erythroplakia [34]. Such progression has not been identified in feline oral SCC, although inflammatory conditions like periodontal disease and stomatitis are common [39]. It is possible that there are similar pre-malignant lesions in cats which, if identified, may be models for chemoprevention or other intervention strategies. In both humans and cats, head and neck SCC is locally invasive, often diagnosed late, and is challenging to treat [33,34,40]. In cats, local disease is typically life-limiting and metastasis is less commonly reported than in humans, though may be underestimated since survival times are short because of advanced stage at diagnosis and poor response to local therapies [33,40]. The most common laboratory models for HHNC are induced tumors in the oral cavity of hamsters or rats, which have shed light on tumor initiation by carcinogens such as tobacco or betel nut, and subcutaneous xenograft models [41]. Feline oral SCC more closely mimics the natural behavior of HHNC and likely more accurately predicts response to treatment than induced tumors in laboratory animals.

As well as clinical features, feline oral SCC shares many molecular features with HHNC, including high frequency of epidermal growth factor (EGFR) over-expression (although not proven to be prognostic in cats) [34,42,43,44,45,46], altered p53 expression [34,47,48], dysregulated CK2 expression [49,50], markers of angiogenesis [34,46,51,52] and cyclooxygenase and lipoxygenase enzyme overexpression [34,53,54,55,56].

Feline oral SCC (either in clinical patients, cell lines or immunohistochemical studies) has been used as a model for tumor hypoxia (which may be targeted to improve responses to chemo- or radio-therapy) [57] and mechanisms and treatment of bone invasion [51,58,59,60,61]. EGFR is a druggable target in HHNC [42], and the feline and human EGFR sequences are highly homologous [10]. The EGFR small molecule inhibitor gefitinib is approved for use in HHNC, but has only a modest effect as monotherapy and, even in patients that initially respond, resistance commonly develops after long-term treatment [62]. Gefitinib resistance has been evaluated in a feline SCC cell line [10,63] and the cat could be a useful model for studying mechanisms of, and strategies to circumvent, EGFR-inhibitor resistance (e.g., RNA interference) [10]. Increased polyamine content is a feature of many tumors in humans, including HNC, and targeting polyamine synthesis with ornithine decarboxylase (ODC) inhibitors has been proposed as a possible therapeutic strategy [64]. A combination of alpha difluoromethylornithine (DFMO), an ODC inhibitor, with a novel membrane transport inhibitor to increase intracellular DFMO concentrations showed positive results in a murine model, with a 71% complete response rate [65]. In feline patients with naturally occurring oral SCC there was some indication of activity, but results were more modest (16.7% partial response rate, 50% stable disease). This may offer more realistic expectation of what might be expected from this type of therapy in people [66]. Inhibition of CK2 is effective in rodent xenograft models of human prostate and head and neck cancers [67,68,69] and small molecule CK2 inhibitors are in early clinical trials. *In vitro* results in feline SCC show similar results to human cell lines [50], and a clinical trial of RNA interference targeting CK2 is underway in cats with oral SCC, which may inform future human studies.

Overall, current standard treatments for feline oral SCC (surgery, radiation and chemotherapy) have almost universally poor outcomes, with median survival times in the order of a few months [40,70,71]. Better results are seen in small tumors [71], but as most patients have advanced disease at the time of diagnosis, treatment is typically palliative. With the grave prognosis and lack of effective standard of care, it is reasonable to offer experimental therapies to cats and owners at the time of diagnosis, and therapies can be assessed in a treatment-naïve population who may be more likely to respond. Potential avenues for comparative investigations in feline SCC include new EGFR inhibitors, including in the setting of gefitinib-resistance, CK2 inhibition alone and in combination with chemo- or radio-therapy, novel COX/LOX inhibitors, methods to reverse hypoxia in combination with other therapies, and anti-angiogenic therapies. Toceranib phosphate (Palladia, Zoetis) is a multi-kinase inhibitor which has shown some anecdotal efficacy in feline oral SCC. It does not inhibit EGFR, so the mechanism of its activity is currently unknown, and an investigation currently underway evaluating expression of toceranib targets in feline oral SCC [72] may identify new targets in HHNC as well.

FELINE MAMMARY GLAND TUMORS

In cats, unlike dogs, the vast majority of mammary gland tumors are malignant, and multiple tumors and metastasis are common at diagnosis [73,74,75,76]. Thus, cats with mammary cancer may offer a larger population of aggressive malignancies to study. The epidemiology of mammary gland tumors in cats and people is similar, with age [23,74] and hormone exposure [73,77] being major risk factors. There is a breed predisposition in Siamese cats, which are more likely to develop mammary tumors and at a younger age than other cat breeds [23,73]. Now that the feline genome is available, Siamese cats may be a model for genetic risk of breast cancer and other neoplasia, given their increased risk of several tumor types. Germline mutations in BRCA1 and BRCA2 genes are associated with familial breast cancer risk in women, although the majority of breast cancers are sporadic in nature [78]. BRCA mutations have not been found in cats with mammary cancer [79]. Since there is a breed predisposition (if not a proven inherited risk), studying Siamese cats specifically may be more likely to identify these or other genetic abnormalities predisposing to mammary cancer.

In contrast to breast cancer in women, feline mammary tumors are more likely to be hormone (estrogen and progesterone) receptor negative, though differing methodologies and scoring makes comparisons between studies challenging [80,81,82,83,84]. Epidermal growth factor receptor 2 (HER2, neu, erbb2) is commonly over-expressed in human breast cancer and is a druggable target, with trastuzumab (Herceptin®, Genentech) improving outcome in women with HER2-expressing breast cancer [85]. Increased HER2 expression and activity, demonstrated by increased downstream AKT activation, is also seen in feline mammary carcinomas, though there is variation among studies with regard to the rate of HER2 expression and methodologies used [79,84,86,87,88,89,90]. Recent studies have used the human standard methodology (HercepTest™, Dako) for evaluation of HER2 in feline mammary tumors [87,90,91] which may offer a useful standard for future studies. Concurrent evaluation of HER2 mRNA expression (as well as protein expression) may add to the understanding of its role in feline mammary gland tumors, though currently published studies are discrepant in terms of relative HER2 expression between normal and neoplastic tissues [11,84,91]. There appears to be a significant proportion of feline mammary carcinomas which are 'triple-negative' *i.e.*, hormone receptor negative and not over-expressing HER2 [79,84]. This phenotype is generally associated with a poorer prognosis in humans and is challenging to treat because of a lack of specific targets. Additional molecular analyses distinguish several other subtypes of breast cancer, e.g., luminal A, luminal B and claudin low, and similar subtypes may exist in cats [84,92]. The overall increased likelihood of aggressive mammary cancer in cats compared to humans offers opportunities to study factors such as drivers of metastasis and potential treatments for triple-negative tumors. Cats may also be a useful model for evaluating new HER2-targeted therapies. A recent study vaccinated healthy cats with HER2 DNA and induced specific T cell responses to self-HER2 in four out of 10 cats [93]. Cats with naturally occurring mammary cancer could be used for rapid pre-clinical assessment of efficacy of HER2 vaccination as well as to assess determinants of response, given the variability in induced immunity. When considering cats as a model for HER2-targeted therapies however, strong consideration needs to be given to the methodologies used to assess HER2 protein expression due to variability between studies, as well as the recently identified sequence variants in HER2 which may impact its affinity for targeted therapies such as trastuzumab, as is seen in humans [91].

INJECTION SITE SARCOMA

Inflammation is well-established as a risk factor for several cancers in people and similar risk factors likely exist in dogs and cats [94,95]. Although there are sporadic cases of sarcomas associated with various implants and injections in humans and animals [96,97,98,99,100], cats appear to have a unique propensity for sarcomagenesis associated with trauma and/or inflammation. Injection site sarcoma (ISS) is a well-recognized phenomenon in cats, especially in association with vaccine administration. Estimates in the US and UK range from one case of ISS per 1,000–12,500 cats vaccinated [101,102]. Most ISS in cats are fibrosarcomas, and common histologic features include multinucleate giant cells, myofibroblastic differentiation and inflammatory infiltrate (lymphocytes and macrophages), which are not typically seen in feline non-injection site fibrosarcomas [103,104,105,106]. Intra-ocular sarcoma formation following trauma or other ocular disease is also recognized in cats [107]. No risk factors have been identified to determine why some cats develop sarcomas following trauma or injection. It is hypothesized that in these cats the immune response to injection or trauma is inappropriate and excessive, resulting in chronic inflammation causing proliferation and malignant transformation of fibroblasts. Chronic inflammation increases the risk for many carcinomas in people, though the only clear association between sarcomagenesis and chronic inflammation is in the case of Kaposi's sarcoma (KS).

KS is frequently associated with inflammatory infiltrate and Kaposi sarcoma-associated herpesvirus (KSHV) proteins activate factors including Th2 lymphocytes, cyclooxygenase 2 and NFκB resulting in a pro-tumor inflammatory microenvironment [108]. ISS in cats may model inflammation-associated tumorigenesis in general, which likely has common pathways in many different tumor histologies. As not every cat vaccinated develops ISS, not every person with chronic inflammatory disease develops associated cancer. Given that lifestyle factors such as environment and diet are likely more controllable in cats than in people, genomic screening in cats that develop ISS may identify features of the immune system or other factors related to tumor development. Such features may also be present in humans, and could identify individuals who may benefit from early intervention or more frequent monitoring. As well as a model for identifying risk factors, ISS may be a model for prevention or therapy. A recent development in ISS treatment is the approval of feline interleukin-2 recombinant canarypox virus (Oncept Il-2) to reduce local recurrence following standard-of-care therapy [109], indicating that manipulation of the immune system in this, and other inflammation-driven tumors, may be of therapeutic benefit. Further elucidation of the nature of feline ISS-associated inflammation (e.g., assessing cytokine profiles, T cell subtypes, and tumor-infiltrating macrophages) may be a first step in identifying strategies to reduce tumor-promoting inflammation and/or promote anti-tumor inflammation. Potential chemoprevention strategies could likely be evaluated in a relatively timely fashion since it appears that most ISS develop within 3 years of vaccination, though latent periods of up to 10 years are reported [110,111].

CONCLUSIONS

Although a decade behind their canine counterparts, cats have great potential to contribute to comparative oncology. Areas of especial focus may include head and neck squamous cell carcinoma, aggressive mammary tumors and inflammation-associated tumorigenesis. Areas for progress in order to exploit the full potential of the feline model include standardization of target assessments, development of efficient genome-wide analyses (e.g., feline-specific microarrays) and education of the public and veterinary communities about clinical trials and other comparative opportunities.

Table 1: Feline squamous cell carcinoma, mammary gland carcinoma and injection-site sarcoma cell lines used in published research

Tumor Type	Cell Line
Head and neck squamous cell carcinoma	SCCF1 [112] SCCF1-Luc (luciferase-expressing) [47] SCCF1G (gefitinib-resistant) [10]
	SCCF2 [58] SCCF2-Luc
	SCCF3 [58] SCCF3-Luc
Mammary gland tumor	K12 [113]
	JM [114]
	FYMp (primary) [115]
	FKNp [115]
	FNNm (metastatic) [115]
	FONp [116] FONm [116]
	FMCp1 [115] FMCp2 [115] FMCm [115]
	FRM [117]
	NAC [118]
	K248C [119]
	K248P [119]
	DT09/06 [120]
Injection site sarcoma	FSA [121]
	FSB [121]
	FS1 [122]
	FS2 [122]
	FS3 [122]
	FS4 [122]
	VAS-1 [123]
	VAS-2 [123]
	VAS-3 [123]
	VAS-4 [123]
	VAS-5 [123]
	JB [124]
	JBLM [124]

REFERENCES

1. Henson, M.S.; O'Brien, T.D. Feline models of type 2 diabetes mellitus. *ILAR J.* 2006, *47*, 234–242.
2. Narfstrom, K.; Deckman, K.H.; Menotti-Raymond, M. Cats: A gold mine for ophthalmology. *Ann. Rev. Anim. Biosci.* 2013, *1*, 157–177.
3. Gordon, I.; Paoloni, M.; Mazcko, C.; Khanna, C. The Comparative Oncology Trials Consortium: Using spontaneously occurring cancers in dogs to inform the cancer drug development pathway. *PLoS Med.* 2009, *6*, e1000161.
4. Gordon, I.K.; Khanna, C. Modeling opportunities in comparative oncology for drug development. *ILAR J.* 2010,*51*, 214–220.
5. Tamazian, G.; Simonov, S.; Dobrynin, P.; Makunin, A.; Logachev, A.; Komissarov, A.; Schevchenko, A.; Brukhin, V.; Cherkasov, N.; Svitin, A.; *et al.* Annotated features of domestic cat —Felis catus genome.*GigaScience*, 2014, 3. Available online: http://www.gigasciencejournal.com/content/3/1/13 (accessed on 25 June 2015).
6. Lindblad-Toh, K.; Wade, C.M.; Mikkelsen, T.S.; Karlsson, E.K.; Jaffe, D.B.; Kamal, M.; Clamp, M.; Chang, J.L.; Kulbokas, E.J., 3rd; Zody, M.C.; *et al.* Genome sequence, comparative analysis and haplotype structure of the domestic dog. *Nature* 2005, *438*, 803–819.
7. Butler, L.M.; Bonnett, B.N.; Page, R.L. *Withrow and MacEwen's Small Animal Clinical Oncology*, 5th ed.; Withrow, S.J., Vail, D.M., Page, R.L., Eds.; Elsevier Saunders: St Louis, MO, USA, 2012; pp. 68 82.
8. MacVean, D.W.; Monlux, A.W.; Anderson, P.S., Jr.; Silberg, S.L.; Roszel, J.F. Frequency of canine and feline tumors in a defined population. *Vet. Pathol.* 1978, *15*, 700–715.
9. Paoloni, M.; Khanna, C. Translation of new cancer treatments from pet dogs to humans. *Nat. Rev. Cancer* 2008,*8*, 147–156.
10. Bergkvist, G.T.; Argyle, D.J.; Pang, L.Y.; Muirhead, R.; Yool, D.A. Studies on the inhibition of feline EGFR in squamous cell carcinoma: Enhancement of radiosensitivity and rescue of resistance to small molecule inhibitors. *Cancer Biol. Therapy* 2011, *11*, 927–937.
11. De Maria, R.; Olivero, M.; Iussich, S.; Nakaichi, M.; Murata, T.; Biolatti, B.; Di Renzo, M.F. Spontaneous feline mammary carcinoma is a model of HER2 overexpressing poor prognosis human breast cancer. *Cancer Res.*2005, *65*, 907–912.
12. Santos, S.; Bastos, E.; Baptista, C.S.; Sá, D.; Caloustian, C.; Guedes-Pinto, H.; Gärtner, F.; Gut, I.G.; Chaves, R. Sequence variants and haplotype analysis of cat ERBB2 gene: A survey on spontaneous cat mammary neoplastic and non-neoplastic lesions. *Int. J. Mol. Sci.* 2012, *13*, 2783–2800.
13. Thomas, R. Cytogenomics of Feline Cancers: Advances and Opportunities. *Vet. Sci.* 2015. in preparation.

14. Bartlett, P.C.; Van Buren, J.W.; Neterer, M.; Zhou, C. Disease surveillance and referral bias in the veterinary medical database. *Prev. Vet. Med.* 2010, *94*, 264–271.

15. Teclaw, R.; Mendlein, J.; Garbe, P.; Mariolis, P. Characteristics of pet populations and households in the Purdue Comparative Oncology Program catchment area, 1988. *J. Amer. Vet. Med. Assoc.* 1992, *201*, 1725–1729.

16. Volk, J.O.; Felsted, K.E.; Thomas, J.G.; Siren, C.W. Executive summary of phase 2 of the Bayer veterinary care usage study. *J. Amer. Vet. Med. Assoc.* 2011, *239*, 1311–1316.

17. Volk, J.O.; Felsted, K.E.; Thomas, J.G.; Siren, C.W. Executive summary of the Bayer veterinary care usage study.*J. Amer. Vet. Med. Assoc.* 2011, *238*, 1275–1282.

18. American Veterinary Medical Association. U.S. Pet Ownership Statistics. 2012. Available online: https://www.avma.org/KB/Resources/Statistics/Pages/Market-research-statistics-US-pet-ownership.aspx (accessed on 19 March 2015).

19. Gruen, M.E.; Jiamachello, K.N.; Thomson, A.; Lascelles, B.D. Clinical trials involving cats: What factors affect owner participation? *J. Feline Med. Surg.* 2014, *16*, 727–735.

20. Thamm, D.H.; Grunerud, K.K.; Rose, B.J.; Vail, D.M.; Bailey, S.M. DNA repair deficiency as a susceptibility marker for spontaneous lymphoma in golden retriever dogs: A case-control study. *PLoS ONE* 2013, *8*, e69192.

21. Lipinski, M.J.; Froenicke, L.; Baysac, K.C.; Billings, N.C.; Leutenegger, C.M.; Levy, A.M.; Longeri, M.; Niini, T.; Ozpinar, H.; Slater, M.R.; *et al.* The ascent of cat breeds: Genetic evaluations of breeds and worldwide random-bred populations. *Genomics* 2008, *91*, 12–21.

22. Kurushima, J.D.; Lipinski, M.J.; Gandolfi, B.; Froenicke, L.; Grahn, J.C.; Grahn, R.A.; Lyons, L.A. Variation of cats under domestication: Genetic assignment of domestic cats to breeds and worldwide random-bred populations. *Anim. Genet.* 2013, *44*, 311–324.

23. Egenvall, A.; Bonnett, B.N.; Haggstrom, J.; Ström Holst, B.; Möller, L.; Nødtvedt, A. Morbidity of insured Swedish cats during 1999–2006 by age, breed, sex, and diagnosis. *J. Feline Med. Surg.* 2010, *12*, 948–959.

24. Egenvall, A.; Nødtvedt, A.; Haggstrom, J.; Ström Holst, B.; Möller, L.; Bonnett, B.N. Mortality of life-insured Swedish cats during 1999–2006: Age, breed, sex, and diagnosis. *J. Vet. Intern. Med.* 2009, *23*, 1175–1183.

25. Rissetto, K.; Villamil, J.A.; Selting, K.A.; Tyler, J.; Henry, C.J. Recent trends in feline intestinal neoplasia: An epidemiologic study of 1,129 cases in the veterinary medical database from 1964 to 2004. *J. Am. Anim. Hosp. Assoc.* 2011, *47*, 28–36.

26. Ebner, T.; Schänzle, G.; Weber, W.; Sent, U.; Elliott, J. *In vitro* glucuronidation of the angiotensin II receptor antagonist telmisartan in the cat: A comparison with other species. *J. Vet. Pharmacol. Therapeut.* 2013, *36*, 154–160.

27. van Beusekom, C.D.; Fink-Gremmels, J.; Schrickx, J.A. Comparing the glucuronidation capacity of the feline liver with substrate-specific glucuronidation in dogs. *J. Vet. Pharmacol. Therapeut.* 2014, *37*, 18–24.
28. Knapp, D.W.; Richardson, R.C.; DeNicola, D.B.; Long, G.G.; Blevins, W.E. Cisplatin toxicity in cats. *J. Vet. Intern. Med.* 1987, *1*, 29–35.
29. Saba, C.F.; Schmiedt, C.W.; Freeman, K.G.; Edwards, G.L. Indirect assessment of dihydropyrimidine dehydrogenase activity in cats. *Vet. Compar. Oncol.* 2013, *11*, 265–271.
30. Musser, M.L.; Quinn, H.T.; Chretin, J.D. Low apparent risk of CCNU (lomustine)-associated clinical hepatotoxicity in cats. *J. Feline Med. Surg.* 2012, *14*, 871–875.
31. Gustafson, D.L.; Page, R.L. Cancer Chemotherapy. In *Withrow and MacEwen's Small Animal Clinical Oncology*, 5th ed.; Withrow, S.J., Vail, D.M., Page, R.L., Eds.; Elsevier Saunders: St Louis, MO, USA, 2012; pp. 157–179.
32. Bertone, E.R.; Snyder, L.A.; Moore, A.S. Environmental and lifestyle risk factors for oral squamous cell carcinoma in domestic cats. *J. Vet. Intern. Med.* 2003, *17*, 557–562.
33. Belcher, R.; Hayes, K.; Fedewa, S.; Chen, A.Y. Current treatment of head and neck squamous cell cancer. *J. Surg. Oncol.* 2014, *110*, 551–574.
34. Huber, M.A.; Tantiwongkosi, B. Oral and oropharyngeal cancer. *Med. Clin. North Amer.* 2014, *98*, 1299–1321.
35. Munday, J.S.; Aberdein, D. Loss of retinoblastoma protein, but not p53, is associated with the presence of papillomaviral DNA in feline viral plaques, Bowenoid *in situ* carcinomas, and squamous cell carcinomas. *Vet. Pathol.* 2012, *49*, 538–545.
36. Munday, J.S.; Fairley, R.A.; Mills, H.; Kiupel, M.; Vaatstra, B.L. Oral Papillomas Associated With Felis catus Papillomavirus Type 1 in 2 Domestic Cats. *Vet. Pathol.* 2015. Available online: http://vet.sagepub.com/content/early/2015/01/02/0300985814565133 (accessed on 26 June 2015).
37. Munday, J.S.; Howe, L.; French, A.; Squires, R.A.; Sugiarto, H. Detection of papillomaviral DNA sequences in a feline oral squamous cell carcinoma. *Res. Vet. Sci.* 2009, *86*, 359–361.
38. Munday, J.S.; French, A.F. Felis catus papillomavirus types 1 and 4 are rarely present in neoplastic and inflammatory oral lesions of cats. *Res. Vet. Sci.* 2015. Available online: http://www.sciencedirect.com/science/article/pii/S0034528815000569.
39. Farcas, N.; Lommer, M.J.; Kass, P.H.; Verstraete, F.J. Dental radiographic findings in cats with chronic gingivostomatitis (2002–2012). *J. Amer. Vet. Med. Assoc.* 2014, *244*, 339–345.
40. Liptak, J.M.; Withrow, S.J. Cancer of the Gastrointestinal Tract. In *Withrow and MacEwen's Small Animal Clinical Oncology*, 5th ed.; Withrow, S.J., Vail, D.M., Page, R.L., Eds.; Elsevier Saunders: St Louis, MO, USA, 2012; pp. 381–431.
41. Mognetti, B.; Di Carlo, F.; Berta, G.N. Animal models in oral cancer research. *Oral Oncol.* 2006, *42*, 448–460.

42. Ribeiro, F.A.; Noguti, J.; Oshima, C.T.; Ribeiro, D.A. Effective targeting of the epidermal growth factor receptor (EGFR) for treating oral cancer: A promising approach. *Anticancer Res.* 2014, *34*, 1547–1552.

43. Bergkvist, G.T.; Argyle, D.J.; Morrison, L.; MacIntyre, N.; Hayes, A.; Yool, D.A. Expression of epidermal growth factor receptor (EGFR) and Ki67 in feline oral squamous cell carcinomas (FOSCC). *Vet. Compar. Oncol.* 2011, *9*, 106–117.

44. Looper, J.S.; Malarkey, D.E.; Ruslander, D.; Proulx, D.; Thrall, D.E. Epidermal growth factor receptor expression in feline oral squamous cell carcinomas. *Vet. Compar. Oncol.* 2006, *4*, 33–40.

45. Sabattini, S.; Marconato, L.; Zoff, A.; Morini, M.; Scarpa, F.; Capitani, O.; Bettini, G. Epidermal growth factor receptor expression is predictive of poor prognosis in feline cutaneous squamous cell carcinoma. *J. Feline Med. Surg.* 2010, *12*, 760–768.

46. Yoshikawa, H.; Ehrhart, E.J.; Charles, J.B.; Thamm, D.H.; Larue, S.M. Immunohistochemical characterization of feline oral squamous cell carcinoma. *Amer. J. Vet. Res.* 2012, *73*, 1801–1806.

47. Tannehill-Gregg, S.H.; Levine, A.L.; Rosol, T.J. Feline head and neck squamous cell carcinoma: A natural model for the human disease and development of a mouse model. *Vet. Compar. Oncol.* 2006, *4*, 84–97.

48. Snyder, L.A.; Bertone, E.R.; Jakowski, R.M.; Booner, M.S.; Jennings-Ritchie, J.; Moore, A.S. p53 expression and environmental tobacco smoke exposure in feline oral squamous cell carcinoma. *Vet. Pathol.* 2004, *41*, 209–214.

49. Faust, R.A.; Gapany, M.; Tristani, P.; Davis, A.; Adams, G.L.; Ahmed, K. Elevated protein kinase CK2 activity in chromatin of head and neck tumors: Association with malignant transformation. *Cancer Lett.* 1996, *101*, 31–35.

50. Cannon, C.M.; Trembley, J.H.; Modiano, J.F.; Cespedes Gomez, O.; Kren, B.; Unger, G.; Ahmed, K. CK2 inhibition in feline cancer cell lines using synthetic oligonucleotides. In Proceedings of the American Veterinary Internal Medicine Forum, Seattle, WA, USA, June 2013.

51. Wypij, J.M.; Fan, T.M.; Fredrickson, R.L.; Barger, A.M.; de Lorimier, L.P.; Charney, S.C. *In vivo* and *in vitro*efficacy of zoledronate for treating oral squamous cell carcinoma in cats. *J. Vet. Intern. Med.* 2008, *22*, 158–163.

52. Moriyama, M.; Kumagai, S.; Kawashiri, S.; Kojima, K.; Kakihara, K.; Yamamoto, E. Immunohistochemical study of tumour angiogenesis in oral squamous cell carcinoma. *Oral Oncol.* 1997, *33*, 369–374.

53. Hayes, A.; Scase, T.; Miller, J.; Murphy, S.; Sparkes, A.; Adams, V. COX-1 and COX-2 expression in feline oral squamous cell carcinoma. *J. Compar. Pathol.* 2006, *135*, 93–99.

54. Wakshlag, J.J.; Peters-Kennedy, J.; Bushey, J.J.; Loftus, J.P. 5-lipoxygenase expression and tepoxalin-induced cell death in squamous cell carcinomas in cats. *Amer. J. Vet. Res.* 2011, *72*, 1369–1377.

55. Wang, Z.M.; Liu, J.; Liu, H.B.; Ye, M.; Zhang, Y.F.; Yang, D.S. Abnormal COX2 protein expression may be correlated with poor prognosis in oral cancer: A meta-analysis. *BioMed Res. Int.* 2014. Available online: http://www.hindawi.com/journals/bmri/2014/364207/ (accessed on 25 June 2015).

56. Celenk, F.; Bayramoglu, I.; Yilmaz, A.; Menevse, A.; Bayazit, Y. Expression of cyclooxygenase-2, 12-lipoxygenase, and inducible nitric oxide synthase in head and neck squamous cell carcinoma. *J. Craniofac. Surg.*2013, *24*, 1114–1117.

57. Ballegeer, E.A.; Madrill, N.J.; Berger, K.L.; Agnew, D.W.; McNiel, E.A. Evaluation of hypoxia in a feline model of head and neck cancer using ^{64}Cu-ATSM positron emission tomography/computed tomography. *BMC Cancer*, 2013, 13. Available online: http://www.biomedcentral.com/1471–2407/13/218 (accessed on 25 June 2015).

58. Martin, C.K.; Dirksen, W.P.; Shu, S.T.; Werbeck, J.L.; Thudi, N.K.; Yamaguchi, M.; Wolfe, T.D.; Heller, K.N.; Rosol, T.J. Characterization of bone resorption in novel *in vitro* and *in vivo* models of oral squamous cell carcinoma. *Oral Oncol.* 2012, *48*, 491–499.

59. Martin, C.K.; Tannehill-Gregg, S.H.; Wolfe, T.D.; Rosol, T.J. Bone-invasive oral squamous cell carcinoma in cats: Pathology and expression of parathyroid hormone-related protein. *Vet. Pathol.* 2011, *48*, 302–312.

60. Martin, C.K.; Dirksen, W.P.; Carlton, M.M.; Lanigan, L.G.; Pillai, S.P.; Werbeck, J.L.; Simmons, J.K.; Hildreth, B.E., 3rd; London, C.A.; Toribio, R.E.; Rosol, T.J. Combined zoledronic acid and meloxicam reduced bone loss and tumour growth in an orthotopic mouse model of bone-invasive oral squamous cell carcinoma. *Vet. Compar. Oncol.* 2013. Available online: http://onlinelibrary.wiley.com/doi/10.1111/vco.12037/epdf (accessed on 25 June 2015).

61. Martin, C.K.; Werbeck, J.L.; Thudi, N.K.; Lanigan, L.G.; Wolfe, T.D.; Toribio, R.E.; Rosol, T.J. Zoledronic acid reduces bone loss and tumor growth in an orthotopic xenograft model of osteolytic oral squamous cell carcinoma. *Cancer Res.* 2010, *70*, 8607–8616.

62. Chen, L.F.; Cohen, E.E.; Grandis, J.R. New strategies in head and neck cancer: Understanding resistance to epidermal growth factor receptor inhibitors. *Clin. Cancer Res.* 2010, *16*, 2489–2495.

63. Pang, L.Y.; Bergkvist, G.T.; Cervantes-Arias, A.; Yool, D.A.; Muirhead, R.; Argyle, D.J. Identification of tumour initiating cells in feline head and neck squamous cell carcinoma and evidence for gefitinib induced epithelial to mesenchymal transition. *Vet. J.* 2012, *193*, 46–52.

64. Battaglia, V.; DeStefano Shields, C.; Murray-Stewart, T.; Casero , R.A., Jr. Polyamine catabolism in carcinogenesis: Potential targets for chemotherapy and chemoprevention. *Amino Acids* 2014, *46*, 511–519.

65. Chen, Y.; Weeks, R.S.; Burns, M.R.; Boorman, D.W.; Klein-Szanto, A.; O'Brien, T.G. Combination therapy with 2-difluoromethylornithine and a polyamine transport inhibitor against murine squamous cell carcinoma. *Int. J. Cancer* 2006, *118*, 2344–2349.

66. Skorupski, K.A.; O'Brien, T.G.; Guerrero, T.; Rodrigeuz, C.O.; Burns, M.R. Phase I/II clinical trial of 2-difluoromethyl-ornithine (DFMO) and a novel polyamine transport inhibitor (MQT 1426) for feline oral squamous cell carcinoma. *Vet. Compar. Oncol.* 2011, *9*, 275–282.

67. Trembley, J.H.; Unger, G.M.; Korman, V.L.; Tobolt, D.K.; Kazimierczuk, Z.; Pinna, L.A.; Kren, B.T.; Ahmed, K. Nanoencapsulated anti-CK2 small molecule drug or siRNA specifically targets malignant cancer but not benign cells. *Cancer Lett.* 2012, *315*, 48–58.

68. Unger, G.M.; Kren, B.T.; Korman, V.L.; Kimbrough, T.G.; Vogel, R.I.; Ondrey, F.G.; Trembley, J.H.; Ahmed, K. Mechanism and efficacy of sub-50-nm tenfibgen nanocapsules for cancer cell-directed delivery of anti-CK2 RNAi to primary and metastatic squamous cell carcinoma. *Mol. Cancer Ther.* 2014, *13*, 2018–2029.

69. Pierre, F.; Chua, P.C.; O'Brien, S.E.; Siddiqui-Jain, A.; Bourbon, P.; Haddach, M.; Michaux, J.; Nagasawa, J.; Schwaebe, M.K.; Stefan, E.; *et al.* Pre-clinical characterization of CX-4945, a potent and selective small molecule inhibitor of CK2 for the treatment of cancer. *Mol. Cell. Biochem.* 2011, *356*, 37–43.

70. Marconato, L.; Buchholz, J.; Keller, M.; Bettini, G.; Valenti, P.; Kaser-Hotz, B. Multimodal therapeutic approach and interdisciplinary challenge for the treatment of unresectable head and neck squamous cell carcinoma in six cats: A pilot study. *Vet. Compar. Oncol.* 2013, *11*, 101–112.

71. Poirier, V.J.; Kaser-Hotz, B.; Vail, D.M.; Straw, R.C. Efficacy and toxicity of an accelerated hypofractionated radiation therapy protocol in cats with oral squamous cell carcinoma. *Vet. Radiol. Ultrasound* 2013, *54*, 81–88.

72. VetCancerTrials.org. Available online: http://www.vetcancertrials.org/studies/analysis-of-vegfr-pdgfr-and-c-kit-in-feline-oral-squamous-cell-carcinoma (accessed on 12 May 2015).

73. Hayes, H.M., Jr.; Milne, K.L.; Mandell, C.P. Epidemiological features of feline mammary carcinoma. *Vet. Rec.* 1981, *108*, 476–479.

74. Sorenmo, K.U.; Worley, D.R.; Goldschmidt, M.H. Tumors of the Mammary Gland. In *Withrow and MacEwen's Small Animal Clinical Oncology*, 5th ed.; Withrow, S.J., Vail, D.M., Page, R.L., Eds.; Elsevier Saunders: St Louis, MO, USA, 2012; pp. 538–556.

75. Benjamin, S.A.; Lee, A.C.; Saunders, W.J. Classification and behavior of canine mammary epithelial neoplasms based on life-span observations in beagles. *Vet. Pathol.* 1999, *36*, 423–436.

76. Sorenmo, K.U.; Kristiansen, V.M.; Cofone, M.A.; Shofer, F.S.; Breen, A.M.; Langeland, M.; Mongil, C.M.; Grondahl, A.M.; Teige, J.; Goldschmidt, M.H. Canine mammary gland tumours; A histological continuum from benign to malignant; Clinical and histopathological evidence. *Vet. Compar. Oncol.* 2009, *7*, 162–172.

77. Overley, B.; Shofer, F.S.; Goldschmidt, M.H.; Sherer, D.; Sorenmo, K.U. Association between ovarihysterectomy and feline mammary carcinoma. *J. Vet. Intern. Med.* 2005, *19*, 560–563.

78. Taylor, M.R. Genetic testing for inherited breast and ovarian cancer syndromes: Important concepts for the primary care physician. *Postgraduate Med. J.* 2001, *77*, 11–15.

79. Wiese, D.A.; Thaiwong, T.; Yuzbasiyan-Gurkan, V.; Kiupel, M. Feline mammary basal-like adenocarcinomas: A potential model for human triple-negative breast cancer (TNBC) with basal-like subtype. *BMC Cancer* 2013, *13*, 403.

80. Beha, G.; Muscatello, L.V.; Brunetti, B.; Asproni, P.; Millanta, F.; Poli, A.; Benazzi, C.; Sarli, G. Molecular phenotype of primary mammary tumours and distant metastases in female dogs and cats. *J. Compar. Pathol.*2014, *150*, 194–197.

81. Brunetti, B.; Asproni, P.; Beha, G.; Muscatello, L.V.; Millanta, F.; Benazzi, C.; Sarli, G. Molecular phenotype in mammary tumours of queens: Correlation between primary tumour and lymph node metastasis. *J. Compar. Pathol.* 2013, *148*, 206–213.

82. Martin de las Mulas, J.; Van Niel, M.; Millán, Y.; Ordás, J.; Blankenstein, M.A.; Van Mil, F.; Misdorp, W. Progesterone receptors in normal, dysplastic and tumourous feline mammary glands. Comparison with oestrogen receptors status. *Res. Vet. Sci.* 2002, *72*, 153–161.

83. Millanta, F.; Calandrella, M.; Vannozzi, I.; Poli, A. Steroid hormone receptors in normal, dysplastic and neoplastic feline mammary tissues and their prognostic significance. *Vet. Rec.* 2006, *158*, 821–824.

84. Caliari, D.; Zappulli, V.; Rasotto, R.; Cardazzo, B.; Frassineti, F.; Goldschmidt, M.H.; Castagnaro, M. Triple-negative vimentin-positive heterogeneous feline mammary carcinomas as a potential comparative model for breast cancer. *BMC Vet. Res.* 2014, *10*, 185.

85. Carlson, R.W.; Allred, D.C.; Anderson, B.O.; Burstein, H.J.; Carter, W.B.; Edge, S.B.; Erban, J.K.; Farrar, W.B.; Goldstein, L.J.; Gradishar, W.J.; *et al.* Breast cancer. Clinical practice guidelines in oncology. *J. Nat. Compr. Cancer Network* 2009, *7*, 122–192.

86. Millanta, F.; Calandrella, M.; Citi, S.; Della Santa, D.; Poli, A. Overexpression of HER-2 in feline invasive mammary carcinomas: An immunohistochemical survey and evaluation of its prognostic potential. *Vet. Pathol.*2005, *42*, 30–34.

87. Rasotto, R.; Caliari, D.; Castagnaro, M.; Zanetti, R.; Zappulli, V. An immunohistochemical study of HER-2 expression in feline mammary tumours. *J. Compar. Pathol.* 2011, *144*, 170–179.

88. Soares, M.; Correia, J.; Rodrigues, P.; Simões, M.; de Matos, A.; Ferreira, F. Feline HER2 protein expression levels and gene status in feline mammary carcinoma: Optimization of immunohistochemistry (IHC) and *in situ*hybridization (ISH) techniques. *Microsc. Microanal.* 2013, *19*, 876–882.

89. Winston, J.; Craft, D.M.; Scase, T.J.; Bergman, P.J. Immunohistochemical detection of HER-2/neu expression in spontaneous feline mammary tumours. *Vet. Compar. Oncol.* 2005, *3*, 8–15.

90. Maniscalco, L.; Iussich, S.; de Las Mulas, J.M.; Millán, Y.; Biolatti, B.; Sasaki, N.; Nakagawa, T.; De Maria, R. Activation of AKT in feline mammary carcinoma: A new prognostic factor for feline mammary tumours. *Vet. J.*2012, *191*, 65–71.

91. Gibson, H.M.; Veenstra, J.; Jones, R.F.; Vaishampayan, U.; Sauerbrey, M.; Bepler, G.; Lum, L.; Reyes, J.; Weise, A.; Wei, W.Z. Induction of HER2 Immunity in Outbred Domestic Cats by DNA Electrovaccination. *Cancer Immunol. Res.* 2015. Available online: http://www.biomedcentral.com/1471-2407/13/218 (accessed on 25 June 2015).

92. Santos, S.; Baptista, C.S.; Abreu, R.M.; Bastos, E.; Amorim, I.; Gut, I.G.; Gärtner, F.; Chaves, R. ERBB2 in cat mammary neoplasias disclosed a positive correlation between RNA and protein low expression levels: a model for erbB-2 negative human breast cancer. *PLoS ONE*, 2013, 8. Available online: http://journals.plos.org/plosone/article?id=10.1371/journal.pone.0083673 (accessed on 25 June 2015).

93. Malhotra, G.K.; Zhao, X.; Band, H.; Band, V. Histological, molecular and functional subtypes of breast cancers.*Cancer Biol. Therapy* 2010, *10*, 955–960.

94. Morrison, W.B. Inflammation and cancer: A comparative view. *J. Vet. Intern. Med.* 2012, *26*, 18–31.

95. Grivennikov, S.I.; Greten, F.R.; Karin, M. Immunity, inflammation, and cancer. *Cell* 2010, *140*, 883–899.

96. Vascellari, M.; Melchiotti, E.; Bozza, M.A.; Mutinelli, F. Fibrosarcomas at presumed sites of injection in dogs: Characteristics and comparison with non-vaccination site fibrosarcomas and feline post-vaccinal fibrosarcomas. *J. Vet. Med. A Physiol. Pathol. Clin. Med.* 2003, *50*, 286–291.

97. Vascellari, M.; Melchiotti, E.; Mutinelli, F. Fibrosarcoma with typical features of postinjection sarcoma at site of microchip implant in a dog: Histologic and immunohistochemical study. *Vet. Pathol.* 2006, *43*, 545–548.

98. Vascellari, M.; Mutinelli, F.; Cossettini, R.; Altinier, E. Liposarcoma at the site of an implanted microchip in a dog. *Vet. J.* 2004, *168*, 188–190.

99. Murray, J. Vaccine injection-site sarcoma in a ferret. *J. Amer. Vet. Med. Assoc.* 1998, *213*, 955.

100. Keel, S.B.; Jaffe, K.A.; Petur Nielsen, G.; Rosenberg, A.E. Orthopaedic implant-related sarcoma: A study of twelve cases. *Modern Pathol.* 2001, *14*, 969–977.

101. Liptak, J.M.; Forrest, L.J. Soft Tissue Sarcomas. In *Withrow and MacEwen's Small Animal Clinical Oncology*, 5th ed.; Withrow, S.J., Vail, D.M., Page, R.L., Eds.; Elsevier Saunders: St Louis, MO, USA, 2012; pp. 356–380.

102. Dean, R.S.; Pfeiffer, D.U.; Adams, V.J. The incidence of feline injection site sarcomas in the United Kingdom.*BMC Vet. Res.* 2013, *9*, 17.

103. Doddy, F.D.; Glickman, L.T.; Glickman, N.W.; Janovitz, E.B. Feline fibrosarcomas at vaccination sites and non-vaccination sites. *J. Compar. Pathol.* 1996, *114*, 165–174.

104. Couto, S.S.; Griffey, S.M.; Duarte, P.C.; Madewell, B.R. Feline vaccine-associated fibrosarcoma: Morphologic distinctions. *Vet. Pathol.* 2002, *39*, 33–41.

105. Hendrick, M.J.; Brooks, J.J. Postvaccinal Sarcomas in the Cat: Histology and Immunohistochemistry. *Vet. Pathol.*1994, *31*, 126–129.

106. Aberdein, D.; Munday, J.S.; Dyer, C.B.; Knight, C.G.; French, A.F.; Gibson, I.R. Comparison of the histology and immunohistochemistry of vaccination-site and non-vaccination-site sarcomas from cats in New Zealand.*New Zealand Vet. J.* 2007, *55*, 203–207.

107. Dubielzig, R.R.; Everitt, J.; Shadduck, J.A.; Albert, D.M. Clinical and morphologic features of post-traumatic ocular sarcomas in cats. *Vet. Pathol.* 1990, *27*, 62–65.

108. Douglas, J.L.; Gustin, J.K.; Moses, A.V.; Dezube, B.J.; Pantanowitz, L. Kaposi Sarcoma Pathogenesis: A Triad of Viral Infection, Oncogenesis and Chronic Inflammation. *Transl. Biomed.* 2010, 1. Available online: http://www.ncbi.nlm.nih.gov/pmc/articles/PMC3472629/ (accessed on 25 June 2015).

109. Jourdier, T.M.; Moste, C.; Bonnet, M.C.; Delisle, F.; Tafani, J.P.; Devauchelle, P.; Tartaglia, J.; Moingeon, P. Local immunotherapy of spontaneous feline fibrosarcomas using recombinant poxviruses expressing interleukin 2 (IL2). *Gene Therapy* 2003, *10*, 2126–2132.

110. Banerji, N.; Kanjilal, S. Somatic alterations of the p53 tumor suppressor gene in vaccine-associated feline sarcoma. *Amer. J. Vet. Res.* 2006, *67*, 1766–1772.

111. McEntee, M.C.; Page, R.L. Feline vaccine-associated sarcomas. *J. Vet. Intern. Med.* 2001, *15*, 176–182.

112. Tannehill-Gregg, S.; Kergosien, E.; Rosol, T.J. Feline head and neck squamous cell carcinoma cell line: characterization, production of parathyroid hormone-related protein, and regulation by transforming growth factor-beta. *In Vitro Cell. Dev. Biol. Anim.* 2001, *37*, 676–683.

113. Modiano, J.F.; Kokai, Y.; Weiner, D.B.; Pykett, M.J.; Nowell, P.C.; Lyttle, C.R. Progesterone augments proliferation induced by epidermal growth factor in a feline mammary adenocarcinoma cell line. *J. Cell. Biochem.* 1991, *45*, 196–206.

114. Norval, M.; Maingay, J.; Else, R.W. Characteristics of a feline mammary carcinoma cell line. *Res. Vet. Sci.* 1985,*39*, 157–164.

115. Uyama, R.; Hong, S.H.; Nakagawa, T.; Yazawa, M.; Kadosawa, T.; Mochizuki, M.; Tsujimoto, H.; Nishimura, R.; Sasaki, N. Establishment and characterization of eight feline mammary adenocarcinoma cell lines. *J. Vet. Med. Sci.* 2005, *67*, 1273–1276.

116. Takauji, S.R.; Watanabe, M.; Uyama, R.; Nakagawa, T.; Miyajima, N.; Mochizuki, M.; Nishimura, R.; Sugano, S.; Sasaki, N. Expression and subcellular localization of E-cadherin, alpha-catenin, and beta-catenin in 8 feline mammary tumor cell lines. *J. Vet. Med. Sci.* 2007, *69*, 831–834.

117. Muleya, J.S.; Nakaichi, M.; Sugahara, J.; Taura, Y.; Murata, T.; Nakama, S. Establishment and characterization of a new cell line derived from feline mammary tumor. *J. Vet. Med. Sci.* 1998, *60*, 931–935.

118. Muleya, J.S.; Nakaichi, M.; Taura, Y.; Yamaguchi, R.; Nakama, S. *In-vitro* anti-proliferative effects of some anti-tumour drugs on feline mammary tumour cell lines. *Res. Vet. Sci.* 1999, *66*, 169–174.

119. Minke, J.M.; Schuuring, E.; van den Berghe, R.; Stolwijk, J.A.; Boonstra, J.; Cornelisse, C.; Hilkens, J.; Misdorp, W. Isolation of two distinct epithelial cell lines from a single feline mammary carcinoma with different tumorigenic potential in nude mice and expressing different levels of epidermal growth factor receptors.*Cancer Res.* 1991, *51*, 4028–4037.

120. Adelfinger, M.; Gentschev, I.; Grimm de Guibert, J.; Weibel, S.; Langbein-Laugwitz, J.; Härtl, B.; Murua Escobar, H.; Chen, N.G.; Aguilar, R.J.; Yu, Y.A.; *et al.* Evaluation of a new recombinant oncolytic vaccinia virus strain GLV-5b451 for feline mammary carcinoma therapy. *PLoS ONE*, 2014, 9. Available online: http://journals.plos.org/plosone/article?id=10.1371/journal.pone.0104337 (accessed on 25 June 2015).

121. Williams, L.E.; Banerji, N.; Klausner, J.S.; Kapur, V.; Kanjilal, S. Establishment of two vaccine-associated feline sarcoma cell lines and determination of *in vitro* chemosensitivity to doxorubicin and mitoxantrone. *Amer. J. Vet. Res.* 2001, *62*, 1354–1357.

122. Banerji, N.; Li, X.; Klausner, J.S.; Kapur, V.; Kanjilal, S. Evaluation of *in vitro* chemosensitivity of vaccine-associated feline sarcoma cell lines to vincristine and paclitaxel. *Amer. J. Vet. Res.* 2002, *63*, 728–732.

123. Katayama, R.; Huelsmeyer, M.K.; Marr, A.K.; Kurzman, I.D.; Thamm, D.H.; Vail, D.M. Imatinib mesylate inhibits platelet-derived growth factor activity and increases chemosensitivity in feline vaccine-associated sarcoma. *Cancer Chemother. Pharmacol.* 2004, *54*, 25–33.

124. Lawrence, J.; Saba, C.; Gogal, R., Jr.; Lamberth, O.; Vandenplas, M.L.; Hurley, D.J.; Dubreuil, P.; Dobbin, K.; Turek, M. Masitinib demonstrates anti-proliferative and pro-apoptotic activity in primary and metastatic feline injection-site sarcoma cells. *Vet. Compar. Oncol.* 2012, *10*, 143–154.

11
CHAPTER

CYTOGENOMICS OF FELINE CANCERS: ADVANCES AND OPPORTUNITIES

Rachael Thomas

Department of Molecular Biomedical Sciences, College of Veterinary Medicine & Center for Comparative Medicine and Translational Research, North Carolina State University, Raleigh NC 27607, USA;

ABSTRACT

Relative to the dog, integration of the cat into the "One Health" concept has been more restricted, particularly in the field of molecular oncology. Beyond the continual need to enhance the sophistication of feline healthcare per se, the unique spectrum of naturally-occurring cancers in the cat offers tremendous opportunities for comparative and translational advances that may have mutual benefit for human and veterinary medicine. The study of feline cancers additionally may generate new insight into underexplored aspects of tumor biology that are less accessible in other species, such as the relationship between chronic inflammation and neoplasia, and the role of viruses in malignant transformation. Several factors that have hindered molecular studies of feline cancers have now been surmounted, with the most fundamental step forward coming from the development of a high-quality reference genome sequence assembly for the cat. This article reviews landmark studies that have led to our current appreciation of feline genome architecture, and outlines techniques used in cancer cytogenomics, from conventional karyotyping analysis through to the development of genomic microarrays and beyond. A summary of progress in the identification and characterization of chromosomal aberrations in feline cancers is provided using examples from studies of injection-site sarcomas, lymphomas and mammary tumors.

INTRODUCTION

The domestic cat offers a diverse range of opportunities to contribute to the "One Health" concept, which capitalizes on the integration of complementary human and

Citation: Rachael Thomas, Cytogenomics of Feline Cancers: Advances and Opportunities, Vet. Sci. 2015, 2(3), 246-258; doi:10.3390/vetsci2030246

veterinary biomedical research efforts for synergistic gain. Cats continue to grow in popularity as family-owned pets and benefit from increasingly comprehensive medical surveillance [1]. It has been estimated that one in three U.S. households owns at least one cat, equating to a total U.S. cat population of approximately 74 million and a total annual expenditure of approximately $7.4 billion on veterinary services [2]. Cats exhibit approximately 200 genetic diseases that are considered analogous to human disorders, many of which are rarely encountered in any other widely studied species [3]. The cat has served as a particularly powerful model system for studying facets of neuroscience, reproduction and both heritable and infectious disease, and the field of feline oncology offers several novel angles to the comparative medicine arena. The ability to explore these attributes from a molecular standpoint has become possible only relatively recently through intensive efforts to characterize domestic cat genome organization in detail. The combination of data from complementary approaches now allows us to explore the cat genome directly in context with that of humans and other key players in comparative biomedical research. In turn we may now begin to investigate in earnest the causes and consequences of genomic abnormalities associated with heritable and spontaneous disease in our feline companions.

GROSS KARYOTYPIC ORGANIZATION IN THE DOMESTIC CAT

The genome of the domestic cat (*Felis catus*, FCA) is organized into 18 pairs of autosomes and two sex chromosomes. Unlike in other mammals, where autosomes are numbered consecutively in descending order of size, standardized nomenclature in the cat takes into account both chromosome size and morphology. The karyotype comprises six autosomal subgroups termed A-F, with between two and four members in each. All but two autosomal pairs, cat chromosomes (FCA) F1 and F2, are biarmed, as are both sex chromosomes. There is substantial variation in chromosome size throughout the karyotype, from the largest (FCA A1, 240Mb) to the smallest (FCA E3, 43Mb) [4,5]. This marked diversity in size and morphology, broadly comparable to that of the human karyotype, means that chromosome identification in the cat is generally less challenging than in other key model species that exhibit more limited karyotypic variation. Gross similarity in the architecture of the human and domestic cat karyotypes has long been evident through direct comparison of their chromosome banding patterns [6,7]. These observations were reinforced by a series of molecular cytogenetic studies that indicated a remarkably limited degree of divergent evolution between the human and domestic cat genomes over the 92 million years since they shared a common ancestor, compared to the more extensive reshuffling evident in other model species [4,8,9,10,11]. The passage towards development of whole genome sequence assemblies for diverse mammals has since provided a far more comprehensive appreciation of conserved genome organization and potential mechanisms for karyotypic evolution.

GENERATION OF A REFERENCE CAT GENOME SEQUENCE ASSEMBLY

The potential role of the domestic cat in comparative biomedical research was boosted substantially by the generation of a light (~two-fold) coverage feline genome sequence assembly of "Cinnamon", a female Abyssinian, which captured ~65% of euchromatic sequence [12]. This formed part of a broader initiative funded by the National Human Genome Research Institute (NHGRI) to aid interpretation of the human genome sequence assembly, and to investigate patterns of sequence conservation, divergence and rearrangement between rodents, primates and other carnivores [13]. These studies showed that genome evolution in canine, ursine and murine lineages was driven strongly by interchromosomal translocation events, while intrachromosomal inversions were predominant in felids and also most primates [10,12]. A ~14x coverage whole genome assembly has recently become available for "Cinnamon", spanning 2.35 Gb, with sequence annotation for almost 22,000 putative protein-coding cat genes [4,5]. This resource affords a fascinating insight into the genomic factors that provide the unique phenotypic attributes of the domestic cat, and firmly equips the cat to contribute to, and benefit from, a "One Health" approach to biomedical research. Among the most rapid and exciting advances in feline molecular medicine are now being made in the area of oncology.

FUNDAMENTALS OF CANCER CYTOGENOMICS

It is well established that the onset of a malignant phenotype is associated with the accumulation of both random and non-random genomic abnormalities [14,15]. Molecular characterization of numerous diverse human cancers has identified vast numbers of recurrent somatic abnormalities, of which a proportion have been shown to correlate with discrete clinicopathologic criteria [16]. The ability to screen individual patients for these genomic markers has revolutionized diagnostic and prognostic capabilities, refining historically broad tumor classifications into clinically predictive subcategories and paving the way towards personalized disease management strategies. "Genomic profiling" also provides insight into the molecular pathogenesis of disease, identifying gene dosage imbalances associated with functional disruption of regulatory pathways, revealing key mechanistic processes underlying neoplastic transformation and progression and highlighting opportunities for targeted therapeutics.

Techniques for molecular cytogenomic evaluation of tumors fall broadly into two categories (see [17] for a detailed review). Direct techniques, such as fluorescence *in situ* hybridization (FISH) analysis, enable both structural and numerical assessment of small numbers of discrete genomic loci (typically < five) within individual cells. In contrast, indirect methods, such as comparative genomic hybridization (CGH) analysis, permit semi-quantitative measurement of mean DNA copy number within a tumor cell population at many thousands of defined intervals selected throughout the genome, but cannot detect balanced structural rearrangements. Since cancers typically exhibit a combination of both structural and numerical aberrations coupled with cell-to-cell heterogeneity, these highly complementary approaches are often used in tandem. Modified protocols allow their application to challenging specimens, such as those where the availability of clinical material is limited, or where the integrity of the sample is compromised, such as archived histologic specimens. This opens up a multitude of possibilities for retrospective studies of case materials for which detailed clinical histories are available.

The concepts of cancer cytogenomics are well established in human medicine, and enormous strides have been made in translating the same fundamental principles to domestic dog cancers. This has revealed remarkable conservation of discrete molecular alterations in human and canine counterparts of the same cancer (reviewed in [18,19]), providing strong evidence in support of a shared pathogenesis. Progress in the feline field is now gaining momentum, particularly in those areas in which the cat offers a novel perspective that has not been explored in other model species.

INJECTION-SITE SARCOMA

It is now 25 years since concerns were first raised over the increasing number of reports of malignant lesions arising at routine vaccination sites in cats [20]. The masses, predominantly fibrosarcomas, were observed most commonly in association with inflammatory reactions following the use of adjuvanted vaccines against rabies and feline leukemia virus. Vaccine-site sarcomas typically exhibit a rapid, aggressive clinical course and a bleak long-term prognosis. Treatment often involves radical surgical intervention due to the highly invasive nature of the disease, despite which localized post-surgical recurrence is common [21]. Since wide surgical margins markedly reduce the risk of tumor regrowth, there has been widespread encouragement for a transition away from traditional interscapular and femoral vaccination sites where adequate resection is highly challenging. The introduction of non-adjuvanted vaccines has also gone some way to limit the impact of vaccine-site sarcoma; however it remains a substantial clinical concern in feline medicine [22].

Interestingly, histopathologically similar tumors have also been described, infrequently, in dogs, ferrets and rabbits [23,24]. Furthermore, this phenomenon is not restricted to vaccination, since there are reports, albeit rare, of apparently related tumors manifesting in conjunction with injection of other fluids, in response to non-absorbable suture materials and even following microchipping procedures [21]. This has led to increased usage of the term "injection-site sarcoma" (ISS). Additionally, ISS shares many features with lesions occurring following ocular trauma in cats, and also with tumors arising in people in response to prolonged contact with foreign materials, such as artificial implants [22,25]. Taken in combination, these observations provide intriguing evidence for an association between persistent inflammation and malignant transformation. More than two decades after the first description of ISS, however, there remains no solid, detailed explanation for their underlying etiology, and they remain somewhat of an enigma [26,27].

Recognition of the etiology, incidence and impact of feline ISS has been challenged by difficulty in conclusive distinction between these sarcomas and those arising spontaneously without an apparent underlying injection-related origin. ISS typically are more locally invasive and prone to local recurrence than fibrosarcomas of spontaneous origin (non-ISS). Consequently, ISS generally warrant highly extensive surgical margins followed by regular and meticulous monitoring for recurrence, while non-ISS tumors may respond favorably to more conservative clinical management [27,28]. The ability to distinguish ISS from non-ISS at diagnosis therefore has far-reaching implications for patient, owner and clinician; however their extensive clinicopathologic similarity often confounds prompt and unequivocal identification. Distinction between these subtypes currently involves combinatorial consideration of multiple histopathologic features in context with clinical history and anatomical location, and often remains subjective and inconclusive. Currently there are no robust and broadly consistent diagnostic features for distinction between these subtypes. Advances in feline genomics now offer a potential molecular means to address this need and comprehend the factors that underlie the differences in their biological behavior.

Prior to the genomics era, conventional cytogenetic studies identified highly disrupted karyotypic organization in feline fibrosarcomas, with frequent hyperdiploidy and broad cell-to-cell heterogeneity [29,30,31,32]. A putative link has since been reported between amplification of feline satellite DNA sequences and the onset of genomic instability in fibrosarcomas, likely through disruption of normal centromere activity and the formation of aberrant marker chromosomes [33]. A subsequent study of five established ISS cell lines by classical enumeration of banded chromosome preparations also showed tremendously complex karyotypic reorganization, with a range of 19 to 155 chromosomes per cell, as compared to the normal 2n = 38 [34]. None of these studies, however, included detailed assessment of the composition of these aberrant chromosome structures.

Towards this goal, a microarray platform was developed to permit CGH-based identification of recurrent genomic DNA copy number aberrations (CNAs) in feline tumors [35]. This "aneuploidy array" comprised 210 large-insert clones representing loci anchored at ~15 Mb intervals throughout the initial 2x-coverage cat genome sequence assembly. Microarray-based profiling of 46 retrospective primary feline fibrosarcomas identified an extensive range of highly recurrent CNAs, consistent with the high level of genomic instability identified in earlier chromosome-based studies. Targeted FISH analysis of tumor chromosome preparations demonstrated broad heterogeneity in the patterns of structural and numerical aberrations evident both within and between cases. Remarkably, combined CGH and FISH analyses showed that a subset of genomic regions exhibited in excess of 30 copies within individual tumor cells, which were distributed across as many as ten different chromosome structures. Also of note, ISS cases showed non-random reorganization of FCA E1 in conjunction with copy number amplification of a discrete region on FCA E1p12 [35], consistent with the location of a nucleolar organizing region (NOR) [36]. Elevated argyrophilic nucleolar organizing region (AgNOR) scores, as defined by silver staining analysis, are common indicators of increased cellular proliferation, and have been associated with decreased overall survival for canine soft tissue sarcomas [37]. It is tempting to consider that this may reflect the inferior outcome that is typically associated with ISS. Statistical comparison of genomic profiles across the cohort identified two subchromosomal regions that showed significant differences in DNA copy number status in ISS *versus* non-ISS cases. While providing support for molecular discrimination, the limited resolution capabilities of the aneuploidy array confounded the ability to refine the boundaries of these regions and in turn to assess their gene content [35].

A higher-density second-generation cat CGH microarray platform has since been developed utilizing the 14x coverage cat genome sequence assembly, comprising

~110,000 oligonucleotide probes distributed at mean intervals of ~21kb. This provides a >300-fold increase in resolution over the aneuploidy array, bringing feline resources closely in line with those of other model systems for the first time. Evaluation of the same cohort of feline fibrosarcomas with this more comprehensive platform [38] identified homozygous deletions of the tumor-suppressor gene *PTEN* and recurrent amplifications of the *KIT* proto-oncogene. Elevated *KIT* protein expression has been reported as a persistent finding in both ISS and non-ISS tumors [39]; however it is not yet clear whether upregulation is a direct consequence of increased *KIT* gene dosage, nor whether this confers potential for utilizing targeted therapies directed towards this receptor tyrosine kinase. ISS and non-ISS tumors showed grossly comparable profiles of DNA copy number imbalance; however ISS cases exhibited elevated levels of global genomic disruption, consistent with their typically more aggressive behavior and poorer outcome. Among these lay a subset of discrete regions with promise as discriminatory markers [38]. With focus on the most clinicopathologically compelling genomic regions, in combination with assessment of transcriptional and translational status, there is great promise for a more detailed definition of the molecular pathogenesis of feline fibrosarcomas, and in turn, for refinement of diagnostic and therapeutic modalities for both subtypes. In a broader sense, genomic characterization of ISS also may aid elucidation of molecular mechanisms involved in the passage from chronic inflammation to neoplastic transformation, which continues to challenge human medicine.

LYMPHOMA

Lymphoma is the most common hematopoietic malignancy of cats and the third most common feline cancer overall, comprising approximately one third of all cancer diagnoses. Moreover, cats are considered to show the highest relative incidence of lymphoma among all species studied to date (reviewed in [40]), offering another promising angle for comprehending key facets of tumor biology. Historically, cytogenetic studies of feline lymphomas have focused heavily on established cell lines, primarily those developed from tumors associated with infection by feline leukemia virus, which often are nodal or mediastinal in origin. Common observations from these reports include hyperdiploidies resulting from low amplitude copy number increases of a variety of chromosomes, with no strongly recurrent features. These investigations have greatly expanded our understanding of the mechanisms by which clonal proviral integration into a host genome can initiate tumorigenesis and genomic instability through oncogenic activation [41,42]. With the diminished incidence of retrovirus-associated feline lymphoma since the 1980's, as a result of increased testing, vaccination and global vigilance, the focus has since shifted toward subtypes that offer opportunities for a more comparative approach.

Extensive volumes of clinically predictive cytogenomic data are accumulating for nodal lymphomas in human patients, and more recently also in dogs [43,44]. In contrast, gastrointestinal (GI) lymphoma, which represents the most common extranodal form in people and comprises more than 50% of all feline lymphomas, remains vastly understudied at the molecular level [45,46,47,48]. Given the high incidence of the disease in cats there is an opportunity for feline studies to pave the way forward for mutual benefit. In cats, the overall survival time for low-grade small-cell GI-lymphomas is generally four-fold greater than for high-grade large-cell tumors, following standard of care chemotherapy [45,49]. The relative frequency of these histologic subtypes in different anatomical locations varies widely in prior reports [40,45,50,51,52], in part due to the logistical challenges of performing diagnostic evaluation of GI lesions by surgical biopsy [40,53]. This invites assessment of a genomic approach for comprehensive DNA-based subclassification. Initial observations from microarray-based CGH analysis have indicated that feline GI-lymphoma exhibits a relatively subtle degree of genomic copy number instability, with no evidence for recurrent high-level amplifications or homozygous deletions. The majority of aberrations are shared by fewer than 30% of cases, and include defects involving key cancer-associated genes, such as elevated copy number of the *MYC* proto-oncogene and deletion of *PTEN*. Efforts to identify candidates for molecular distinction between histologic and immunophenotypic subtypes are now underway [54].

MAMMARY CARCINOMA

Mammary tumors represent the third most commonly diagnosed feline neoplasm, the vast majority of which (in contrast to dogs) are malignant, primarily simple carcinomas. Feline mammary carcinomas (FMCs) generally are highly aggressive, infiltrative and metastatic and show extensive heterogeneity in outcome that is not readily predicted at the time of diagnosis [55]. FMC shares extensive clinicopathologic, demographic and epidemiological similarity with human breast carcinoma (HBC), the most frequently diagnosed cancer in women [56]. While there is evidence for steroid hormone involvement in some FMCs, 80%–90% are estrogen- and progesterone-receptor negative [57,58,59]. FMC therefore offers a particularly powerful spontaneous model of the ~30% of "basal-like" late-stage HBCs that are highly aggressive and unresponsive to hormone-antagonist therapies, with a lack of targeted treatments and a poor prognosis.

Diagnostic and prognostic descriptions for FMC frequently are limited in detail since there is little evidence to associate specific histomorphologic subtypes with outcome. In HBC histologic grade, typically defined using the Elston and Ellis scoring system, is one of the most robust prognostic factors [60]. Although inconclusive in dogs, it has been shown recently, using this same grading system, that invasive FMC also shows a significant incremental association between histologic grade and outcome [61]. In both human and feline patients, intermediate grade tumors show the lowest concordance in routine diagnosis and the broadest heterogeneity in outcome [60,61], and thus the greatest need for improved subclassification.

Genome-wide surveys of HBC have identified discrete genomic signatures that define clinically predictive subtypes, leading to effective treatment strategies based on molecular pathogenesis [62]. Assessment of evidence for corresponding molecular subtypes in FMC may confer potential to extrapolate these advances rapidly to feline patients. To date, the search for prognostic factors for FMC from a molecular perspective has been targeted to individual candidate genes known to be associated with HBC. Of particular note, approximately 25% of HBCs exhibit upregulation of the *ERBB2* gene encoding the receptor tyrosine kinase HER2/neu, of which >90% exhibit DNA copy number amplification of this region [63]. This aberration, historically considered to be an indicator of poor prognosis, also confers susceptibility to Trastuzamab (Herceptin®), a monoclonal antibody targeted against the HER2/neu receptor. Published estimates of HER2-positive FMCs by immunohistochemistry show tremendous variation between studies, largely due to the use of diverse patient cohorts and contrasting analytical techniques [64]. Consequently the true frequency of HER2-positive FMC, and the relationship between protein expression and gene copy number, is yet to be determined.

At the genome-wide level, early conventional chromosome banding studies of FMC identified highly disrupted karyotypes, including recurrent deletions of FCA B2 and gains of FCA E3 [65,66]. These long predated the "genomics era", precluding detailed interpretation in terms of their significance in disease pathogenesis. Microarray-based molecular profiling of FMC is now yielding more substantial insight. Preliminary results with the second-generation CGH array have demonstrated moderate DNA copy number instability in FMC that is distributed broadly throughout the genome, with very few CNAs shared by more than 50% of cases surveyed [67]. Overall, higher-grade tumors exhibit an elevated incidence of genomic imbalance, suggesting that increased chromosome instability may itself represent an indicator of inferior outcome. Interestingly, copy number gain of *ERBB2* was >3-fold more common in high-grade *versus* intermediate-grade tumors. The incidence of *PTEN* deletion was also increased in high-grade tumors, correlating with an earlier study that showed inferior outcome in FMC cases with decreased PTEN protein expression [68]. Gain of *ERBB2* and deletion of *PTEN* are among the most recurrent genomic imbalances in HBC and are associated with concomitant disregulation of gene expression and anti-apoptotic activity, and in turn with inferior outcome [69]. Continued efforts should offer new insight into the degree to which the clinicopathologic similarities between HBC and FMC are recapitulated at the genomic level, highlighting disrupted pathways and potential therapeutic targets for FMC.

CONCLUSIONS

The domestic cat is becoming increasingly well placed to stimulate new advances in molecular medicine. The unique range and distribution of cancers diagnosed in our feline companions fills a series of critical niches that have confounded progress in human medicine. Included among this diverse spectrum are those with direct human counterparts that have remained understudied due to their rarity in people, while others offer a means to study discrete facets of tumor biology that are largely peculiar to the cat. We are now in a position to perform rapid and comprehensive interrogation of normal and aberrant feline genomes and to interpret our observations directly in terms of gene content and potential dysfunction. In turn we have the ability to extrapolate with relative ease between the genomes of different species in the search for conserved molecular features that suggest a common disease mechanism. Given the gross similarity in the structural organization and evolutionary history of the human and cat genomes, it is conceivable that an integrated cytogenomic approach may help to reveal as yet unrecognized mechanisms of tumor-associated chromosome instability.

The field of personalized medicine continues to make tremendous strides in the human field, and opportunities to integrate similar concepts into the veterinary arena are gradually becoming a reality. Cytogenomic techniques are continuing to evolve, with increases in resolution, sensitivity, flexibility, throughput and cost-effectiveness, coupled with the ability to combine related techniques into single platforms that allow synergistic acquisition of data from complementary approaches in a single experiment. In the human field, cancer cytogenomic discovery is gradually transitioning from chromosome- and microarray-based techniques toward the use of next generation sequencing approaches [17]. These strategies provide substantially increased resolution capabilities and have the advantage of permitting concomitant assessment of both structural and numerical aberrations in conjunction with detection of sequence mutations. At the present time, however, their integration into the veterinary arena is constrained by high costs and intensive computational needs, and limited access to dedicated reagents and analytical tools for non-human species. Ten years ago, the same limitations applied to the use of microarray-based technologies such as those described here. Given that the field of veterinary molecular oncology is now well established, and its comparative and translational value is continually being proven, one must hope that the delay in widespread introduction of next generation sequencing strategies for use in companion animal medicine will be less profound.

REFERENCES

1. Cannon, C. Cats, cancer and comparative oncology. *Vet. Sci.* 2015, *2*, 111–126.
2. American Veterinary Medical Association (AVMA). *U.S. Pet Ownership and Demographics Sourcebook*; AVMA: Schaumburg, IL, USA, 2012.
3. Online Mendelian Inheritance in Animals (OMIA). Faculty of Veterinary Science, University of Sydney. Available online: http://omia.angis.org.au (accessed on 28 May 2015).
4. Montague, M.J.; Li, G.; Gandolfi, B.; Khan, R.; Aken, B.L.; Searle, S.M.; Minx, P.; Hillier, L.W.; Koboldt, D.C.; Davis, B.W.; *et al.* Comparative analysis of the domestic cat genome reveals genetic signatures underlying feline biology and domestication. *Proc. Natl. Acad. Sci. USA* 2014, *111*, 17230–17235.
5. Tamazian, G.; Simonov, S.; Dobrynin, P.; Makunin, A.; Logachev, A.; Komissarov, A.; Shevchenko, A.; Brukhin, V.; Cherkasov, N.; Svitin, A.; *et al.* Annotated features of domestic cat-*Felis catus* genome. *Gigascience* 2014, *3*.
6. Nash, W.G.; O'Brien, S.J. Conserved regions of homologous G-banded chromosomes between orders in mammalian evolution: Carnivores and primates. *Proc. Natl. Acad. Sci. USA* 1982, *79*, 6631–6635.
7. Yang, F.; Graphodatsky, A.S.; O'Brien, P.C.; Colabella, A.; Solanky, N.; Squire, M.; Sargan, D.R.; Ferguson-Smith, M.A. Reciprocal chromosome painting illuminates the history of genome evolution of the domestic cat, dog and human. *Chromosome Res.* 2000, *8*, 393–404.

8. Rettenberger, G.; Klett, C.; Zechner, U.; Bruch, J.; Just, W.; Vogel, W.; Hameister, H. Zoo-FISH analysis: Cat and human karyotypes closely resemble the putative ancestral mammalian karyotype. *Chromosome Res.* 1995, *3*, 479–486.

9. Stanyon, R.; Yang, F.; Cavagna, P.; O'Brien, P.C.; Bagga, M.; Ferguson-Smith, M.A.; Wienberg, J. Reciprocal chromosome painting shows that genomic rearrangement between rat and mouse proceeds ten times faster than between humans and cats. *Cytogenet. Cell Genet.* 1999, *84*, 150–155.

10. O'Brien, S.J.; Johnson, W.; Driscoll, C.; Pontius, J.; Pecon-Slattery, J.; Menotti-Raymond, M. State of cat genomics. *Trends Genet.* 2008, *24*, 268–279.

11. Graphodatsky, A.S.; Trifonov, V.A.; Stanyon, R. The genome diversity and karyotype evolution of mammals.*Mol. Cytogenet.* 2011, *4*.

12. Pontius, J.U.; Mullikin, J.C.; Smith, D.R.; Lindblad-Toh, K.; Gnerre, S.; Clamp, M.; Chang, J.; Stephens, R.; Neelam, B.; Volfovsky, N.; *et al.* Initial sequence and comparative analysis of the cat genome. *Genome Res.* 2007,*17*, 1675–1689.

13. Lindblad-Toh, K.; Garber, M.; Zuk, O.; Lin, M.F.; Parker, B.J.; Washietl, S.; Kheradpour, P.; Ernst, J.; Jordan, G.; Mauceli, E.; *et al.* A high-resolution map of human evolutionary constraint using 29 mammals. *Nature* 2011,*478*, 476–482.

14. Bernheim, A. Cytogenomics of cancers: From chromosome to sequence. *Mol. Oncol.* 2010, *4*, 309–322.

15. Sandberg, A.A.; Meloni-Ehrig, A.M. Cytogenetics and genetics of human cancer: Methods and accomplishments. *Cancer Genet. Cytogenet.* 2010, *203*, 102–126.

16. Mitelman, F.; Johansson, B.; Mertens, F. Mitelman Database of Chromosome Aberrations and Gene Fusions in Cancer. Available online: http://cgap.nci.nih.gov/chromosomes/mitelman (accessed on 31 May 2015).

17. Le Scouarnec, S.; Gribble, S.M. Characterising chromosome rearrangements: Recent technical advances in molecular cytogenetics. *Heredity (Edinb)* 2012, *108*, 75–85.

18. Breen, M. Comparative Cytogenetics. Available online: http://www.els.net (accessed on 22 July 2015).

19. Schiffman, J.D.; Breen, M. Comparative oncology: What dogs and other species can teach us about humans with cancer. *Phil. Trans. Roy. Soc. B-Biol. Sci.* 2015, *370*.

20. Hendrick, M.J.; Goldschmidt, M.H. Do injection site reactions induce fibrosarcomas in cats? *J. Amer. Vet. Med. Assoc.* 1991. Avaiable online: http://europepmc.org/abstract/med/1748617 (accessed 28 August 2015).

21. Martano, M.; Morello, E.; Buracco, P. Feline injection-site sarcoma: Past, present and future perspectives. *Vet. J.*2011, *188*, 136–141.

22. Woodward, K.N. Origins of injection-site sarcomas in cats: The possible role of chronic inflammation—A review. *ISRN Vet. Sci.* 2011, *2011*.

23. Munday, J.S.; Stedman, N.L.; Richey, L.J. Histology and immunohistochemistry of seven ferret vaccination-site fibrosarcomas. *Vet. Pathol.* 2003, *40*, 288–293.

24. Vascellari, M.; Melchiotti, E.; Bozza, M.A.; Mutinelli, F. Fibrosarcomas at presumed sites of injection in dogs: Characteristics and comparison with non-vaccination site fibrosarcomas and feline post-vaccinal fibrosarcomas. *J. Vet. Med. A-Physiol. Pathol. Clin. Med.* 2003, *50*, 286–291.

25. Moizhess, T.G. Carcinogenesis induced by foreign bodies. *Biochemistry (Mosc.)* 2008, *73*, 763–775.

26. Hendrick, M.J. Musings on feline injection site sarcomas. *Vet. J.* 2011, *188*, 130–131.

27. Ladlow, J. Injection site-associated sarcoma in the cat: Treatment recommendations and results to date. *J. Feline Med. Surg.* 2013, *15*, 409–418.

28. Dobson, J.M.; Demetriou, J.; Seguin, B. Chapters 20: Skin tumors and 22: Injection site sarcomas. In *Feline Soft Tissue and General Surgery*, 1st ed.; Langley-Hobbs, S., Demetriou, J., Ladlow, J., Eds.; Saunders Elsevier: Philadelphia, PA, USA, 2013; pp. 209–242.

29. Kalat, M.; Mayr, B.; Schleger, W.; Wagner, B.; Reifinger, M. Chromosomal hyperdiploidy in a feline sarcoma.*Res. Vet. Sci.* 1991, *51*, 227–228.

30. Mayr, B.; Bockstahler, B.; Loupal, G.; Reifinger, M.; Schleger, W. Cytogenetic variation between four cases of feline fibrosarcoma. *Res. Vet. Sci.* 1996, *61*, 268–270.

31. Mayr, B.; Eschborn, U.; Kalat, M. Near triploidy in a feline fibrosarcoma. *Zentralbl. Veterinarmed. A* 1991, *38*, 617–620.

32. Mayr, B.; Hofstadler, E.; Schleger, W.; Reifinger, M.; Eisenmenger, E. Trisomy D1, marker F1: New cytogenetic findings in two cases of feline fibrosarcoma. *Zentralbl. Veterinarmed. A* 1994, *41*, 197–201.

33. Santos, S.; Chaves, R.; Adega, F.; Bastos, E.; Guedes-Pinto, H. Amplification of the major satellite DNA family (FA-SAT) in a cat fibrosarcoma might be related to chromosomal instability. *J. Hered.* 2006, *97*, 114–118.

34. von Erichsen, J.; Hecht, W.; Lohberg-Gruene, C.; Reinacher, M. Cell lines derived from feline fibrosarcoma display unstable chromosomal aneuploidy and additionally centrosome number aberrations. *Vet. Pathol.* 2012,*49*, 648–657.

35. Thomas, R.; Valli, V.E.; Ellis, P.; Bell, J.; Karlsson, E.K.; Cullen, J.; Lindblad-Toh, K.; Langford, C.F.; Breen, M. Microarray-based cytogenetic profiling reveals recurrent and subtype-associated genomic copy number aberrations in feline sarcomas. *Chromosome Res.* 2009, *17*, 987–1000.

36. Szczerbal, I.; Michalak, E. FISH-localization of the nucleolar organizer region on the feline E1p12 chromosome.*Anim. Genet.* 2003, *34*, 386–387.

37. Ettinger, S.N.; Scase, T.J.; Oberthaler, K.T.; Craft, D.M.; McKnight, J.A.; Leibman, N.F.; Charney, S.C.; Bergman, P.J. Association of argyrophilic nucleolar organizing regions, Ki-67, and proliferating cell nuclear antigen scores with histologic grade and survival in dogs with soft tissue sarcomas: 60 cases (1996–2002). *J. Am. Vet. Med. Assoc.* 2006, *228*, 1053–1062.

38. Thomas, R.; Pontius, J.; Borst, L.; Lamm, C.; Breen, M. Development Of A Genome-Anchored Microarray Platform for Identification of Clinically Predictive Somatic DNA Copy Number Aberrations in Feline Cancers. In Proceedings of the 7th International Conference on Advances in Canine and Feline Genomics and Inherited Diseases, Cambridge, MA, USA, 23–27 September 2013.

39. Smith, A.J.; Njaa, B.L.; Lamm, C.G. Immunohistochemical expression of c-KIT protein in feline soft tissue fibrosarcomas. *Vet. Pathol.* 2009, *46*, 934–939.

40. Moore, P.F.; Rodriguez-Bertos, A.; Kass, P.H. Feline gastrointestinal lymphoma: Mucosal architecture, immunophenotype, and molecular clonality. *Vet. Pathol.* 2011, *49*, 658–668.

41. Wu, F.Y.; Iijima, K.; Tsujimoto, H.; Tamura, Y.; Higurashi, M. Chromosomal translocations in two feline T-cell lymphomas. *Leuk. Res.* 1995, *19*, 857–860.

42. Fujino, Y.; Ma, Z.; Satoh, H.; Mizuno, T.; Hisasue, M.; Baba, K.; Masuda, K.; Ohno, K.; Onishi, T.; Tsujimoto, H. Characterization of a newly established nonproducer lymphoma cell line for feline leukemia virus. *Vet. Immunol. Immunopathol.* 2004, *102*, 429–439.

43. Breen, M.; Modiano, J.F. Evolutionarily conserved cytogenetic changes in hematological malignancies of dogs and humans—Man and his best friend share more than companionship. *Chromosome Res.* 2008, *16*, 145–154.

44. Thomas, R.; Seiser, E.L.; Motsinger-Reif, A.; Borst, L.; Valli, V.E.; Kelley, K.; Suter, S.E.; Argyle, D.; Burgess, K.; Bell, J.; *et al.* Refining tumor-associated aneuploidy through "genomic recoding" of recurrent DNA copy number aberrations in 150 canine non-Hodgkin lymphomas. *Leuk. Lymphoma* 2011, *52*, 1321–1335.

45. Wilson, H.M. Feline alimentary lymphoma: Demystifying the enigma. *Top. Companion Anim. Med.* 2008, *23*, 177–184.

46. Vail, D.M. Chapter 324: Hematopoetic tumors. In *Textbook of Veterinary Internal Medicine*, 7th ed.; Ettinger, S.N., Feldman, E.C., Eds.; Saunders: Philadelphia, PA, USA, 2009; p. 2148.

47. Rissetto, K.; Villamil, J.A.; Selting, K.A.; Tyler, J.; Henry, C.J. Recent trends in feline intestinal neoplasia: An epidemiologic study of 1129 cases in the veterinary medical database from 1964 to 2004. *J. Am. Anim. Hosp. Assoc.* 2011, *47*, 28–36.

48. Jasdanwala, S.; Pitchumoni, C. Epidemiological spectrum of gastrointestinal lymphoma. *Pract. Gastroenterol.*2014, *38*, 8–28.

49. Moore, P.F.; Woo, J.C.; Vernau, W.; Kosten, S.; Graham, P.S. Characterization of feline T cell receptor gamma (TCRG) variable region genes for the molecular diagnosis of feline intestinal T cell lymphoma. *Vet. Immunol. Immunopathol.* 2005, *106*, 167–178.

50. Waly, N.E.; Gruffydd-Jones, T.J.; Stokes, C.R.; Day, M.J. Immunohistochemical diagnosis of alimentary lymphomas and severe intestinal inflammation in cats. *J. Comp. Pathol.* 2005, *133*, 253–260.

51. Briscoe, K.A.; Krockenberger, M.; Beatty, J.A.; Crowley, A.; Dennis, M.M.; Canfield, P.J.; Dhand, N.; Lingard, A.E.; Barrs, V.R. Histopathological and immunohistochemical evaluation of 53 cases of feline lymphoplasmacytic enteritis and low-grade alimentary lymphoma. *J. Comp. Pathol.* 2011, *145*, 187–198.

52. Pohlman, L.M.; Higginbotham, M.L.; Welles, E.G.; Johnson, C.M. Immunophenotypic and histologic classification of 50 cases of feline gastrointestinal lymphoma. *Vet. Pathol.* 2009, *46*, 259–268.

53. Scott, K.D.; Zoran, D.L.; Mansell, J.; Norby, B.; Willard, M.D. Utility of endoscopic biopsies of the duodenum and ileum for diagnosis of inflammatory bowel disease and small cell lymphoma in cats. *J. Vet. Intern. Med.*2011, *25*, 1253–1257.

54. Thomas, R.; *et al.* Genomic profiling of feline gastrointestinal lymphoma (To be submitted).

55. Hughes, K.; Dobson, J.M. Prognostic histopathological and molecular markers in feline mammary neoplasia.*Vet. J.* 2012, *194*, 19–26.

56. Siegel, R.; Naishadham, D.; Jemal, A. Cancer statistics, 2013. *CA Cancer J. Clin.* 2013, *63*, 11–30.

57. Burrai, G.P.; Mohammed, S.I.; Miller, M.A.; Marras, V.; Pirino, S.; Addis, M.F.; Uzzau, S.; Antuofermo, E. Spontaneous feline mammary intraepithelial lesions as a model for human estrogen receptor- and progesterone receptor-negative breast lesions. *BMC Cancer* 2010, *10*.

58. Gimenez, F.; Hecht, S.; Craig, L.E.; Legendre, A.M. Early detection, aggressive therapy: Optimizing the management of feline mammary masses. *J. Feline Med. Surg.* 2010, *12*, 214–224.

59. Zappulli, V.; De Zan, G.; Cardazzo, B.; Bargelloni, L.; Castagnaro, M. Feline mammary tumours in comparative oncology. *J. Dairy Res.* 2005, *72*, 98–106.

60. Rakha, E.A.; Reis-Filho, J.S.; Baehner, F.; Dabbs, D.J.; Decker, T.; Eusebi, V.; Fox, S.B.; Ichihara, S.; Jacquemier, J.; Lakhani, S.R.; *et al.* Breast cancer prognostic classification in the molecular era: The role of histological grade. *Breast Cancer Res.* 2010, *12*, 207.

61. Seixas, F.; Palmeira, C.; Pires, M.A.; Bento, M.J.; Lopes, C. Grade is an independent prognostic factor for feline mammary carcinomas: A clinicopathological and survival analysis. *Vet. J.* 2011, *187*, 65–71.

62. Curtis, C.; Shah, S.P.; Chin, S.F.; Turashvili, G.; Rueda, O.M.; Dunning, M.J.; Speed, D.; Lynch, A.G.; Samarajiwa, S.; Yuan, Y.; *et al.* The genomic and transcriptomic architecture of 2000 breast tumours reveals novel subgroups. *Nature* 2012, *486*, 346–352.

63. Kiyose, S.; Igarashi, H.; Nagura, K.; Kamo, T.; Kawane, K.; Mori, H.; Ozawa, T.; Maeda, M.; Konno, K.; Hoshino, H.; *et al.* Chromogenic *in situ* hybridization (CISH) to detect HER2 gene amplification in breast and gastric cancer: Comparison with immunohistochemistry (IHC) and fluorescence *in situ* hybridization (FISH). *Pathol. Int.* 2012, *62*, 728–734.

64. Rasotto, R.; Caliari, D.; Castagnaro, M.; Zanetti, R.; Zappulli, V. An immunohistochemical study of HER-2 expression in feline mammary tumours. *J. Comp. Pathol.* 2011, *144*, 170–179.

65. Mayr, B.; Jugl, M.; Brem, G.; Reifinger, M.; Loupal, G. Cytogenetic variation in six cases of feline mammary tumours. *Zentralbl. Veterinarmed. A* 1999, *46*, 367–377.

66. Mayr, B.; Ortner, W.; Reifinger, M.; Loupal, G. Loss of chromosome B2-material in three cases of feline mammary tumours. *Res. Vet. Sci* 1995, *59*, 61–63.

67. Thomas, R.; Seixas, F.; Borst, L.; Breen, M. Landscapes of Genomic Copy Number Aberrations in Feline Mammary Cancer. In Proceedings of the 8th International Conference on Advances in Canine and Feline Genomics and Inherited Diseases, Cambridge, UK; Available online: http://www.caninefelinegenomicsconference.org/ (accessed on 22–26 June 2015).

68. Ressel, L.; Millanta, F.; Caleri, E.; Innocenti, V.M.; Poli, A. Reduced pten protein expression and its prognostic implications in canine and feline mammary tumors. *Vet. Pathol.* 2009, *46*, 860–868.

69. Curtis, C.; Lynch, A.G.; Dunning, M.J.; Spiteri, I.; Marioni, J.C.; Hadfield, J.; Chin, S.F.; Brenton, J.D.; Tavare, S.; Caldas, C. The pitfalls of platform comparison: DNA copy number array technologies assessed. *BMC Genom.*2009, *10*

12

CHAPTER

ANIMAL MODELS OF ALLERGIC DISEASES

Domenico Santoro and Rosanna Marsella

Department of Small Animal Clinical Sciences, College of Veterinary Medicine, University of Florida, Gainesville, FL 32610, USA

ABSTRACT

Allergic diseases have great impact on the quality of life of both people and domestic animals. They are increasing in prevalence in both animals and humans, possibly due to the changed lifestyle conditions and the decreased exposure to beneficial microorganisms. Dogs, in particular, suffer from environmental skin allergies and develop a clinical presentation which is very similar to the one of children with eczema. Thus, dogs are a very useful species to improve our understanding on the mechanisms involved in people's allergies and a natural model to study eczema. Animal models are frequently used to elucidate mechanisms of disease and to control for confounding factors which are present in studies with patients with spontaneously occurring disease and to test new therapies that can be beneficial in both species. It has been found that drugs useful in one species can also have benefits in other species highlighting the importance of a comprehensive understanding of diseases across species and the value of comparative studies. The purpose of the current article is to review allergic diseases across species and to focus on how these diseases compare to the counterpart in people.

INTRODUCTION

Several types of allergic diseases affect the skin in both humans and animals. One of the most common is atopic dermatitis (AD), also referred to as eczema in human medicine. Atopic disease is genetically inherited in all species and results from complex interactions between genetic and environmental factors. In a subset of patients, AD is linked to allergies. In people, the first manifestation of atopic disease is cutaneous and

Citation: Domenico Santoro and Rosanna Marsella, Animal Models of Allergic Diseases, Vet. Sci. 2014, 1(3), 192-212; doi:10.3390/vetsci1030192

is frequently first triggered by food allergens. The disease is chronic and relapsing in nature with acute exacerbations frequently associated with allergen exposure. Many studies have shown evidence of various mutations affecting skin barrier function highlighting the fact that sensitization occurs first through defective skin. Due to the increased permeability of the skin, allergens are more readily absorbed and this increased exposure leads to the development of allergic sensitization. As the disease progresses, sensitizations may develop against a variety of environmental allergens and not just foods. Some patients appear to progress from the cutaneous phase to respiratory signs such as asthma as part of the "atopic march", although debate still exists in human medicine regarding the existence of this phenomenon. Atopic disease has become very common in industrialized countries possibly due to changes in lifestyle and diet and much effort has been devoted to identifying the causes and mechanisms to either prevent or minimize this epidemic of allergies. For this reason many animal models have been studied for both environmental and food allergies. Many similarities, yet some differences exist in the manifestation of AD across species. Some of these differences can be leveraged to improve our understanding regarding the mechanisms involved in the pathogenesis of this complex disease and, in the future, to improve our understanding on why some individuals have multiple manifestations of atopic disease and some only have one clinical sign. In this review, we will discuss the various models by focusing on the primary manifestation of allergy that they were attempting to reproduce and study.

ATOPIC DERMATITIS: COMPARATIVE OBSERVATIONS

With this term in veterinary medicine, we refer to a recurrent chronic pruritic dermatitis with a characteristic distribution and most often associated with allergen specific IgE against environmental allergens [1]. People also suffer from AD. The term eczema is frequently used interchangeably with AD in human medicine while it has been abandoned in veterinary medicine. Eczema has become quite common in children in westernized countries and it is estimated to affect approximately 40% of preschool children in the USA and the UK [2,3]. This increase has a major impact both medically and financially and it has been referred to as an epidemic of allergies.

The clinical distribution of AD is very similar between children and dogs. Lesions are erythematous, pruritic and prone to be secondarily infected with *Staphylococcus spp.* Areas that are typically affected are folds and flexural surfaces such as the antebrachial area, axillary, and groin area. The perioral and periocular regions, hands and feet are also commonly involved.

In both species, AD is frequently *but not always* linked to an allergic sensitization. There is indeed a subset of patients in both humans and dogs in which the disease is not linked to allergies. This form of AD is called "intrinsic" or "not allergic" to differentiate it from the more classic "extrinsic" or "allergic" form of the disease in which allergen specific IgE are detectable [4,5,6]. Approximately 10% of people with AD are affected by the "intrinsic" form. Although the intrinsic form has been considered by some as a step toward the development of extrinsic form, it is becoming increasingly clear that it may actually represent a different subtype [5]. No difference in severity of disease is typically observed between the two subsets of patients although different frequency in distribution of lesions has been described [7]. The intrinsic form tends to develop in older patients and filaggrin mutations are not a characteristic of this form [8]. Studies investigating skin barrier function in patients diagnosed with intrinsic AD have shown that normal function and sensory reactivity to external stimuli is retained in these individuals, which is different from patients with the extrinsic form [9]. Immunologically, lower expression of T helper (Th)2 cytokines such as Interleukin (IL)-4, 5, and 13 are found in affected individuals. The same distinction has been proposed in the dog and the term atopic-like dermatitis" has been proposed for individuals in which no detectable IgE can be found. Multiple immune dysregulations have been reported in AD. It is generally accepted that AD may in part be due to defective immune tolerance [10]. Regulatory mechanisms are necessary to maintain peripheral tolerance by the immune system [11]. Regulatory T cells (Tregs) are a diverse subset of T cells capable of dampening inflammatory cell responses [12,13]. Several studies have shown that Tregs are dysfunctional in atopic patients [5,14] leading to aberrant immune response after allergen exposure. Other immune dysregulations described in allergic skin diseases have highlighted the role of basophils [15] and mast cells [16]. Interestingly, no increased skin mast cells' releasability [17] and no increased circulating levels of histamine have been reported in human AD patients [18]. Additionally, the usefulness of antihistamines H1 receptor blockers is limited [12]. More interest now exists in the role of H4 receptors and other mast cell products such as tryptase [19,20]. In particular, the histamine H4 receptor has been demonstrated to mediate inflammation and Th2-dependent inflammation and is a potential target for future therapies [21,22,23,24].

In dogs with AD, studies examining number of mast cells and the histamine release between normal and atopic dogs showed no differences or even a lower mast cell density in lesional and non-lesional atopic skin compared to healthy control skin [25]. In addition, studies evaluating serum histamine concentrations revealed that levels are similar [26] or lower [27] in dogs with AD compared to healthy controls, thus the role of histamine is still under debate. Interestingly, the few studies evaluating the effect of antihistamines, including H4 blockers, have failed to report a beneficial effect [28,29]. In a subset of human patients with AD, genetically inherited skin barrier defects are demonstrable and further skin barrier impairment occurs once sensitization develops and inflammation is triggered [30]. Thus, skin barrier impairment can be both primary and secondary and it plays some role in all patients at some point during the course of the disease. One of the most documented genetically inherited mutations is in the filaggrin gene. Filaggrin is very important for proper keratinization (the process of differentiation of cutaneous epithelial cells). Mutations in the filaggrin gene have been extensively studied and reported in people with AD to the point that null mutations in this gene, leading to a decrease expression of filaggrin, are considered one of the strongest risk factors for the development of the disease [31,32]. It is important to note that not all patients with AD have filaggrin mutations and that some patients with them do not necessarily develop the disease, highlighting the fact that the development of AD is multifactorial resulting from a complex interaction between genetics and environmental conditions. As primary skin barrier defect may not be present in all patients with AD, it is important to point out that AD may actually represent a clinical syndrome that could result from different mechanisms.

Recent research in dogs has highlighted that skin barrier impairment may be one of the mechanisms of allergic sensitization also in this species [33,34] when allergens come in contact with a more permeable and disrupted skin which results in a Th2 polarization and production of allergen specific IgE. Although it is not clear yet whether the skin barrier defect is primary in dogs, it is clear that the skin barrier function is impaired [35,36] in atopic dogs and it plays a role in the aggravation of the disease.

Interestingly, in people, AD is typically the first step in a progression of events called "atopic march" which starts in the skin and progresses in many, but not all cases, into respiratory signs (rhinitis and later on asthma) [37]. As mentioned above, it is important to point out that although this progression is noted in individual patients, debate exists on the evidence of this phenomenon. Some publications have questioned the existence of an actual atopic march [38,39] while more recent studies have provided renewed support of an actual temporal pattern of progression from eczema to allergic rhinitis and asthma and a correlation between early eczema and childhood asthma [40,41,42].

In dogs, atopic disease typically only manifests in the skin, without progression to respiratory signs in the vast majority of cases. On the contrary, in other domestic animals, such as cats and horses, the atopic disease can manifest as both dermatitis and respiratory disease. It is currently unclear why allergies have different forms of manifestations in various species and why some species are prone to skin manifestations while others are prone to respiratory disease. Allergic diseases have very complex pathogenesis and many genes have been considered as possible candidates to explain development of allergies. It is very likely that many different pathways can lead to the development of allergies and that even within one species allergies should be considered more like a syndrome rather than one disease. It is interesting to note that even within the canine species, different gene mutations may play a role in various breeds and various geographical areas [43]. As the recent literature has emphasized the role of increased penetration of allergens as one of the mechanisms to explain increased risk for sensitization, it is possible that different aberrations in the skin *versus* the respiratory epithelium may be one of the reasons for the various clinical manifestations of allergic disease in different species. The similarities and yet differences across species may actually constitute a key to understanding what determines the progression of the disease and hopefully allow early identification of the individuals that are at increased risk for the development of asthma.

Histologically and immunologically the similarity of AD between dogs and people is striking, making dogs the closest naturally occurring animal model to study this disease in people [44]. Atopy patch test reactions in dogs mimic naturally occurring lesions and are very similar to what is reported in human medicine [45]. AD type lesions may be experimentally induced in mice, but this species does not spontaneously develop the disease and the experimental models only reproduce limited aspects of the disease [46] and recent literature has questioned the value of mouse models [47] as mice appear to only reproduce a very simplistic approach to allergies as a Th2 mediated disease and fail to reproduce more complex aspects of the human condition [48]. Dogs, on the other hand, are genetically closer to people, they are spontaneously affected by AD, and they also share the same environment with their owners constituting a precious and better tool to fully understand this complex disease in people.

Dog Models of Atopic Dermatitis

A few canine models of AD have been identified and validated. One model is composed by a colony of high IgE producing atopic Beagles [49]. These dogs have skin barrier defects demonstrated by ultrastructural studies showing an abnormally organized lipid lamellae and retained lamellar bodies [50]. These changes are similar to what reported in human atopic patients in which disorganized intercellular lipids, decreased ceramides and defects of extrusion of lamellar bodies have been described [51,52]. The abnormalities in the skin barrier do not only affect lipids but also epidermal proteins. Filaggrin has also been studied in dogs, in particular in the atopic beagle colony mentioned above, and an irregular, patchy staining for filaggrin was found in immunohistochemical and immunofluorescence studies [53,54]. In addition, in histochemical studies, morphological differences have been identified when comparing the keratohyalin granules (granules where the filaggrin and its precursor are stored before complete keratinization) in the atopic beagles with age matched healthy controls. In people, the decreased expression of filaggrin is not always linked to genetic mutations, but it can also be caused by increased degradation of the protein. More specifically, two enzymes—caspase-14 and calpain-1—are responsible for the degradation of filaggrin into amino acids fundamental for proper miniaturization of the skin (natural moisturizing factors) [55]. A decreased expression of caspase-14 has been found in both people [56,57] and in the atopic Beagle [58] colony showing the relevance and the similarities between the canine model and the atopic condition in human patients.

In this Beagle model, the skin barrier defects are not only ultrastructural but also functional as demonstrated by an increased transepidermal water loss (TEWL) compared to age matched healthy controls [36]. Measurement of this parameter is a non-invasive approach to test skin permeability. Atopic people have increased TEWL when compared to healthy controls and skin barrier dysfunction correlates with disease activity [59]. It is believed that younger skin is more susceptible to sensitizations and interestingly puppies from this atopic colony have higher TEWL than adults of the same colony and age matched healthy Beagles kept in the same living conditions [36]. These findings seem to emphasize the existence of a window of opportunity of allergic sensitization. This leads to the fascinating hypothesis that maybe the development of AD could be prevented or at last minimized if skin barrier repair is enacted at a young age, before sensitization sets in. Indeed, pilot studies in infants showed a decrease sensitization in children at high risk for the atopic disease due to genetic predisposition in which emollients and occlusive therapy was started in the first few months of life [60,61]. Preventative studies are difficult to accomplish in people or in pet dogs with naturally occurring disease due to the variable environmental conditions which tend to make design and interpretation of studies quite challenging. That is where animal models can provide useful information that can benefit multiple species. One example of that is the proactive use of probiotics with the intention of preventing or at least lessening the severity of disease in highly predisposed individuals. One of the ideas behind this strategy is that allergies are partly due to improved hygiene conditions leading to less opportunity to have bacterial and parasitic exposure which helps to modulate the immune response toward a more protective cell mediated response. The exact mechanisms of probiotics in allergies are still under investigation and are more complex than the direct modulation of the immune response. With the development of methodologies targeting the 16S rRNA, knowledge of the importance of the microbiome in healthy and disease states is rapidly growing. It is becoming evident that loss of biodiversity can predispose to the development of allergies while high biodiversity can have a protective effect [62,63,64,65,66]. Oral assumption of probiotics can modulate gut microbiota [67] and this can be an additional mechanism by which probiotic can affect the immune response [68], although this mechanism has not be confirmed in recent clinical trials in infants. In one study, skin and gut microbiome was investigated after oral administration of*Lactobacillus rahmnosus GG* (LGG) but no significant changes were detected when compared to the control group [69]. When studies on probiotic have been done in people, the results of clinical efficacy have been mixed [70] probably because it was not possible to control for genetic differences, variable diets and environmental conditions. In animal models, this can be done and even studies with a relatively low number of subjects can produce useful information. Using the colony of atopic Beagles, it was possible to breed the same parents twice, producing two litters, one used as control and the other one as probiotic litter. Puppies were raised under the same housing and dietary conditions, they were all exposed to house dust mites using the exact same doses and protocols and the only difference was the administration of LGG, which is a probiotic for both dogs and people. The results showed that prenatal and postnatal (for the first 6 months of life) exposure to LGG had a protective effect in decreasing the severity of sensitization [71]. Even more interestingly, the protective effect was long lasting and carried out for at least 3 years after the discontinuation of the LGG [72]. The probiotic litter continued to show significantly lower severity of clinical signs and was associated with increased regulatory cytokines such as transforming growth factor (TGF)-β. In the canine study, no investigation on the effects of LGG on skin or gut microbiome was done. This is an area that should be investigated further as preliminary studies on skin microbiome in allergic and normal dogs have shown that atopic dogs have less biodiversity and increased colonization by Staphylococcus compared to the healthy controls [73]. The preventative effects of this study echoed more recent metanalyses in human medicine that support a prophylactic role for probiotics, but not the therapeutic role once the disease has already been established [74].

A model for AD in dogs has also been described in Maltese-Beagles. In this model, pruritus and dermatitis can be elicited after epicutaneous application of house dust mites [75]. Lesions are consistent with naturally occurring AD lesions [76,77] making it a suitable model to test new therapies. No skin barrier defect has been described in this model compared to a control population. Ceramide reductions have been described as an effect of allergen exposure and development of inflammation [78]. Another well described but older model of AD and asthma was the one of Basenji-Greyhound dogs. While dogs typically do not develop asthma as progression of their skin disease, in this model both manifestations (skin and respiratory) of atopic disease were described [79] making them an appealing model to study the human condition [80,81]. No recent publications have been reported on this model.

Mouse Models of Atopic Dermatitis

Many different mouse models of AD have been described over time. The Nishiki-nezumi Cinnamon/Nagoya (NC/Nga) was the first AD-like murine model that spontaneously develops AD-like dermatitis only if raised under air-uncontrolled conventional conditions [82,83,84]. This model has been useful to test new treatments [85] although the fact that the NC/Nga mice exposure to only conventional environments is not enough to induce human AD-like clinical symptoms questions the relevance of such model to the human condition.

Other mouse models have been described by epicutaneous stimulation with certain environmental allergens [86]. SKH-1 hairless mice have been shown to be easily sensitized epicutaneously with allergens due to skin barrier impairment and reported to be helpful to test strategies such as probiotics [87]. Mice with a null mutation in the filaggrin gene develop flaky tails and that has been used as model for AD although this model may only represent one subset of AD [88,89].

FOOD ALLERGY

Food allergy is also becoming quite common in people. In people, food allergy is defined as "a pattern of immune reactivity to the ingestion of natural food components resulting in IgE mediated [reaction], which by nature routinely results in tolerance". In non-allergic individuals, the normal immune response to dietary protein is associated with a natural tolerance; on the contrary, in allergic patients, an excessive complex immune response against food proteins may occur. Several immune responses including an immediate and a delayed hypersensitivity have been associated with food allergy explaining the highly variable time of reaction after the ingestion of an allergen. Food allergy is extremely important in people due to the high variability of the clinical signs associated with it; the spectrum of clinical signs can range from mildly irritating to life-threatening conditions [90].

Food allergy is a substantial and evolving public health issue [91,92] with an increasing prevalence in the last decades [93] due to environmental changes [94]. In the USA, up to 8% of children and 4% of adults have food allergy [92]. Of major concern is the fact that, while previous generations of children would typically outgrow food allergies (particularly if not peanuts related), the new generations appear less able to outgrow food allergy. It is proposed that environmental factors have significant effect on this phenomenon and that "westernization" plays a role [95]. The most serious allergic response to food allergy is anaphylaxis [96,97]. More than 3 million Americans are allergic to peanuts and this is the leading cause of death by anaphylaxis [98]. In children, the most common foods able to trigger an immunological response include, but are not limited to, cow's milk, hen's egg, peanut, soybeans, wheat, fish, and tree nuts. Whereas, in adults, the most common food allergies are due to ingestion of peanuts, tree nuts, fish, and shellfish [99,100,101]. In people, most commonly food allergy started in the first 3 years of life; however, several studies have shown that most allergies that begin early in life (e.g., milk, egg, soy, and wheat) are generally outgrown. On the contrary, allergies to peanut, tree nuts, fish and shellfish tend to persist for life [102,103].

To better determine the immunological mechanisms and in order to develop safe therapeutic options for children and adults affected by food allergy, the use of animal models is fundamental. To date, animal models have been identified with some success in small animals (mice, rats, and guinea pigs) as well as in large animals (dogs, pigs, and sheep). Those species have been fundamental to assess routes of administration to induce sensitization and to better identify the gastrointestinal allergic response. However, each model has benefits and limitations.

Rodent Models of Food Allergy

Examples of murine model include strains like the BALB/c, DBA/2, C3H/HeJ, BDF-1, A/J, and the C57/Bl6. Of those, the most studied have been the C3H/HeJ and the BALB/c able to produce IgE and IgG1 anaphylactic antibodies [104,105]. The former has been used to investigate potential immunotherapeutic approaches to treat food allergy through intragastric administration of peanut and milk proteins [106,107]. The BALB/c mice have instead been used to evaluate the potential to predict the allergenicity of a novel protein for people through intraperitoneal administration of several proteins including ovalbumin, peanut agglutinin, and bovine serum albumin [108]. Due to the artificial sensitization methods it is unclear how well representative mouse models are for the natural disease in people and their usefulness in predicting efficacy of therapies [109].

Rats have also been used as an animal model for food allergy. The most commonly used strain is the brown Norway able to produce allergen specific IgE after oral sensitization and able to predict the allergenicity of novel proteins [110,111]. Other strains like Wistar, Hooded Lister, and Piebald Virol Glaxo have been studied, but not commonly used due to the inability to detect quantifiable levels of antigen specific IgE [112].

An alternative to mice and rats is the guinea pig. Indeed, these rodents are able to display fatal anaphylaxis after sensitization to cow's milk proteins. However, due to the technical difficulties (e.g., inability to directly quantify IgE production) and for the limited tools to study their immune system, guinea pigs have been abandoned as an animal model for food allergy [113].

Dog Models of Food Allergy

Dogs have been recently identified as a spontaneous model for food allergy in people. In fact, as in people, up to 8%–15% of the canine population is spontaneously affected by food allergy and it manifests more commonly during puppyhood [114]. Like in people, dogs may present with skin and gastrointestinal clinical signs, although these latter involves up to 10%–15% of the affected patients [113,115]. Contrary to the rodent models, dogs and people share the same food allergens: beef, dairy, wheat, lamb, egg, chicken, soy, oats, and pork [116]. In addition, they share similar gut anatomy and physiology, as well as nutritional requirements. On dogs, it is easier performing repeated endoscopic analysis, high IgE dogs are easy to identify, and the large size of immune organs along with larger blood volume facilitate certain analyses [104]. To date, three canine models have been well validated [117,118,119]. All the models include mixed breed atopic dogs. Two models are constituted by the same colony of inbred, high IgE producing, atopic spaniel/basenji dogs [117,118], whereas the other one is constituted by a colony of Maltese/Beagles atopic dogs [104,120]. The first generation of the spaniel/basenji model was developed by subcutaneous injection of wheat, cow's milk and beef extract showing signs of vomiting, diarrhea, or more rarely constipation [118]. The second generation was instead sensitized by subcutaneous injection of peanut, walnut, Brazil nut, wealth or barley developing vomiting and lethargy after oral challenge [117]. On the contrary, the Maltese/Beagle colony spontaneously developed food allergy (pruritus, diarrhea, and/or vomiting) to cow's milk, dairy products, corn, and soy without any experimental sensitization [104]. In all three models, the investigators were able to show clinical response to oral challenge between 1 h and 12 h, a higher production of total and allergen-specific serum IgE, and positive intradermal test [104,117,118]. Using the canine model for food allergy, the investigators proposed the hypothesis that in genetically predisposed children an early infection may stimulate the immune system to respond to "bystander" antigens more aggressively than healthy individuals. In the affected patients, the inflamed gut becomes more permeable to food allergens (proteins) leading to their exposure to the local immune system inducing sensitization of otherwise innocuous food proteins [105].

A recently described model for peanut allergy has been reported in atopic Beagles [121]. In this model, dogs were sensitized after epicutaneous application of a peanut paste and developed macular, popular dermatitis after oral challenge. No systemic effects were detected after oral challenge making it a safe model to test therapies. An IgE mediated response was detected on intradermal test and skin biopsies. This model could be useful to test new allergy vaccines to treat peanut allergy in children. The epicutaneous sensitization is very relevant to what is believed to occur in young atopic children where the perioral region is frequently one of the first affected areas, most likely due to increased penetration of food allergens through an impaired skin barrier [122].

Other Large Animal Models for Food Allergy

Another large animal model proposed for food allergy is constituted by neonatal pigs. This model, although very similar to the canine model, is much less commonly used due to several limitations. The major benefits of this model over the others include the strong similarity in anatomy and physiology of the gastrointestinal tract and the development of mucosal immunity between pigs and people [105]. Neonatal piglets have been used as an animal model for sensitization to cow's milk, soy, and peanuts. Sensitized piglets show a very similar immunological response occurring in sensitized children [105]. The induction of food sensitization in piglets involves the use of intraperitoneal injections (peanut extract) in the presence of cholera toxin as adjuvant and later on repeated oral challenges with sensitizing food allergen [105,123]. After challenge the pigs show clinical signs including vomiting, lethargy, diarrhea, bleeding, weight loss, and respiratory distress [123]. Finally, like in dogs, the clinical signs are associated with an increase in allergen-specific IgE and IgG, and a positive passive cutaneous anaphylaxis showing the involvement of IgE as cause of the allergic symptoms [105].

The last large animal model proposed for food allergy in people involves the use of sheep. Like dogs and pigs, also sheep are very similar in size and physiology to people. Sheep have been successfully used as model for peanut allergy [111]. Similarly to other animal models, sheep were sensitized by multiple subcutaneous injections of crude peanut extract and ovalbumin. As outcome the investigators were able to show the presence of Ara h 1- and Ara h 2-specific serum IgE in 100% and 80%, respectively, of the sensitized sheep and a positive intradermal test in 80% of the high-IgE producing sheep [111].

ASTHMA

Asthma in people is defined as "a [multiphenotypic] chronic inflammatory disorder of the airways associated with airway hyper-responsiveness [leading] to recurrent episodes of wheezing, breathlessness, chest tightness, coughing, [and] airflow obstruction often reversible with or without treatment" [124,125,126]. Asthma affects more than 10% of the North American population with the age of onset, pathophysiology, and response to treatment extremely variable [127,128]. In addition, a correlation between chronic obstructive pulmonary disease (COPD) has also been proven in patients with asthma [129].

Due to the high heterogeneity and the ethical problems in analyzing the pathomechanism of asthma in children, many disease models have been developed (mathematical modelling system as well as *in vitro* and *in vivo* models) [130]. The mathematical model has been used to describe patterns of flow limitations in the airways [131], whereas understanding of cell signaling, cellular responses under Th2 conditions, and wound repair have been facilitated by the use of primary or immortalized cell lines [132,133,134]. Although these two model systems have been largely used and are fundamental to unravelling the physical and immunological processes at a cellular and molecular level, their major limitation is the impossibility to evaluate such processes in a dynamic immunological milieu present in the asthmatic patient [130]. For this reason, the only model system able to reproduce the asthma in people is the animal (*in vivo*) model. In the past 100 years, the use of animal models have largely contributed to the identification of important immunological alterations in the lungs of asthmatic patients (e.g., the importance of Th2 phenotype in the progression and perpetuation of an inflammatory response in allergic asthma) as well as the development, safety, and efficacy of new drugs (e.g., montelukast, integrin antibodies, and tryptase inhibitors) [130].

Contrarily to AD and food allergy, an appropriate animal model for human asthma is lacking. Indeed, to date, a laboratory animal that spontaneously develops a disease with characteristics present in asthma has not been identified [135]. However, different species have diseases with some similarities to the human disease; cats spontaneously develop a bronchial disease similar to chronic asthma, horses are affected by a neutrophilic-dominated airway disease more close to COPD than asthma, sheep and dogs are naturally susceptible to allergen sensitization [135].

Mouse models have also been developed and use for identification of immunological alterations leading to pulmonary inflammation in asthmatic people; however, this model is not ideal for testing of new drugs due to the significant anatomic and immunological differences between mice and people [135,136]. Like mice, rats have also been largely used as animal model due to the abundance of reagents available, the ease handling and sensitization protocols, as well as the low maintenance expense. However, one advantage over mice is their larger size which determines an increase in sampling volume and possibility of testing compared with mice [135]. In addition, rats are able to develop an early- and a late-phase response as well as airway hyperresponsiveness to non-specific bronchoconstricting agents present in people but not in mice [135,137]. Although extremely useful to investigate the acute allergic reaction in asthma, the murine models have been largely criticized for their ability to easily develop tolerance following allergen sensitization limiting the use of such models for the investigation of chronic allergic response in asthmatic patients [135].

Contrary to the murine models, pet cats are spontaneously affected by a syndrome similar to human asthma [138]. In the past 10 years, such similarities have led to the development of two feline asthma models for preclinical studies [139,140,141]. Like in people, in cats asthma is extremely common and triggered by aeroallergens and the clinical manifestations include cough, wheeze and episodic expiratory respiratory distress [138]. In addition, cats with asthma have important features of asthma in people including recurrent and variable symptoms of chronic airway disease, airflow restriction, bronchial hyperresponsiveness, and airway inflammation [142]. However, contrarily to people in which airway hyperresponsiveness is triggered by drugs, pollutants, occupational factors, exercise, emotional stress, infections, and allergens; in cats the predominant triggers seem to be aeroallergens [138].

Like the feline models, the canine model has been identified as a better model due to the natural predisposition of dogs to develop allergic disease after exposure to allergens clinically relevant for people. However, naturally-occurring asthma is very uncommon in allergic dogs [143]. In fact, the most common clinical manifestations of allergy in dogs include dermatitis, otitis, and conjunctivitis [144]. However, many naturally or actively sensitized dogs to*Ascasis suum* larvae or ragweed have been used as canine model for asthma [134]. Although an increase in eosinophils have been identified in the airways of allergic dogs, this does not seem to be associated with an increase in responsiveness of the airways probably due to the significant anatomical difference of dogs with the other species; proportionally larger airways and less prone to bronchoconstriction [145]. Nevertheless, anatomical and clinical differences are evident between dogs and people; such model has been largely used due to the unique ability of dogs to show persistent sensitization (prolonged airways hyperresponsiveness) up to 5 months post challenge with *A. suum* [146]. The main drawback for this model is that dogs are labor intense and expensive, but these difficulties are easily overridden by the usefulness of such model to identify pathomechanisms and long term pulmonary changes related to the asthmatic disease [134]. The canine model has also been used as animal model for COPD in people. Although, no as much research as in asthma has been involved using the canine model, three model systems have been identified in dogs: inhalation of cigarette smoke, exposure to SO_2 gas and intratracheal or aerosolization of proteolytic enzymes [125].

Finally, the last animal model system used for asthma is sheep. Like dogs, sheep are naturally sensitized to *A. suum*and house dust mite [135,147,148]; although an inter-individual variability to mount an allergic physiological response to the allergen is present among sheep [149]. Similar to dogs, after challenges sheep develop an early- and late-phase as well as airway hyperresponsiveness [135]. In term of drug response, cromolyn and corticosteroids are highly effective in sheep with an allergic airway response [147]. In addition, sheep are more similar in size and physiology to people, they are very docile, and fewer ethical constraints are taken [147,150]. For all the reasons abovementioned sheep represent a very useful model system for asthma in people; however, relevant differences between sheep and people may affect the use of such model for development and testing of new drugs. One example is the efficacy of platelet activating factors extremely useful to modulate the inflammatory response in the sheep model, but not at all effective in people [151]. As in dogs, the main difficulties to work with sheep are the expense and the labor intensity; however, like for the canine model, such difficulties are easily overridden by the advantages of such model. Some key advantages of using large animal models include their outbred nature, allowing studies that are more comparable to humans, the ability to conduct serial experiments within the same cohort of animals, and their relative longevity, allowing more relevant investigations into chronic disease as well as the long-term evaluation of specific therapies.

CONCLUSIONS

Animals and people share many important allergic diseases, and animals have proven to be the key to improve our understanding on the mechanisms involved across species for the mutual benefit of people and animals. Animals and people share the same environment and are inextricably linked. A comparative approach to medicine has improved our appreciation of similarities and differences of diseases that affect multiple species and how that can be leveraged to improve our knowledge of the mechanisms involved. It is hoped that by improving our understanding on how we are all connected, veterinarians and physicians can collaborate across species to improve the lives of all species and develop therapies than can benefit multiple species.

ACKNOWLEDGMENTS

The authors would like to acknowledge Ahrens for helping with the editing of the manuscript.

AUTHOR CONTRIBUTIONS

Domenico Santoro and Rosanna Marsella equally contributed to the writing, revisions and editing of the paper. They are both veterinary dermatologists with extensive experience in animal models of allergy.

REFERENCES

1. Olivry, T.; DeBoer, D.J.; Griffin, C.E.; Halliwell, R.E.; Hill, P.B.; Hillier, A.; Marsella, R.; Sousa, C.A. The ACVD task force on canine atopic dermatitis: Forewords and lexicon. *Vet. Immunol. Immunopathol.* 2001, *81*, 143–146.
2. Thestrup-Pedersen, K. Atopic eczema. What has caused the epidemic in industrialised countries and can early intervention modify the natural history of atopic eczema? *J. Cosmet. Dermatol.* 2003, *2*, 202–210.
3. Giannetti, A.; Girolomoni, G. Skin diseases with high public health impact. Atopic dermatitis. *Eur. J. Dermatol.*2007, *17*, 566.
4. Wüthrich, B.; Schmid-Grendelmeier, P. The atopic eczema/dermatitis syndrome. Epidemiology, natural course, and immunology of the IgE-associated ("extrinsic") and the nonallergic ("intrinsic") AEDS. *J. Investig. Allergol. Clin. Immunol.* 2003, *13*, 1–5.
5. Roguedas-Contios, A.M.; Misery, L. What is intrinsic atopic dermatitis? *Clin. Rev. Allergy Immunol.* 2011, *41*, 233–236.
6. Fujimura, M. The study of canine atopic dermatitis involving the isolation of dogs. *Pol. J. Vet. Sci.* 2011, *14*, 273–277.
7. Kulthanan, K.; Boochangkool, K.; Tuchinda, P.; Chularojanamontri, L. Clinical features of the extrinsic and intrinsic types of adult-onset atopic dermatitis. *Asia Pac. Allergy.* 2011, *1*, 80–86.
8. Tokura, Y. Extrinsic and intrinsic types of atopic dermatitis. *J. Dermatol. Sci.* 2010, *58*, 1–7.
9. Mori, T.; Ishida, K.; Mukumoto, S.; Yamada, Y.; Imokawa, G.; Kabashima, K.; Kobayashi, M.; Bito, T.; Nakamura, M.; Ogasawara, K.; *et al.* Comparison of skin barrier function and sensory nerve electric current perception threshold between IgE-high extrinsic and IgE normal intrinsic types of atopic dermatitis. *Br. J. Dermatol.* 2010, *162*, 83–90.
10. Stelmaszczyk-Emmel, A.; Zawadzka-Krajewska, A.; Szypowska, A.; Kulus, M.; Demkow, U. Frequency and activation of CD4+CD25 FoxP3+ regulatory T cells in peripheral blood from children with atopic allergy. *Int. Arch. Allergy Immunol.* 2013, *162*, 16–24.
11. Rouse, B.T. Regulatory T cells in health and disease. *J. Intern. Med.* 2007, *262*, 78–95.
12. Bilate, A.M.; Lafaille, J.J. Induced CD4+Foxp3+ regulatory T cells in immune tolerance. *Annu. Rev. Immunol.*2012, *30*, 733–758.
13. Daniel, C.; von Boehmer, H. Extrathymic generation of regulatory T cells—Chances and challenges for prevention of autoimmune disease. *Adv. Immunol.* 2011, *112*, 177–213.
14. Samochocki, Z.; Alifier, M.; Bodera, P.; Jeziorkowska, R.; Rosiak, E.; Jurkiewicz, B.; Glińska, O.; Gliński, W.; Stankiewicz, W. T-regulatory cells in severe atopic dermatitis: Alterations related to cytokines and other lymphocyte subpopulations. *Arch. Dermatol. Res.* 2012, *304*, 795–801.

15. Falcone, F.H.; Knol, E.F.; Gibbs, B.F. The role of basophils in the pathogenesis of allergic disease. *Clin. Exp. Allergy* 2011, *41*, 939–947.

16. Ohsawa, Y.; Hirasawa, N. The role of histamine H1 and H4 receptors in atopic dermatitis: From Basic Research to Clinical Study. *Allergol. Int.* 2014.

17. Wahlgren, C.F.; Hägermark, O.; Bergström, R. Patients' perception of itch induced by histamine, compound 48/80 and wool fibres in atopic dermatitis. *Acta. Derm. Venereol.* 1991, *71*, 488–494.

18. Amon, U.; Menz, U.; Wolff, H.H. Investigations on plasma levels of mast cell mediators in acute atopic dermatitis. *J. Dermatol. Sci.* 1994, *7*, 63–67.

19. Sher, L.G.; Chang, J.; Patel, I.B.; Balkrishnan, R.; Fleischer, A.B., Jr. Relieving the pruritus of atopic dermatitis: A meta-analysis. *Acta. Derm. Venereol.* 2012, *92*, 455–461.

20. Darsow, U.; Pfab, F.; Valet, M.; Tölle, T.R.; Ring, J. Itch and eczema. *Chem. Immunol. Allergy* 2012, *96*, 81–88.

21. Cowden, J.M.; Zhang, M.; Dunford, P.J.; Thurmond, R.L. The histamine H4 receptor mediates inflammation and pruritus in Th2-dependent dermal inflammation. *J. Invest. Dermatol.* 2010, *130*, 1023–1033.

22. Gutzmer, R.; Mommert, S.; Gschwandtner, M.; Zwingmann, K.; Stark, H.; Werfel, T. The histamine H_4 receptor is functionally expressed on T_H2 cells. *J. Allergy Clin. Immunol.* 2009, *123*, 619–625.

23. Kollmeier, A.; Francke, K.; Chen, B.; Dunford, P.J.; Greenspan, A.J.; Xia, Y.; Xu, X.L.; Zhou, B.; Thurmond, R.L. The histamine H4 receptor antagonist, JNJ 39758979, is effective in reducing histamine-induced pruritus in a randomized clinical study in healthy subjects. *J. Pharmacol. Exp. Ther.* 2014, *350*, 181–187.

24. Dunford, P.J.; Williams, K.N.; Desai, P.J.; Karlsson, L.; McQueen, D.; Thurmond, R.L. Histamine H_4 receptor antagonists are superior to traditional antihistamines in the attenuation of experimental pruritus. *J. Allergy Clin. Immunol.* 2007, *119*, 176–183.

25. Welle, M.M.; Olivry, T.; Grimm, S.; Suter, M. Mast cell density and subtypes in the skin of dogs with atopic dermatitis. *J. Comp. Pathol.* 1999, *120*, 187–197.

26. Nimmo-Wilkie, J.S.; Yager, J.A.; Eyre, P.; Parker, W.M. Morphometric analyses of the skin of dogs with atopic dermatitis and correlations with cutaneous and plasma histamine and total serum IgE. *Vet. Pathol.* 1990, *27*, 179–186.

27. Helton-Rhodes, K.; Kerdel, F.; Soter, N.A.; Chinnici, R. Investigation into the immunopathogenesis of canine atopy. *Semin. Vet. Med. Surg. (Small Anim.)* 1987, *2*, 199–201.

28. Bäumer, W.; Stahl, J.; Sander, K.; Petersen, L.J.; Paps, J.; Stark, H.; Kietzmann, M.; Olivry, T. Lack of preventing effect of systemically and topically administered histamine H_1 or H_4 receptor antagonists in a dog model of acute atopic dermatitis. *Exp. Dermatol.* 2011, *20*, 577–581.

29. Olivry, T.; Mueller, R.S. International Task Force on Canine Atopic Dermatitis. Evidence-based veterinary dermatology: A systematic review of the pharmacotherapy of canine atopic dermatitis. *Vet. Dermatol.* 2003, *14*, 121–146.

30. Agrawal, R.; Woodfolk, J.A. Skin barrier defects in atopic dermatitis. *Curr. Allergy Asthma Rep.* 2014, *14*.

31. Kawasaki, H.; Kubo, A.; Sasaki, T.; Amagai, M. Loss-of-function mutations within the filaggrin gene and atopic dermatitis. *Curr. Probl. Dermatol.* 2011, *41*, 35–46.

32. O'Regan, G.M.; Sandilands, A.; McLean, W.H.; Irvine, A.D. Filaggrin in atopic dermatitis. *J. Allergy Clin. Immunol.* 2008, *122*, 689–693.

33. Olivry, T.; Wofford, J.; Paps, J.S.; Dunston, S.M. Stratum corneum removal facilitates experimental sensitization to mite allergens in atopic dogs. *Vet. Dermatol.* 2011, *22*, 188–196.

34. Marsella, R.; Olivry, T.; Carlotti, D.N.; International Task Force on Canine Atopic Dermatitis. Current evidence of skin barrier dysfunction in human and canine atopic dermatitis. *Vet. Dermatol.* 2011, *22*, 239–248.

35. Yoon, J.S.; Nishifuji, K.; Sasaki, A.; Ide, K.; Ishikawa, J.; Yoshihara, T.; Iwasaki, T. Alteration of stratum corneum ceramide profiles in spontaneous canine model of atopic dermatitis. *Exp. Dermatol.* 2011, *20*, 732–736.

36. Hightower, K.; Marsella, R.; Flynn-Lurie, A. Effects of age and allergen exposure on transepidermal water loss in a house dust mite-sensitized beagle model of atopic dermatitis. *Vet. Dermatol.* 2010, *21*, 88–95.

37. Shaker, M. New insights into the allergic march. *Curr. Opin. Pediatr.* 2014, *26*, 516–520.

38. Williams, H.; Flohr, C. How epidemiology has challenged 3 prevailing concepts about atopic dermatitis. *J. Allergy Clin. Immunol.* 2006, *118*, 209–213.

39. Curtiss, F.R. Atopic march to a dead end or does the theory really have legs? *J. Manag. Care Pharm.* 2007, *13*, 810–811.

40. Ker, J.; Hartert, T.V. The atopic march: What's the evidence? *Ann. Allergy Asthma Immunol.* 2009, *103*, 282–289.

41. Spergel, J.M. From atopic dermatitis to asthma: The atopic march. *Ann. Allergy Asthma Immunol.* 2010, *105*, 99–106.

42. Saunes, M.; Øien, T.; Dotterud, C.K.; Romundstad, P.R.; Storrø, O.; Holmen, T.L.; Johnsen, R. Early eczema and the risk of childhood asthma: A prospective, population-based study. *BMC Pediatr.* 2012, *12*.

43. Wood, S.H.; Ollier, W.E.; Nuttall, T.; McEwan, N.A.; Carter, S.D. Despite identifying some shared gene associations with human atopic dermatitis the use of multiple dog breeds from various locations limits detection of gene associations in canine atopic dermatitis. *Vet. Immunol. Immunopathol.* 2010, *138*, 193–197.

44. Marsella, R.; Girolomoni, G. Canine models of atopic dermatitis: A useful tool with untapped potential. *J. Invest. Dermatol.* 2009, *129*, 2351–2357.

45. Olivry, T.; Deangelo, K.B.; Dunston, S.M.; Clarke, K.B.; McCall, C.A. Patch testing of experimentally sensitized beagle dogs: Development of a model for skin lesions of atopic dermatitis. *Vet. Dermatol.* 2006, *17*, 95–102.

46. Amagai, Y.; Matsuda, H.; Tanaka, A. Abnormalities in itch sensation and skin barrier function in atopic NC/Tnd mice. *Biol. Pharm. Bull.* 2013, *36*, 1248–1252.

47. Takeda, K.; Gelfand, E.W. Mouse models of allergic diseases. *Curr. Opin. Immunol.* 2009, *21*, 660–665.

48. Graham, M.T.; Nadeau, K.C. Lessons learned from mice and man: Mimicking human allergy through mouse models. *Clin. Immunol.* 2014, *155*, 1–16.

49. Marsella, R.; Olivry, T.; Nicklin, C.; Lopez, J. Pilot investigation of a model for canine atopic dermatitis: Environmental house dust mite challenge of high-IgE-producing beagles, mite hypersensitive dogs with atopic dermatitis and normal dogs. *Vet. Dermatol.* 2006, *17*, 24–35.

50. Marsella, R.; Samuelson, D.; Doerr, K. Transmission electron microscopy studies in an experimental model of canine atopic dermatitis. *Vet. Dermatol.* 2010, *21*, 81–88.

51. Fartasch, M.; Bassukas, I.D.; Diepgen, T.L. Disturbed extruding mechanism of lamellar bodies in dry non-eczematous skin of atopics. *Br. J. Dermatol.* 1992, *127*, 221–227.

52. Fartasch, M.; Diepgen, T.L. The barrier function in atopic dry skin. Disturbance of membrane-coating granule exocytosis and formation of epidermal lipids? *Acta. Derm. Venereol. Suppl. (Stockh.)* 1992, *176*, 26–31.

53. Marsella, R.; Samuelson, D.; Harrington, L. Immunohistochemical evaluation of filaggrin polyclonal antibody in atopic and normal beagles. *Vet. Dermatol.* 2009, *20*, 547–554.

54. Santoro, D.; Marsella, R.; Ahrens, K.; Graves, T.K.; Bunick, D. Altered mRNA and protein expression of filaggrin in the skin of a canine animal model for atopic dermatitis. *Vet. Dermatol.* 2013, *24*, 329–336.

55. Eckhart, L.; Tschachler, E. Cuts by caspase-14 control the proteolysis of filaggrin. *J. Invest. Dermatol.* 2011, *131*, 2173–2175.

56. Hvid, M.; Johansen, C.; Deleuran, B.; Kemp, K.; Deleuran, M.; Vestergaard, C. Regulation of caspase 14 expression in keratinocytes by inflammatory cytokines—A possible link between reduced skin barrier function and inflammation? *Exp. Dermatol.* 2011, *20*, 633–636.

57. Yamamoto, M.; Kamata, Y.; Iida, T.; Fukushima, H.; Nomura, J.; Saito, M.; Tajima, M.; Okubo, Y.; Momoi, T.; Tsuboi, R.; *et al.* Quantification of activated and total caspase-14 with newly developed ELISA systems in normal and atopic skin. *J. Dermatol. Sci.* 2011, *61*, 110–117.

58. Papastavros, V.; Marsella, R.; Cronin, M.; Ahrens, K.; Kim, H.J.; Santoro, D. Investigation of caspase-14 expression in canine atopic dermatitis. *Vet. Dermatol.* 2014, *25*, 155.

59. Addor, F.A.; Takaoka, R.; Rivitti, E.A.; Aoki, V. Atopic dermatitis: Correlation between non-damaged skin barrier function and disease activity. *Int. J. Dermatol.* 2012, *51*, 672–676.

60. Simpson, E.L.; Berry, T.M.; Brown, P.A.; Hanifin, J.M. A pilot study of emollient therapy for the primary prevention of atopic dermatitis. *J. Am. Acad. Dermatol.* 2010, *63*, 587–593.

61. Williams, H.C.; Chalmers, J.R.; Simpson, E.L. Prevention of atopic dermatitis. *F1000 Med. Rep.* 2012, *4*.

62. Haahtela, T.; Holgate, S.; Pawankar, R.; Akdis, C.A.; Benjaponpitak, S.; Caraballo, L.; Demain, J.; Portnoy, J.; von Hertzen, L.; WAO Special Committee on Climate Change and Biodiversity. The biodiversity hypothesis and allergic disease: World allergy organization position statement. *World Allergy Organ. J.* 2013, *6*.

63. Hanski, I.; von Hertzen, L.; Fyhrquist, N.; Koskinen, K.; Torppa, K.; Laatikainen, T.; Karisola, P.; Auvinen, P.; Paulin, L.; Mäkelä, M.J.; *et al.* Environmental biodiversity, human microbiota, and allergy are interrelated. *Proc. Natl. Acad. Sci. USA* 2012, *109*, 8334–8339.

64. Legatzki, A.; Rösler, B.; von Mutius, E. Microbiome diversity and asthma and allergy risk. *Curr. Allergy Asthma Rep.* 2014, *14*.

65. Sjögren, Y.M., Jenmalm, M.C.; Böttcher, M.F.; Björkstén, B.; Sverremark-Ekström, E. Altered early infant gut microbiota in children developing allergy up to 5 years of age. *Clin. Exp. Allergy* 2009, *39*, 518–526.

66. Sjögren, Y.M.; Tomicic, S.; Lundberg, A.; Böttcher, M.F.; Björkstén, B.; Sverremark-Ekström, E., Jenmalm, M.C. Influence of early gut microbiota on the maturation of childhood mucosal and systemic immune responses.*Clin. Exp. Allergy* 2009, *39*, 1842–1851.

67. Kwok, L.Y.; Wang, L.; Zhang, J.; Guo, Z.; Zhang, H. A pilot study on the effect of Lactobacillus casei Zhang on intestinal microbiota parameters in Chinese subjects of different age. *Benef. Microbes.* 2014, *5*, 295–304.

68. Geuking, M.B.; Köller, Y.; Rupp, S.; McCoy, K.D. The interplay between the gut microbiota and the immune system. *Gut Microbes.* 2014, *5*, 411–418.

69. Nermes, M.; Kantele, J.M.; Atosuo, T.J.; Salminen, S.; Isolauri, E. Interaction of orally administered *Lactobacillus rhamnosus* GG with skin and gut microbiota and humoral immunity in infants with atopic dermatitis. *Clin. Exp. Allergy.* 2011, *41*, 370–377.

70. Ismail, I.H.; Licciardi, P.V.; Tang, M.L. Probiotic effects in allergic disease. *J. Paediatr. Child. Health.* 2013, *49*, 709–715.

71. Marsella, R. Evaluation of *Lactobacillus rhamnosus* strain GG for the prevention of atopic dermatitis in dogs. *Am. J. Vet. Res.* 2009, *70*, 735–740.

72. Marsella, R.; Santoro, D.; Ahrens, K. Early exposure to probiotics in a canine model of atopic dermatitis has long-term clinical and immunological effects. *Vet. Immunol. Immunopathol.* 2012, *146*, 185–189.

73. Rodrigues Hoffmann, A.; Patterson, A.P.; Diesel, A.; Lawhon, S.D.; Ly, H.J.; Elkins Stephenson, C.; Mansell, J.; Steiner, J.M.; Dowd, S.E.; Olivry, T.; *et al.* The skin microbiome in healthy and allergic dogs. *PLOS ONE* 2014, *9*.

74. Panduru, M.; Panduru, N.M.; Sălăvăstru, C.M.; Tiplica, G.S. Probiotics and primary prevention of atopic dermatitis: A meta-analysis of randomized controlled studies. *J. Eur. Acad. Dermatol. Venereol.* 2014.

75. Pucheu-Haston, C.M.; Jackson, H.A.; Olivry, T.; Dunston, S.M.; Hammerberg, B. Epicutaneous sensitization with Dermatophagoides farinae induces generalized allergic dermatitis and elevated mite-specific immunoglobulin E levels in a canine model of atopic dermatitis. *Clin. Exp. Allergy* 2008, *38*, 667–679.

76. Olivry, T.; Dean, G.A.; Tompkins, M.B.; Dow, J.L.; Moore, P.F. Toward a canine model of atopic dermatitis: Amplification of cytokine-gene transcripts in the skin of atopic dogs. *Exp. Dermatol.* 1999, *8*, 204–211.

77. Pucheu-Haston, C.M.; Shuster, D.; Olivry, T.; Brianceau, P.; Lockwood, P.; McClanahan, T.; de Waal Malefyt, R.; Mattson, J.D.; Hammerberg, B. A canine model of cutaneous late-phase reactions: Prednisolone inhibition of cellular and cytokine responses. *Immunology* 2006, *117*, 177–187.

78. Stahl, J.; Paps, J.; Bäumer, W.; Olivry, T. Dermatophagoides farinae house dust mite allergen challenges reduce stratum corneum ceramides in an experimental dog model of acute atopic dermatitis. *Vet. Dermatol.* 2012, *23*.

79. Butler, J.M.; Peters, J.E.; Hirshman, C.A.; White, C.R., Jr.; Margolin, L.B.; Hanifin, J.M. Pruritic dermatitis in asthmatic basenji-greyhound dogs: A model for human atopic dermatitis. *J. Am. Acad. Dermatol.* 1983, *8*, 33–38.

80. Peters, J.E.; Hirshman, C.A.; Malley, A. The Basenji-Greyhound dog model of asthma: Leukocyte histamine release, serum IgE, and airway response to inhaled antigen. *J. Immunol.* 1982, *129*, 1245–1249.

81. Hirshman, C.A.; Downes, H.; Leon, D.A.; Peters, J.E. Basenji-greyhound dog model of asthma: Pulmonary responses after beta-adrenergic blockade. *J. Appl. Physiol. Respir. Environ. Exerc. Physiol.* 1981, *51*, 1423–1427.

82. Shiohara, T.; Hayakawa, J.; Mizukawa, Y. Animal models for atopic dermatitis: Are they relevant to human disease? *J. Dermatol. Sci.* 2004, *36*, 1–9.

83. Suto, H.; Matsuda, H.; Mitsuishi, K.; Hira, K.; Uchida, T.; Unno, T.; Ogawa, H.; Ra, C. NC/Nga mice: A mouse model for atopic dermatitis. *Int. Arch. Allergy Immunol.* 1999, *120*, S70–S75.

84. Matsuda, H.; Watanabe, N.; Geba, G.P.; Sperl, J.; Tsudzuki, M.; Hiroi, J.; Matsumoto, M.; Ushio, H.; Saito, S.; Askenase, P.W.; *et al.* Development of atopic dermatitis-like skin lesion with IgE hyperproduction in NC/Nga mice. *Int. Immunol.* 1997, *9*, 461–466.

85. Yang, F.; Tanaka, M.; Wataya-Kaneda, M.; Yang, L.; Nakamura, A.; Matsumoto, S.; Attia, M.; Murota, H.; Katayama, I. Topical application of rapamycin ointment ameliorates Dermatophagoides farina body extract-induced atopic dermatitis in NC/Nga mice. *Exp. Dermatol.* 2014.

86. Kim, J.Y.; Jeong, M.S.; Park, M.K.; Lee, M.K.; Seo, S.J. Time-dependent progression from the acute to chronic phases in atopic dermatitis induced by epicutaneous allergen stimulation in NC/Nga mice. *Exp. Dermatol.* 2014,*23*, 53–57.

87. Kim, H.J.; Kim, Y.J.; Kang, M.J.; Seo, J.H.; Kim, H.Y.; Jeong, S.K.; Lee, S.H.; Kim, J.M.; Hong, S.J. A novel mouse model of atopic dermatitis with epicutaneous allergen sensitization and the effect of *Lactobacillus rhamnosus*. *Exp. Dermatol.* 2012, *21*, 672–675.

88. Vercelli, D. Of flaky tails and itchy skin. *Nat. Genet.* 2009, *41*, 512–513.

89. Presland, R.B.; Boggess, D.; Lewis, S.P.; Hull, C.; Fleckman, P.; Sundberg, J.P. Loss of normal profilaggrin and filaggrin in flaky tail (*ft/ft*) mice: An animal model for the filaggrin-deficient skin disease ichthyosis vulgaris. *J. Invest. Dermatol.* 2000, *115*, 1072–1081.

90. NIAID-Sponsored Expert Panel; Boyce, J.A.; Assa'ad, A.; Burks, A.W.; Jones, S.M.; Sampson, H.A.; Wood, R.A.; Plaut, M.; Cooper, S.F.; Fenton, M.J.; *et al.* Guidelines for the diagnosis and management of food allergy in the United States: Report of the NIAID-sponsored expert panel. *J. Allergy Clin. Immunol.* 2010, *126*, S1–S58.

91. Prescott, S.; Allen, K.J. Food allergy: Riding the second wave of the allergy epidemic. *Pediatr. Allergy Immunol.*2011, *22*, 155–160.

92. Amin, A.J.; Davis, C.M. Changes in prevalence and characteristics of IgE-mediated food allergies in children referred to a tertiary care center in 2003 and 2008. *Allergy Asthma Proc.* 2012, *33*, 95–101.

93. Gupta, R.S.; Springston, E.E.; Warrier, M.R.; Smith, B.; Kumar, R.; Pongracic, J.; Holl, J.L. The prevalence, severity, and distribution of childhood food allergy in the United States. *Pediatrics* 2011, *128*, e9–e17.

94. Pałgan, K.; Bartuzi, Z. Gene and environmental interactions of food allergy. *Postepy. Hig. Med. Dosw. (Online)*2012, *66*, 385–391.

95. Chiang, W.C.; Pons, L.; Kidon, M.I.; Liew, W.K.; Goh, A.; Wesley Burks, A. Serological and clinical characteristics of children with peanut sensitization in an Asian community. *Pediatr. Allergy Immunol.* 2010, *21*, e429–e438.

96. Levy, M.B.; Goldberg, M.R.; Nachshon, L.; Tabachnik, E.; Katz, Y. Lessons from cases of mortality due to food allergy in Israel: Cow's milk protein should be considered a potentially fatal allergen. *Isr. Med. Assoc. J.* 2012,*14*, 29–33.

97. Vetander, M.; Helander, D.; Flodström, C.; Ostblom, E.; Alfvén, T.; Ly, D.H.; Hedlin, G.; Lilja, G.; Nilsson, C.; Wickman, M. Anaphylaxis and reactions to foods in children—A population-based case study of emergency department visits. *Clin. Exp. Allergy* 2012, *42*, 568–577.

98. De Leon, M.P.; Rolland, J.M.; O'Hehir, R.E. The peanut allergy epidemic: Allergen molecular characterisation and prospects for specific therapy. *Expert Rev. Mol. Med.* 2007, *9*, 1–18.

99. Hefle, S.; Nordlee, J.A.; Taylor, S.L. Allergenic foods. *Crit. Rev. Food Sci. Nutr.* 1996, *36*, S69–S89.

100. Sicherer, S.H.; Sampson, H.A. Food allergy. *J. Allergy Clin. Immunol.* 2010, *125*, S116–S125.

101. Wang, J.; Sampson, H.A. Food allergy. *J. Clin. Invest.* 2011, *121*, 827–835.

102. Helm, R.M.; Ermel, R.W.; Frick, O.L. Nonmurine animal models of food allergy. *Environ. Health Perspect.* 2003,*111*, 239–244.

103. Maloney, J.M.; Rudengren, M.; Ahlstedt, S.; Bock, S.A.; Sampson, H.A. The use of serum-specific IgE measurements for the diagnosis of peanut, tree nut, and seed allergy. *J. Allergy Clin. Immunol.* 2008, *122*, 145–151.

104. Helm, R.M.; Burks, Q.W. Animal models of food allergy. *Curr. Opin. Allergy Clin. Immunol.* 2002, *2*, 541–546.

105. Helm, R.M. Food allergy animal models: An overview. *Ann. N. Y. Acad. Sci.* 2002, *964*, 139–150.

106. Srivastava, K.D.; Kattan, J.D.; Zou, Z.M.; Li, J.H.; Zhang, L.; Wallenstein, S.; Goldfarb, J.; Sampson, H.A.; Li, X.M. The Chinese herbal medicine formula FAHF-2 completely blocks anaphylactic reactions in a murine model of peanut allergy. *J. Allergy Clin. Immunol.* 2005, *115*, 171–178.

107. Li, X.M.; Schofield, B.H.; Huang, C.K.; Kleiner, G.I.; Sampson, H.A. A murine model of IgE-mediated cow's milk hypersensitivity. *J. Allergy Clin. Immunol.* 1999, *103*, 206–214.

108. Dearman, R.J.; Stone, S.; Caddick, H.T.; Basketter, D.A.; Kimber, I. Evaluation of protein allergenic potential in mice: Dose-response analyses. *Clin. Exp. Allergy.* 2003, *33*, 1586–1594.

109. Gonipeta, B.; Kim, E.; Gangur, V. Mouse models of food allergy: How well do they simulate the human disorder? *Crit. Rev. Food Sci. Nutr.* 2013.

110. Van Gramberg, J.L.; de Veer, M.J.; O'Hehir, R.E.; Meeusen, E.N.T.; Bischof, R.J. Induction of allergic responses to peanut allergen in sheep. *PLOS ONE* 2012, *7*.

111. Ladics, G.S.; Knippels, L.M.; Penninks, A.H.; Bannon, G.A.; Goodman, R.E.; Herouet-Guicheney, C. Review of animal models designed to predict the potential allergenicity of novel proteins in genetically modified crops.*Regul. Toxicol. Pharmacol.* 2010, *56*, 212–224.

112. Knippels, L.M.; Penninks, A.H.; van Meeteren, M; Houben, G.F. Humoral and cellular immune responses in different rat strains on oral exposure to ovalbumin. *Food Chem. Toxicol.* 1999, *37*, 881–888.

113. Van Gramberg, J.L.; de Veer, M.J.; O'Hehir, R.E.; Meeusen, E.N.; Bischof, R.J. Use of animal models to investigate major allergens associated with food allergy. *J. Allergy (Cairo)* 2013.

114. Favrot, C.; Steffan, J.; Seewald, W.; Picco, F. A prospective study on the clinical features of chronic canine atopic dermatitis and its diagnosis. *Vet. Dermatol.* 2010, *21*, 23–31.

115. Carlotti, D.N.; Remy, I.; Prost, C. Food allergy in dogs and cats: A review and report of 43 cases. *Vet. Dermatol.*1990, *1*, 55–62.

116. Verlinden, A.; Hesta, M.; Millet, S.; Janssens, G.P. Food allergy in dogs and cats: A review. *Crit. Rev. Food Sci. Nutr.* 2006, *46*, 259–273.

117. Jackson, H.A.; Jackson, M.W.; Coblentz, L.; Hammerberg, B. Evaluation of the clinical and allergen specific serum immunoglobulin E responses to oral challenge with cornstarch, corn, soy and a soy hydrolysate diet in dogs with spontaneous food allergy. *Vet. Dermatol.* 2003, *14*, 181–187.

118. Teuber, S.S.; del Val, G.; Morigasaki, S.; Jung, H.R.; Eisele, P.H.; Frick, O.L.; Buchanan, B.B. The atopic dog as a model of peanut and tree nut food allergy. *J. Allergy Clin. Immunol.* 2002, *110*, 921–927.

119. Buchanan, B.B.; Frick, O.L. The dog as a model for food allergy. *Ann. N. Y. Acad. Sci.* 2002, *964*, 173–183.

120. Kennis, R.A. Use of atopic dogs to investigate adverse reactions to food. *J. Am. Vet. Med. Assoc.* 2002, *221*, 638–640.

121. Marsella, R.; Ahrens, K. Experimental model of peanut allergy in dogs after epicutaneous sensitization. *Br. J. Dermatol.* 2014, *170*, E4.

122. Matsumoto, K.; Saito, H. Epicutaneous immunity and onset of allergic diseases—Per-"eczema"tous sensitization drives the allergy march. *Allergol. Int.* 2013, *62*, 291–296.

123. McClain, S.; Bannon, G.A. Animal models of food allergy: Opportunities and barriers. *Curr. Allergy Asthma Rep* 2006, *6*, 141–144.

124. Global Strategy for Asthma Management and Prevention. Available online: http://erj.ersjournals.com/content/31/1/143.full.pdf+html (accessed on 10 October 2014).

125. Chapman, R.W. Canine models for asthma and COPD. *Pulm. Pharmacol. Ther.* 2008, *21*, 731–742.

126. Cabana, M.D.; Kunselman, S.J.; Nyenhuis, S.M.; Wechsler, M.E. Researching asthma across the ages: Insights from the National Heart, Lung, and Blood Institute's Asthma Network. *J. Allergy Clin. Immunol.* 2014, *133*, 27–33.

127. Masoli, M.; Fabian, D.; Holt, S.; Beasley, R. The global burden of asthma: Executive summary of the GINA Dissemination Committee Report. *Allergy* 2004, *59*, 469–478.

128. Subbarao, P.; Mandhane, P.J.; Sears, M.R. Asthma: Epidemiology, etiology and risk factors. *CMAJ* 2009, *181*, E181–E190.

129. Gershon, A.; Guan, J.; Victor, J.C.; Wang, C.; To, T. The course of asthma activity: A population study. *J. Allergy Clin. Immunol.* 2012, *129*, 679–686.

130. Zosky, G.R.; Sly, P.D. Animal models of asthma. *Clin. Exp. Allergy* 2007, *37*, 973–988.

131. Bates, J.H.T. Stochastic-model of the pulmonary airway tree and its implications for bronchial responsiveness.*J. Appl. Physiol.* 1993, *75*, 2493–2499.

132. Barnes, P.J. Corticosteroid effects on cell signalling. *Eur. Respir. J.* 2006, *27*, 413–426.

133. Eriksson, U.; Egermann, U.; Bihl, M.P.; Gambazzi, F.; Tamm, M.; Holt, P.G.; Bingisser, R.M. Human bronchial epithelium controls TH2 responses by TH1-induced, nitric oxide-mediated STAT5 dephosphorylation: Implications for the pathogenesis of asthma. *J. Immunol.* 2005, *175*, 2715–2720.

134. Howat, W.J.; Holgate, S.T.; Lackie, P.M. TGF-β isoform release and activation during *in vitro* bronchial epithelial wound repair. *Am. J. Physiol.* 2002, *282*, L115–L123.

135. Szelenyi, I. Animal models of bronchial asthma. *Inflamm. Res.* 2000, *49*, 639–654.

136. Taube, C.; Dakhama, A.; Gelfand, E.W. Insights into the pathogenesis of asthma utilizing murine models. *Int. Arch. Allergy Immunol.* 2004, *135*, 173–186.

137. Turner, D.J.; Myron, P.; Powell, W.S.; Martin, J.G. The role of endogenous corticosterone in the late-phase response to allergen challenge in the brown Norway rat. *Am. J. Respir. Crit. Care Med.* 1996, *153*, 545–550.

138. Reinero, C.; DeClue, A.; Rabinowitz, P. Asthma in humans and cats: Is there a common sensitivity to aeroallergens in shared environments? *Environ. Res.* 2009, *109*, 634–640.

139. Kirschvink, N.; Leemans, J.; Delvaux, F.; Snaps, F.; Clercx, C.; Gustin, P. Non-invasive assessment of airway responsiveness in healthy and allergen sensitized cats by use of barometric whole body plethysmography. *Vet. J.* 2007, *173*, 343–352.

140. Norris Reinero, C.; Decile, K.; Berghaus, R.; Williams, K.; Leutenegger, C.; Walby, W.; Schelegle, E.; Hyde, D.; Gershwin, L. An experimental model of allergic asthma in cats sensitized to house dust mite or Bermuda grass allergen. *Int. Arch. Allergy Immunol.* 2004, *135*, 117–131.

141. Padrid, P.; Snook, S.; Finucane, T. Persistent airway hyperresponsiveness and histologic alterations after chronic antigen challenge in cats. *Am. J. Resp. Crit. Care Med.* 1995, *151*, 184–193.

142. Expert Panel Report 3: Guidelines for the Diagnosis and Management of Asthma. Available online: http://www.nhlbi.nih.gov/health-pro/guidelines/current/asthma-guidelines/full-report (accessed on 20 October 2014).

143. Haliwell, R.E.W.; Schwartzmann, R.M. Atopic diseases in the dog. *Vet. Rec.* 1971, *89*, 209–214.

144. De Weck, A.L.; Mayer, P.; Stumper, B.; Schiessel, B.; Pickat, L. Dog allergy, a model for allergy genetics. *Int. Arch. Allergy Immunol.* 1997, *113*, 55–57.

145. Collie, D.D.; DeBoer, D.J.; Muggenburg, B.A.; Bice, D.E. Evaluation of association of blood and bronchoalveolar eosinophil number and serum total immunoglobulin. *Am. J. Vet. Res.* 1997, *58*, 34–39.

146. Redman, T.K.; Rudolph, K.; Barr, E.B.; Bowan, L.E.; Muggenburg, B.A.; Bice, D.E. Pulmonary immunity to ragweed in a beagle dog model of allergic asthma. *Exp. Lung Res.* 2001, *27*, 433–451.

147. Meeusen, E.N.; Snibson, K.J.; .Hirst, S.J.; Bischof, R.J. Sheep as a model species for the study and treatment of human asthma and other respiratory diseases. *Drug Discov. Today* 2009, *6*, 101–106.

148. Bischof, R.J.; Snibson, K.; Shaw, R.; Meeusen, E.N. Induction of allergic inflammation in the lungs of sensitized sheep after local challenge with house dust mite. *Clin. Exp. Allergy* 2003, *33*, 367–375.

149. Abraham, W.M. Pharmacology of allergen-induced early and late airway responses and antigen-induced airway hyperresponsiveness in allergic sheep. *Pulm. Pharmacol.* 1989, *2*, 33–40.

150. Scheerlinck, J.P.; Snibson, K.J.; Bowles, V.M.; Sutton, P. Biomedical applications of sheep models: From asthma to vaccines. *Trends Biotechnol.* 2008, *26*, 259–266.

151. Gomez, F.P.; Rodriguez-Roisin, R. Platelet-activating factor antagonists—Current status in asthma. *BioDrugs*2000, *14*, 21–30.

13
CHAPTER

RECENT ADVANCES IN REPRODUCTIVE BIOTECHNOLOGIES IN SHEEP AND GOAT

Basil Alexander[1,2], Gabriela Mastromonaco[1,3], and W. Allan King[1]

[1]Department of Biomedical Sciences, Ontario Veterinary College (OVC), University of Guelph, Ontario, Canada

[2]Department of Farm Animal Production and Health, Faculty of Veterinary Medicine and Animal Science, University of Peradeniya, Sri Lanka

[3]Reproductive Physiology, Toronto Zoo, 361A Old Finch Avenue, Scarborough, ON, M1B 5K7

CONTENTS

This review focuses on the platform of recent advances in reproductive biotechnologies in sheep and goat. Here, we discuss some aspects of veterinary and biomedical importance in artificial insemination using sexed semen, in vitro/in vivo fertilization, interspecies in vitro fertilization, multiple ovulation and embryo transfer (MOET), somatic cell nuclear transfer and transgenic animal production in sheep and goat. Some of these technologies are already widely used in the cattle industry, and some are new to the goat and sheep industry.

INTRODUCTION

The world sheep and goat populations in 2006 were recorded as 416 and 489 million, respectively [1]. Reproductive biotechnologies are playing an increasingly important role in the production and management of these species. Animal biotechnology encompasses the application of science and engineering principles to the processing or production of materials to provide services or goods for human use [2]. Examples of current animal biotechnologies include artificial insemination using fresh, frozen or sexed semen, embryo transfer using fresh or frozen in vivo or in vitro produced embryos, cloning using somatic cell nuclear transfer procedures and production of transgenic animals. Recent advances in reproductive biotechnologies have shown important developments in the technologies and their delivery that promise to yield significant benefits for their

Citation: Alexander B, Mastromonaco G, King WA (2010) Recent Advances in Reproductive Biotechnologies in Sheep and Goat. J Veterinar Sci Technol 1:101. doi:10.4172/2157-7579.1000101

application within the livestock industry as well as in biomedical sciences. This review focuses on the recent advances of biotechnologies in sheep and goats.

METHODS

Artificial Insemination (AI)

Artificial insemination is the procedure involving the mechanical deposition of pre-collected semen into the uterus of an estrous female by a technician. The widespread commercial application of AI, a robust tool in livestock breeding, began in earnest in the 1950's after researchers developed methods to successfully freeze cattle semen [3]. This technology, which is the most extensively applied reproductive biotechnology in the world, has many valuable advantages such as reducing venereal diseases, rapidly increasing genetic merits of the production animals through selective breeding and eliminating lethal alleles. The potential to pass high genetic merits of a selected male to thousands of females makes this a far more efficient technology for producing large numbers (1.5 x 108) of offspring per year compared to female based technologies, such as embryo transfer (ET), which can only produce a few progeny from a selected female. More recently, the advent of separation of sperm into X- and Y-chromosome fractions using flow cytometry has added a new dimension to livestock production [4].

Since the first report of live rabbit pups of predetermined sex using X and Y-enriched sorted semen over 20 years ago [5], there have been more than 40,000 births of live animals resulting from the so- called Beltsville sperm sexing technology [4]. This sperm sexing technology has proven to be a reliable and more efficient method of obtaining predetermined sex in animals compared to other relatively wasteful methods of embryo sexing and pre-implantation genetic diagnosis [6 - 8]. Live offspring born from fresh sex- sorted semen have been reported in many species including cattle [9], pigs [10,11], horses [12,13] and sheep [14,15]. As the sorting procedure can separate sperm only at a speed of approximately 10 million per hour, inseminations have to be carried out using limited numbers of sperm in each insemination dose compared to the conventional standards for AI. To obtain high success rates with sorted semen AI, most trials have been carried out using fresh sorted semen, nevertheless, use of frozen sorted semen is ultimately more beneficial to the livestock industry as it can be stored for long duration and easy to transport anywhere in the world.

Semen sexing technology

Semen sexing is the process of separating spermatozoa into two subpopulations containing X-chromosome and Y-chromosome bearing spermatozoa. In theory, use of the X-bearing spermatozoa fraction for insemination will result in female progeny, while the Y-bearing spermatozoa fraction will give male progeny. Considerable efforts have been made in this area over the past 30-40 years, but only recently has there been considerable progress, particularly in cattle [16]. The most commonly applied technique for the separation of a fresh semen sample into X and Y-chromosome bearing fractions is fluorescence activated cell sorting (FACS). The concept behind this technique is described below:

Fluorescence activated cell sorting (FACS)

This technique involves the separation of X- and Y- bearing spermatozoa in small quantities based on the DNA content of the spermatozoa so that they can then be used in in vitro fertilization and AI programs [17]. The procedure is relatively slow and requires expensive infrastructure at least for mass scale commercial application. The technique is based on the biological principle that the DNA content of the X and Y chromosomes as X-chromosome has 3.8% more DNA than Y-chromosome [9]. This difference can, nonetheless, be detected with FACS technique. Before the spermatozoa are passed through the cell sorter, the sample is exposed to a nontoxic DNA dye that specifically binds to DNA to allow measurement of the DNA content of each spermatozoa. The cell suspension is then passed through an extremely fine nozzle that vibrates at high frequency causing the fluid stream to disperse into micro-drops which, optimally holds only one spermatozoa after the conditions are calibrated. When the stream of micro-droplets is passing through a UV laser beam, the already stained DNA will start to glow or emit fluorescence. The strength (intensity) of the florescence is measured by a detector, and if the florescence is in the range designated for the Y bearing spermatozoa, that micro-drop is given an electric charge. Furthermore, if the intensity is within the range for X-bearing spermatozoa, the micro-drop is given an opposite electric charge. The charged micro-drops fall between two charged plates, resulting in two groups of droplets to be separated into different pools (Figure 1). Droplets that fall outside of the fluorescence range for X or Y are collected into a third group where the sex cannot be determined. The disadvantages of the technique are its relatively slow process and increased wastage of unsorted spermatozoa. The advantage is it can give up to 95% purity sexed semen samples.

Application of sexed semen in goat and sheep production

Although the sexed semen technology is gaining in popularity in commercial cattle industries, its use has yet to be developed in the sheep and goat industries. Nevertheless recent attempts to separate the X- and Y-chromosomal fractions using flow cytometry on ram semen has been attempted and yielded fraction purity greater than 90% [18]. In flow cytometry, the sperm extending medium plays a critical role in the efficiency of separation and the viability of the sperm after sorting [17,19,20]. Ram sperm have to be diluted 20- fold before sorting and a further 200-fold dilution takes place when it passes through the cell sorter resulting in capacitation-like changes that lead to reduced fertility of sexed sheep semen [17,20]. It has also been shown that suspension of ram semen in Tris-based medium without egg- yolk, improves the staining of the DNA and efficiency of separation of sperm without reducing its viability [8,18,21].

When working with frozen sex- sorted semen in sheep, it is believed that the semen should be deposited in the oviduct or deep within the uterus to obtain high success rates, although it appears to be not as critical in cattle [16]. In sheep, frozen semen is usually deposited laparoscopically into the uterus and these same methods have been used effectively to produce offspring from frozen sexsorted semen [15]. Oviductal deposition of frozen semen in sheep is not practical if large numbers of sheep are to be inseminated. To our knowledge, there have been no reports of attempts to inseminate sheep or goat using sex- sorted semen in the cervix or transcervically.

The minimum number of sperm in an intrauterine AI dose in sheep varies between 5 x 106 and 25 x 106, but in Australia it has been suggested as 25 x 106 motile spermatozoa. Although it is not known exactly the minimum number of frozen sex-sorted sperm for intrauterine insemination of sheep, it is expected that it should be in the range of standard commercial intrauterine AI semen dose [20]. However, it is acceptable that the number of sperm in frozen sex sorted semen should be increased in line with the negative effects of the sorting process to obtain high efficiency.

The timing of AI also plays a significant role in AI success in sheep but recent findings have suggested that the best results can be achieved with sex–sorted frozen sperm when inseminated just before the expected ovulation time in ovulation-synchronized progesterone treated ewes. Using sex sorted frozen semen (40 million sperm per AI dose), optimal results can be expected when ewes are inseminated at 58 h after sponge removal or 36 h after GnRH injection [20].

Embryo production and transfer

Multiple ovulation and embryo transfer (MOET): This breeding model has been extensively used to multiply genetically superior goats and sheep and many protocols have been developed to optimize its application in research as well as in commercial practice [22-25]. In most domestic farm animals, especially in cattle, the genetic gain is limited on the female side due to low reproductive rate with only one calf being produced per year and also relatively long intervals between generations. To overcome these limitations MOET has been developed. Using this method, a female is hormonally stimulated to have multiple ovulations (superovulation). Most MOET programs in sheep and goat consist of a 14 to 17 day progesterone exposure, with FSH injections beginning 2 days before the removal of the progesterone releasing device. Following six or eight FSH injections given twice daily, the animals are allowed to breed naturally or by artificial insemination. The ovulated ova are allowed to fertilize in vivo following artificial insemination or natural mating. After fertilization and initiation of embryo development, 6-7 day old embryos (morula/ blastocyst stage) are recovered from within the uterus using embryo flushing techniques. In sheep, this is done surgically [26]. These embryos are then transferred to non-pregnant estrus-synchronized recipients 6-7 days post estrus or frozen in liquid nitrogen (-196i° C) for future use.

It is well-known that the superovulation protocols in small ruminants do not guarantee the recovery of quality transferable embryos due to various factors that affect the success of the program [25]. These factors can be listed as extrinsic and intrinsic factors. The extrinsic factors include: a) source and purity of the gonadotrophins, b) protocol of gonadotrophin injection, and c) the type of progesterone treatment protocol [25]. Intrinsic factors include: age, breed, nutrition and reproductive status of the animals [25]. However, despite all the achievements in the MOET programs in small ruminants so far, the success of obtaining high quality transferable embryos still remains Figure 1:

Schematic representation of the concept behind the Florescent Activated Cell Sorting technique used in separation of X- and Y-bearing chromosomes in a fresh semen sample low and more studies are needed to investigate the optimization of these programs.

Embryo transfer (ET)

According to the available data from the International Embryo Transfer Society (IETS), the number of embryo transfers carried out in small ruminants is shown in Table 1. In sheep and goat, ET is usually carried out by laparoscopic surgery 6-7 days post estrus [27], (Figure 2). Estrus is generally synchronized in sheep as follows. On day-1 of the program, progesterone releasing intravaginal sponges (Veramix®, 60mg medroxyprogesterone acetate, Pharmacia & Upjohn, Orangeville, Canada) are inserted in to the vagina. On day- 14, the sponges are removed and 300 IU PMSG (Folligon®, Intervet) are injected intramuscularly to each ewe at the time of sponge withdrawal. Vasectomised rams are introduced on day-15 and ewes in estrus are identified between 12-36 h post PMSG injections. Surgical embryo transfer is then performed on day-22 of the program [27].

The embryos are usually evaluated for morphology according to the IETS criteria [28] and only the excellent quality blastocysts/ morulae are transferred into recipient ewes. Ewes are anesthetized using xylazine (0.2mg/kg) injection intravenously, and are secured on a laparoscopic cradle. An incision of approximately 1 cm is made in the skin approximately 3 cm to the left of the mid line and approximately 5 cm from the udder, using a scalpel blade (Figure 2B-D). A trochar and cannula are inserted into the abdominal cavity through the incision made in the skin (Figure 2E-F). The uterine horns and the ovaries with corpora lutea are visualized using a laparoscope (Figure 2G). The uterine horn is punctured close to the utero-tubular junction using a blunt 18-gauge needle and the embryos are loaded into an embryo transfer catheter and transferred into the lumen of the uterine horn (Figure 2H). The ewes are then monitored postoperatively for a few hours and released to the paddocks.

Recently, a goat ET group in Sri Lanka reported that they have produced ET born goat kids (Figure 2B) from fresh embryos in a field embryo transfer program without using sophisticated equipment [22], thus validating the field application of the technique in veterinary practice to multiply genetically valuable goats to establish an elite goat herd under local production conditions. Moreover, ET in small ruminants is still carried out using the conventional ET techniques employing laparoscopic techniques with an average pregnancy rate of 60% with fresh embryo transfers. The pregnancy rates can vary due to many factors such as donor, recipient, embryo and operator. The transcervical ET procedure seems to be not practical in these species due to the problems associated with handling of the cervix and its anatomy. Recently, a research group [29] reported that anestrus sheep cervix can be dilated using prostaglandin 12 h prior to the insertion of AI gun into the uterus suggesting possibility of transcervical ET in sheep. However, more studies are needed to optimize this technique in small ruminants to obtain high success rates.

In vitro embryo production in sheep and goat

In vitro embryo production in sheep and goat provides an alternate source of low cost embryos for transfer in breeding programs such as MOET. The process consists of 3 main steps: 1) oocyte collection and In vitro maturation (IVM) of cumulus-oocyte complexes (COCs), 2) In vitro fertilization (IVF) and 3) in vitro culture of embryos. These steps have been reviewed in detail by others [30 - 33]. Here we will highlight the important differences between species.

Oocyte collection and In vitro maturation

Prior to in vitro fertilization, COCs are collected either by minimally invasive laparoscopic ovum pick up (LOPC) or postmortem from slaughtered females [32,34]. Cumulus-oocyte complexes are collected from live sheep by a laparotomy followed by aspiration of oocytes from ovaries using an aspiration pump. This method is often called as laparoscopic ovum pick-up (LOPU) and seems to be very efficient for the recovery and quality of the COCs obtained in sheep and goats. Usually, in sheep, a short repeated gonadotrophin treatment is followed by LOPU [35-38]. In contrast, goats can be stimulated with a 'one shot' regime of gonadotrophins (one shot of follicular stimulating hormone (FSH) plus equine chorionic gonadotrophin (eCG), compared to the traditional multi-dose gonadotrophin regimes. The results revealed no differences in the efficiency of COCs recovered and their quality [36,39]. It has also been shown that 'one shot' regime can be performed as a 4-day treatment regime followed by LOPU in sheep and goats without reducing the efficiency in oocyte recovery and quality [40]. The most common method of oocyte collection is from abattoir derived ovaries from sheep or goat. Ovaries are transported to the laboratory at 37°C in phosphate buffered saline (PBS) after which they are finely sliced with a scalpel blade and rinsed in oocyte collection medium consisting of 2% steer serum in Ham's F10 medium [34].

In vitro maturation of abattoir derived oocytes from sheep and goats (for comprehensive reviews see 32, 31) rely on methods based on bi-carbonate buffered TCM 199 medium supplemented with L-glutamine, ovine FSH (10 μg/ml), ovine LH (10 μg/ml, estrogen (1 μg/ml) and 10% fetal bovine serum [34]. Some researchers have used mature follicular fluid supplementation in the IVM medium to enhance the maturation of sheep oocytes [31]. Under these conditions, goat and sheep oocytes tend to extrude first polar body between 16-24 h of in vitro maturation [41]. In contrast, it is accepted that supplementation of the glutathione precursor cysteamine (100 μM) in IVM medium enhances the in vitro maturation process of goat oocytes [41]. In addition, a recent study [42] showed that cysteamine and BSA added to IVM medium for sheep, resulted in high blastocyst rates (42% blastocyst rate from total cultured oocytes) and high survival rate of blastocysts after embryo transfer. It is obvious that artificial oocyte maturation and culture systems have detrimental effects on embryo development compared to their in vivo counterparts. Recent fluorescent in situ hybridization cytogenetic studies from our laboratory using whole chromosome painting probes have revealed that high incidence of chromosomal abnormalities in sheep blastocysts derived from IVP systems, compared to in vivo derived blastoctsts [43] emphasizing the inherent differences in the two production methods.

In vitro fertilization

In vitro fertilization of the oocytes is usually carried out following 24 h maturation in the IVM medium. Surrounding cumulus cells are removed by gentle pippetting and washing in fertilization medium and groups of 40-50 oocytes are placed in 4-well dishes in 500 μl of synthetic oviductal fluid (SOF) covered by 200 μl of mineral oil [31,43]. Motile sperm are obtained by centrifugation of frozen-thawed semen in Percoll gradient (45%/90%) at 500 g for 10 min in room temperature. Percoll gradient separation of spermatozoa seems to be an effective means of yielding motile sperm from frozen-thawed semen [44]. Motile sperm are collected from the bottom of the 90% fraction and diluted to a concentration of 107 spermatozoa/ml in media. Recent studies have shown that incubation of spermatozoa for a further 1 h period in media supplemented with heat-inactivated estrus serum enhances the capacitation process of spermatozoa (sheep and goat : [41]; deer : [45,46]). In our laboratory we routinely add heat – inactivated sheep serum (2%) to the IVF medium and incubate oocytes with motile spermatozoa for 17 hours resulting acceptable levels of blastocyst development [43]. Although 17 h co-incubation is practiced in IVF, it has been shown that even 4 h co-incubation was enough to obtain acceptable cleavage and blastocyst rates in sheep [41]. Further application of in vitro fertilization in obtaining sex pre-determined offspring will be an advantage for the livestock industry [20,47]. In vitro fertilization of prepubertal oocytes and oocytes recovered from LOPU [37] are also important areas to be developed further.

In vitro culture

Following in vitro fertilization, embryos are washed several times and then placed in in vitro culture (IVC) media for further development. There are 3 methods available for embryo culture after fertilization, such as co-culture with somatic cells, culture in semi-defined media and culture of embryos in in vivo systems (oviducts) of the same or different species [41]. Co-culture systems in sheep and goat are usually based on including oviductal cells in TCM-199 medium. Semi-defined medium is also used often in small ruminant IVC based on the components of the sheep oviductal fluid (SOF), a medium containing essential and non-essential amino acids supplemented with BSA [43,48]. In our laboratory, sheep embryos cultured in SOF medium supplemented with amino acids and BSA at 38°C in 5% O_2, 5% CO_2, 90% N_2 humidified atmosphere resulted in 19.2% blastocyst rates from total oocytes cultured [43]. This rate is confirmed by [38], who showed that SOF culture systems supplemented with BSA and amino acids produce high quality blastocysts in sheep. Addition of fetal bovine serum (FBS) on day 2 or 3 of culture does result in high embryo survival post-embryo transfer and normal viable offspring [41]. However, some studies have reported that sheep embryos reduce their viability by 15%–25% when produced in SOF systems supplemented with serum compared to co-culture [48] or in in vivo systems of culturing the embryos in oviducts [49]. It has been noted that adding steer serum or human serum to sheep and goat IVC media may attribute to many abnormalities in the offspring [50,51].

Interspecies in vitro fertilization

Investigating interspecies fertilization provides valuable insights into the role of cytoplasmic and nuclear events that regulate full term development. Due to species specific molecular, morphological and chronological markers these embryo models are unique for examining the paternal and maternal interactions and their vital role in development. Interesting findings from our laboratory revealed that ram spermatozoa is not able to fertilize bovine oocytes in vivo, however, in vitro fertilization occurs and the resulting hybrid embryos, confirmed by cytogenetic analysis (Figure 3), arrested at 4-8 cell stage [52] even when zygotes were transferred to sheep oviducts for early development. Similar developmental arrest occurs with the reverse cross. Hybridization between sheep and goats through cross or chance breeding like many species, appears to be polar with the success or efficiency dependent of the parent of origin [53]. Goats bred to rams conceive and pregnancies will progress to second trimester while in the case of the reverse cross, sheep oocytes exposed to buck sperm in vivo do not fertilize [52]. However, a few cases of sheep X goat hybrids born to goats have been documented [54]. In vitro sheep and goat oocytes, could be fertilized by buck or ram sperm and embryos developed to the blastocyst stage, hatched and, following transfer into the uteri of sheep or goats, they established pregnancies. However, retarded fetal growth, defects in placentome formation and pregnancy failure during the second month of gestation were observed [52]. The in vitro production of hybrid embryos is particularly amenable to facilitate further study of the reproductive barriers and species differences in imprinted and epigenetic, regulation of early embryo development that are key to embryo survival and development.

Somatic cell nuclear transfer (Cloning)

A new era in reproductive biotechnology began when Wilmut and colleagues produced the first somatic cell nuclear transfer (SCNT) derived viable sheep, “Dolly”, from transplanting an adult somatic cell into an enucleated sheep oocyte [55]. Following this breakthrough, theoretically, it seems to be a promising technology to produce unlimited numbers of genetic copies from an adult animal or a fetus; and so far many species including farm, pet and endangered animals have been cloned using this technology [56]. Obtaining a viable offspring through this technology still imposes a great challenge for researchers due to its relatively low success rate and in some instances compromised health status of offspring [57,58]. At present, cloning is carried out for biomedical and research purposes, and agriculture production. Although extensive reviews are available on animal cloning, here we emphasize some recent findings that are important in small ruminant cloning.

The standard SCNT technique in sheep/goat in most of the laboratories follows some common steps such as oocyte maturation, removal of cumulus cells from oocytes, enucleation, transplantation of the somatic cell into the perivitelline space of the oocyte, electrofusion of the cell couplet, activation of the embryo and in vitro embryo culture. When the embryos develop to blastocyst, they are transplanted into the uteri of estrus-synchronized surrogate animals 6-7 day post estrus [27]. In most cases, the oocytes are collected from abattoir ovaries using the slicing method and undergo IVM for 17h (goat: [59-61], Sheep: [27,34]). Some laboratories that conduct goat SCNT programs preferred in vivo derived oocytes either following ovulation [62,63] or LOPU [64,65]. This may be due to the decreased availability of goat abattoirs in different countries or the higher success rates from in vivo matured oocytes. Following maturation, the cumulus cells are removed by vortexing in 3% Sodium citrate medium [27] for 1-2 minute or in 0.01% hyaluronidase. Cumulus –free oocytes with first polar body extrusion are selected and after a short exposure to cytochalasin B and Hoechst stain, enucleation is carried out in a micromanipulator equipped with UV light [27,61,64,65]. Following oocyte enucleation, cell cycle-synchronized donor cells are transplanted into the perivitelline space of the oocytes in a manner that both cell membranes attach firmly to each other. The cellcouplets are then electrofused in a 0.3 M mannitol fusion medium. One hour following fusion, cell-couplets are activated by culturing for 5 min in ionomycin containing medium followed by culturing them in 6-DMAP or cycloheximide containing medium [27,34,61]. Recent studies in our laboratory revealed that a greater incidence of chromosomal abnormalities occur when SCNT-sheep embryos are cultured in 6-DMAP containing medium compared to cycloheximide [27,34]. After activation, embryos are cultured in IVC medium and are surgically transferred into uteri of estrus –synchronized ewes [27] or into the oviducts of the does [61]. Pregnancy confirmation is done by ultrasound scanning beginning on day 35 of pregnancy. Pregnancy loss in sheep following SCNT-derived embryo transfer can be monitored by ultrasound imaging combined with serum progesterone levels [27].

Recently, there has been some controversy on the biological age of the SCNT-derived offspring, and whether they may susceptible for pre-mature death compared to their age-matched control counterparts [56]. A good example of this was the premature death of "Dolly". The hypothesis behind this is that donor somatic cells from adults may correlate with offspring carrying shortened telomere lengths compared to normal controls. Telomeres are located at the end of the chromosomes and become shorter in each cell cycle when somatic cells replicate. When the telomere length reaches a critical length the cell either enters senescence or enters a 'crisis' state associated with the development of cancer cells. This phenomenon does not happen in the germ line and in embryonic cells as these cells posses telomerase, an enzyme that adds telomere sequences to chromosomes during cell replication thus preventing telomere shortening from occurring. In most somatic cells, the telomerase enzyme is not present, leading to continuous telomere shortening when cells replicate [66].

Recent findings in telomere lengths in animal clones revealed cases of shorter [67, 68] not different [69-71] and surprisingly even longer lengths compared to those measured in their age matched control counterparts [72]. These findings have triggered much speculation on the fate of clones. However, this makes animal clones derived from adult somatic cells appropriate models for studying cellular rejuvenation and aging in vivo since they are generated from aged and culture propagated somatic cells known to contain shorten telomeres. Following SCNT, the differentiated donor nucleus undergoes extensive remodeling and reprogramming by the recipient oocyte cytoplasm [73], which has been shown to cause altered gene expression profiles [74] and chromatin modifications [75] that likely contribute to the high incidence of abnormalities, prenatal and postnatal losses found in clones[73]. Altered expression of telomerase activity

[71] and donor cell type-dependent telomere length differences [76] further support inappropriate genome reprogramming, however, the precise etiology of altered telomere lengths in vivo are not clear for clones. Recent studies from our laboratory on SCNT-derived small ruminants showed that shortened telomere lengths in sheep cloned using adult donor cells compared to controls [67] and a similar phenomenon was observed in SCNTderived goats [77]. Interestingly, the offspring derived from natural breeding between cloned parents, did not show any discrepancies in telomere length [67] suggesting that telomere length was reset in the germ line of the cloned offspring. To date we do not possess enough data on telomere length of clones and "Dolly" cannot be considered the only incidence in this nature, thus more research is needed to investigate the lifespan of cloned offspring; at this stage the data available is inconclusive.

Production of transgenic sheep and goats

Transgenic animals are produced either to carry an exogenous gene or to have a "knock out" gene from their own genome. Many transgenic animals have been produced for biomedical research interests as well as to test their application in livestock production [78]. There are many techniques available for the production of transgenic animals, such as pronuclear microinjection [37,79,80], sperm-mediated transgenesis [81] and somatic cell nuclear transfer[65,82,83]. During the last decade, research has focused on producing transgenic animals which secrete recombinant proteins in their milk. These animals produce relatively high quantities of recombinant proteins compared to other conventional methods due to the physiological nature of the mammary gland for its unique ability to synthesize proteins [78,84,85,86,87,88]. A few examples of transgenic small ruminants producing recombinant proteins in milk for pharmaceutical and biomedical interest are sheep producing human clotting factor VIII [89] and factor IX [82] and goats synthesizing human antithrombin III [90], human alpha-fetoprotein [91], human monoclonal antibodies [92, 93], malaria antigens [94] spider silks [95], human granulocyte colony stimulating factor (96) and human butyryl-cholinesterase [97,98]. Although these animals have shown high expression of the transgene product in the milk, a recent report suggests that the transgene may have some negative effects on the physiology of mammary gland function, leading to a compromised situation [87]. However, the first protein produced by transgenic animals, ATryn, a recombinant human anti-thrombinproduced in transgenic goats' milk, received approval for use in humans in 2009.

CONCLUSIONS

In this review, we have focused on some aspects of reproductive biotechnology that are of veterinary and biomedical importance in sheep and goat that have been reported in the recent past. It is well known that most biotechnologies take many years to come into full practice after enormous amounts of laboratory and field research. Therefore, more focus should be carried out in emerging areas like artificial insemination of sheep and goat using sexed semen, in vitro and in vivo embryo production systems, transgenic animal production and cloning using stem cells.

ACKNOWLEDGEMENTS

The authors gratefully acknowledge the assistance provided by Ed R Reyes, Elizabeth St. John, Pamela Hasson in the University of Guelph, the MITACS Accelerate internship program, Canada, the Canadian Commonwealth Scholarship Plan and the University of Peradeniya in preparation of this manuscript.

REFERENCES

1. Zygoyiannis D (2006) Sheep production in the world and in Greece. Small Rumin Res 62: 143-147.
2. Ghadar F, Spindler H (2005) The growth of biotechnology. Industrial Management 47: 19-26.
3. Polge C (1968) Frozen semen and the A.I. Programme in Proc. 2nd Tech. Conf. Artif. Insem. Reprod. NAAB, Columbia, MO: 46-51.
4. Johnson LA, Rath D, Vazquez JM, Maxwell WMC, Dobrinsky JR (2005) Preselection of sex of offspring in swine for production: current status of the process and its application. Theriogenology 63: 615-624.
5. Johnson LA, Flook JP, Hawk HW (1989) Sex preselection in rabbits: live births from X and Y sperm separated by DNA and cell sorting.Biol Reprod 41: 199-203.
6. Garner DL (2001) Sex-sorting mammalian sperm: concept to application in mammals. J Androl 22: 519-526.
7. Seidel GE Jr, Garner DL (2002) Current status of sexing mammalian spermatozoa. Reproduction 124: 733-743.
8. Evans G, Hollinshead FK, Maxwell WMC (2004) Preservation and artificial insemination of sexed semen in sheep. Reprod Fertil Dev 16: 455-464.
9. Seidel GE, Schenk JL, Hcrickhoff LA, Doyle SP, Brink Z, et al. (1999) Insemination of heifers with sexed sperm. Theriogenology 52: 1407-1420.
10. Vazquez JM, Martinez EA, Parrilla I, Roca J, Gill MA, et al. (2003) Birth of piglets after deep intrauterine insemination with flow cytometrically sorted boar spermatozoa. Theriogenology 59: 1605-1614.
11. Rath D, Ruiz S, Sieg B (2003) Birth of female piglets following intrauterine insemination of a sow using flow cytometrically sexed boar semen. Vet Rec 152: 400-401.
12. Buchanan BR, Seidel GE, McCue PM, Schenk JL, Heickhoff LA, et al. (2000) Insemination of mares with low numbers of either unsexed or sexed spermatozoa. Theriogenology 53: 1333-1344.
13. Lindsey AC, Schenk JL, Graham JK, Bruemmer JE, Squires EL (2002) Hysteroscopic insemination of low numbers of flow sorted fresh and frozen thawed stallion spermatozoa. Equine Vet J 34: 121-127.
14. Catt SL, Catt JW, Gomez MC, Maxwell WMC, Evans G (1996) The birth of a male lamb derived from an in vitro matured oocyte fertilized by intra-cytoplasmic injection of a single presumptive male sperm. Vet Rec 139: 494-495.

15. Hollinshead FK, O'Brien JK, Maxwell WMC, Evans G (2002) Production of lambs of pre-determined sex after the insemination of ewes with low numbers of X- or Y-chromosome bearing spermatozoa. Reprod Fertil Dev 14: 503-508.

16. Garner DL, Seidel GE Jr (2003) Past, present and future perspectives on sexing sperm. Can J Anim Sci 83: 375-384.

17. Maxwell WMC, Johnson LA (1997) Chlortetracycline analysis of boar spermatozoa after incubation, flow cytometric sorting, cooling or cryopreservation. Mol Reprod Dev 46: 408-418.

18. Hollinshead FK, O' Brien JK, Gillan L, Mayers M, Maxwell WMC, et al. (2004) Liquid storage of flow cytometrically sorted ram spermatozoa. Theriogenology 62: 587-605.

19. Catt SL, O'Brian JK, Maxwell WMC, Evans G (1997) Assessment of ram and boar spermatozoa during cell-sorting by flow cytometry. Reprod Domestic Anim 32: 251- 258.

20. Hollinshead FK, Gillan L, O'Brian JK, Evans G, Maxwell WMC (2003) In vitro and in vivo assessment of functional capacity of flow cytometrically sorted ram spermatozoa after freezing and thawing. Reprod Fertil Dev 15: 351-359.

21. De Graaf SP, Gillan L, Evans G, Maxwell WMC, O'Brian JK (2004). The effect of the sheath fluid on the quality of sex-sorted ram spermatozoa. Reprod Fertil Dev 16: 284-285.

22. Perera GDRK, Pushpakumara PGA, De Silva LNA, Alexander B (2008) Production of genetically superior goats through embryo transfer technology in Sri Lanka. Tropi Agri Res 20: 177-184.

23. Bartlewski PM, Alexander BD, Rawlings NC, Barrett DMW, King WA (2008) Ovarian responses, hormonal profiles and embryo yields in anoestrus ewes superovulated with Folltropin-V after pretreatment with medroxyprogesterone acetate (MAP)- releasing vaginal sponges and a single dose of estradiol-17ß (E2-17ß). Reprod Domest Anim 43: 299 – 307.

24. Bartlewski PM, Alexander BD, King WA (2008a) Ovarian and endocrine determinants of superovulatory responses in anestrous ewes.Small Rumin Res 75: 210-216.

25. Gonzalez-Bulnes A, Baird DT, Campbell BK, Cocero MJ, Garcia-Garcia RM, et al. (2004) Multiple factors affecting the efficiency of multiple ovulation and embryo transfer in sheep and goats. Reprod Fertil Dev 16: 421-435.

26. Menchaca A, Vilarino M, Pinczak A, Kmaid S, Saldana JM (2009) Progesterone treatment, FSH plus eCG, GnRH administration, and Day 0 Protocol for MOET programs in sheep. Theriogenology 72: 477-483.

27. Alexander B, Coppola G, Mastromonaco GF, John ES, Reyes ER, et al. (2008) Early Pregnancy Diagnosis by Serum Progesterone and Ultrasound in Sheep Carrying Somatic Cell Nuclear Transfer - Derived Pregnancies. Repro Domest Anim 43: 207-211.

28. String fellow and Seidel (1998) Manual of the International Embryo Transfer Society.

29. Candappa IBR, Bainbridge HC, Price NT, Hourigan KR, Bartlewski PM (2009) A preliminary study on the suitability of Cervidil to induce cervical dilation for artifi cial insemination in ewes. Res Vet Sci 87: 204-206.

30. Garcia-Garcia R, Ward F, Fair S, O'Meara C, Wade M, et al. (2007) Development and quality of sheep embryos cultured in commercial G1.3/G2. 3 sequential media. Anim Reprod Sci 98: 233-240.

31. Cognie Y, Poulin N, Locatelli Y, Mermillod P (2004) State-of-the-art production, conservation and transfer of in-vitro-produced embryos in small ruminants. Reprod Fertil Dev 16: 437-445.

32. Wani NA (2002) In vitro maturation and in vitro fertilization of sheep oocytes. Small Rumin Res 44: 89-95.

33. Wang S, Liu Y, Holyoak GR, Evans RC, Bunch TD (1998) A protocol for in vitro maturation and fertilization of sheep oocytes. Small Rum Res 29: 83-88.

34. Alexander B, Coppola G, Di Berardino D, Rho GJ, St John E, et al. (2006) The effect of 6-dimethylaminopurine (6-DMAP) and cycloheximide (CHX) on the development and chromosomal complement of sheep parthenogenetic and nuclear transfer embryos. Mol Reprod Dev 73: 20-30.

35. Alberio R, Olivera J, Roche A, Alabart J, Folch J (2002) Performance of a modified ovum pick-up system using three different FSH stimulation protocols in ewes. Small Rumin Res 46: 81-87.

36. Baldassarre H, Wang B, Kafi di N, Keefer C, Lazaris A, et al. (2002) Advances in the production and propagation of transgenic goats using laparoscopic ovum pickup and in vitro embryo production technologies. Theriogenology 57: 275-284.

37. Baldassarre H, Wang B, Kafi di N, Gauthier M, Neveu N, et al. (2003) Production of transgenic goats by pronuclear microinjection of in vitro produced zygotes derived from oocytes recovered by laparoscopy. Theriogenology 56: 83-839.

38. Wan PC, Haoa ZD, Zhoub P, Wua Y, Yanga L (2009) Effects of SOF and CR1 media on developmental competence and cell apoptosis of ovine in vitro fertilization embryos. Anim Reprod Sci 114: 279-288.

39. Baldassarre H, Furnus CC, De Matos DG, Pessi H (1996) In vitro production of sheep embryos using laparoscopic folliculocentesis: Alternative gonadotrophin treatments for stimulation of oocyte donors. Theriogenology 45: 707-717.

40. Gibbons A, Bonnet FP, Cueto MI, Catala M, Salamone DF, et al. (2007) Procedure for maximizing oocyte harvest for in vitro embryo production in small ruminants. Reprod Dom Anim 42: 423-440.

41. Cognie Y, Baril G, Poulin N, Mermillod P (2003) Current status of embryo technologies in sheep and goat. Theriogenology 59: 171-188.

42. Accardo C, Dattena M, Pilichi S, Mara L, Chessa B, et al. (2004) Effects of recombinant human FSH and LH on in vitro maturation of sheep oocytes: embryo development and viability. Anim Reprod Sci 81: 77-86.

43. Coppola G, Alexander B, Di Berardino D, St John E, Basrur PK, et al. (2007) Use of cross-species in-situ hybridization (ZOO-FISH) to assess chromosome abnormalities in day-6 in vivo- or in vitro-produced sheep embryos. Chromosome Res 15: 399-408.

44. Rho GJ, Hahnel AC, Betteridge KJ (2001) Comparison of oocyte maturation times and of three methods of sperm preparation for their effects on the production of goat embryos in vitro. Theriogenology 56: 503-516.

45. Comizzoli P, Mermillod P, Cognie Y, Chal N, Legendre X, et al. (2001) Successful in vitro production of embryos in red deer (Cervus elaphus) and the sika deer (Cervus nippon). Theriogenology 55: 649-659.

46. Berg DK, Thompson JG, Asher GW (2002) Development of In Vitro Embryo Production Systems for Red Deer (Cervus Elaphus). Part 3. In Vitro Fertilisation Using Sheep Serum as a Capacitating Agent and the Subsequent Birth of Calves. Anim Reprod Sci 70: 85-98.

47. O' Brien JK, Hollinshead FK, Maxwell WMC (2004) In vivo development capacity of in vitro produced embryos derived from sex-sorted and re-cryopreserved frozen-thawed ram-sperm. Reprod Fertil Dev 16: 286.

48. Hoshi H (2003) In vitro production of bovine embryos and their application for embryo transfer. Theriogenology 59: 675-685.

49. Holm P, Walker SK, Seamark RF (1996) Embryo viability, duration of gestation and birth weight in sheep after transfer of in vitro matured and in vitro fertilized zygotes cultured in vitro or in vivo. J Reprod Fertil 107: 175-181.

50. Sinclair KD, McEvoy TG, Maxfi eld EK, Maltin CA, Young LE, et al. (1999) Aberrant fetal growth and development after in vitro culture of sheep zygotes. J Reprod Fertil 116: 177-186.

51. Walker S, Hill J, Kleeman D, Nancarrow C (1996) Development of ovine embryos in synthetic oviductal fluid containing amino acids at oviductal fluid concentrations. Biol Reprod 55: 703-708.

52. Kelk DA (1997) Development characteristics of interspecific hybrid embryos. PhD Thesis. University of Guelph, Ontario, Canada.

53. Anderson GB (1988) Interspecific pregnancy: barriers and prospects. Biol Reprod 38: 1-15.

54. Pinheiro LEL, Guimaraes SEF, Almeida IL, Mikich AB (1989) The natural occurrence of sheep X goat hybrids. Theriogenology 32: 987 – 994.

55. Wilmut I, Schnieke AE, McWhir J, Kind AJ, Campbell KH (1997) Viable offspring derived from fetal and adult mammalian cells. Nature 385: 810-813.

56. Vajta G, Gjerris M (2006) Science and technology of farm animal cloning: state of the art. Anim Reprod Sci 92: 211-230.

57. Hill JR, Roussel AJ, Cibelli JB, Edwards JF, Hooper NL, et al. (1999) Clinical and pathological features of cloned transgenic calves and fetuses (13 case studies). Theriogenology 51: 1451-1465.

58. Rho GJ, Coppola G, Sosnowski J, Kasimanickam R, Johnson WH, et al. (2007) Use of somatic cell nuclear transfer to study meiosis in female cattle carrying a sex-dependent fertility-impairing X-chromosome abnormality. Cloning Stem Cells 9: 118-29.

59. Ma S, Lan G, Miao Y, Wang Z, Chang Z, et al. (2003) Hypoxanthine (HX) inhibition of in vitro meiotic resumption in goat oocytes. Mol Reprod Dev 66: 306-313.

60. Lan GC, Han D, Wu YG, Han ZB, Ma SF, et al. (2005) Effects of duration, concentration and timing of ionomycin and 6-dimethylaminopurine (6-DMAP) treatment on activation of goat oocytes. Mol Reprod Dev 71: 380-388.

61. Lan GC, Chang ZL, Luo MJ, Jiang YL, Han D, et al. (2006) Production of Cloned Goats by Nuclear Transfer of Cumulus Cells and Long-Term Cultured Fetal Fibroblast Cells Into Abattoir-Derived Oocytes. Mol Reprod Dev 73: 834-840.

62. Zou X, Wang Y, Cheng Y, Yang Y, Ju H, et al. (2002) Generation of cloned goats (Capra hircus) from transfected foetal fibroblast cells, the effect of donor cell cycle. Mol Reprod Dev 61: 164-172.

63. Behboodi E, Memili E, Melican DT, Destrempes MM, Overton SA, et al. (2004) Viable transgenic goats derived from skin cells.Transgenic Res 13: 215-224.

64. Keefer CL, Stone RK, Bhatia B, Lazaris A, Begin I, et al.(2000) Efficient production of viable goat offspring following nuclear transfer using adult somatic cells. Biol Reprod 62: 192.

65. Keefer CL, Baldassarre H, Keyston R, Wang B, Bhatia B, et al. (2001) Generation of dwarf goat (Capra hircus) clones following nuclear transfer with transfected and nontransfected fetal fi broblasts and in vitro-matured oocytes. Biol Reprod 64: 849-856.

66. Xu J, Yang X (2003) Will cloned animals suffer premature aging - the story at the end of clone's chromosomes. Reprod Biol Endocrinol 1: 105-110.

67. Alexander B, Coppola G, Perrault SD, Peura TT, Betts DH, et al. (2007) Telomere length of sheep clones and their offspring. Mol Reprod Dev 74: 1525-1537.

68. Shiels PG, Jardine AG (2003) Dolly, no longer the exception: Telomeres and implications for transplantation. Cloning stem cells 5: 157-160.

69. Jiang L, Carter DB, Xu J, Yang X, Prather RS, et al. (2004) Telomere lengths in cloned transgenic pigs. Biol Reprod 70: 1589-1593.Betts DH, Bordingnon V, Hill JR, Winger Q, Westhusing ME, et al. (2001) Reprogramming of telomerase activity and rebuilding of telomere length in cloned cattle. Proc Natl Acad Sci USA 98: 1077-1082.

70. Betts DH, Bordingnon V, Hill JR, Winger Q, Westhusing ME, et al. (2001) Reprogramming of telomerase activity and rebuilding of telomere length in cloned cattle. Proc Natl Acad Sci USA 98: 1077-1082.

71. Tian XC, Xu J, Yang X (2000) Normal telomere lengths found in cloned cattle. Nat Genet 26: 272-273.

72. Lanza R, Cibelli JB, Blackwell C, Cristofalo VJ, Francis MK, et al. (2000) Extension of cell life- span and telomere length in animals cloned from senescent somatic cells. Science 288: 665-669.

73. Reik W, Dean W (2002) Epigenetic reprogramming: back to the beginning. Nature 420: 127.

74. Humpherys D, Eggan K, Akatsu H, Friedman A, Hoechedlinger K, et al. (2002) Abnormal gene expression in cloned mice derived from embryonic stem cell and cumulus cell nuclei. Proc Natl Acad Sci USA 99: 12889-12894.

75. Dean W, Santos F, Stojkovic M, Zakhartchenko V, Walter J, et al. (2001) Conservation of methylation reprogramming in mammalian development: aberrant reprogramming in cloned embryos. Proc Natl Acad Sci USA 98: 13734-13738.

76. Miyashita N, Shiga K, Yonai M, Keneyama K, Kobayashi S, et al. (2002) Remarkable differences in telomere lengths among cloned calves derived from different cell types. Biol Repro 66: 1649-1655.

77. Betts DH, Perrault SD, Petrik J, Lin L, Favetta LA, et al. (2005) Telomere length analysis in goat clones and their offspring. Mol Reprod Dev 72: 461-470.

78. Wheeler MB, Walters EM, Clark SG (2003) Transgenic animals in biomedicine and agriculture: outlook for the future. Anim Reprod Sci 79: 265-289.

79. Ebert KM, Selgrath JP, DiTullio P, Denman J, Smith TE, et al. (1991) Transgenic production of a variant of human tissue-type plasminogen activator in goat milk: generation of transgenic goats and analysis of expression. Biotechnology 9: 835-838.

80. Baldassarre H, Wang B, Gauthier M (1999) Embryo transfer in a commercial transgenic production program using BELE® goat embryos. Theriogenology 51: 415.

81. Celebi C, Guillaudeux T, Auvray P, Vallet-Erdtmann V, Jegou B (2003) The making of "transgenic spermatozoa". Biol Reprod 68: 1477-1483.

82. Schnieke AE, Kind AJ, Ritchie WA, Mycock K, Scott AR, et al. (1997) Human Factor IX transgenic sheep produced by nuclear transfer of nuclei form transfected fetal fibroblasts. Science 278: 2130-2133.

83. Keefer CL, Lazaris A, Keyston R (2002) Cloning using somatic cells for the production and propagation of transgenic Nigerian dwarf and dwarf-crossed goats. Theriogenology 57: 422.

84. Houdebine LM (2000) Transgenic animal bioreactors Transgenic Res 9: 305-320.

85. Keefer CL (2004) Production of bioproducts through the use of transgenic animal models. Anim Reprod Sci 82: 5-12.

86. Baldassarre H, Wang B, Pierson J, Neveu N, Sneek L, et al. (2004) Prepubertal Propagation of Transgenic Cloned Goats by Laparoscopic Ovum Pick-Up and in Vitro Embryo Production. Cloning Stem Cells 6: 25-29.

87. Baldassarre H, Hockley DK, Dore M, Brochu E, Hakier B, et al. (2008a) Lactation performance of transgenic goats expressing recombinant human butyrylcholinesterase in the milk. Transgenic Res 17: 73-84.

88. Baldassarre H, Hockley DK, Olaniyan B, Brochu E, Zhao X, et al. (2008b) Milk composition studies in transgenic goats expressing recombinant human butyrylcholinesterase in the mammary gland. Transgenic Res 17: 863-872.

89. Niemann H, Halter R, Carnwath JW, Herrmann D, Lemme E, et al. (1999) Expression of blood clotting factor VIII in the mammary gland of transgenic sheep. Transgenic Res 8: 237-247.

90. Zhou Q, Kyazike J, Echelard Y, Meade HM, Higgins E, et al. (2005) Effect of genetic background on glycosylation heterogeneity in human antithrombin produced in the mammary gland of transgenic goats. J Biotechnol 117: 57-72.

91. Parker MH, Birck-Wilson E, Allard G, Masiello N, Day M, et al. (2004) Purification and characterization of a recombinant version of human alpha-fetoprotein expressed in the milk of transgenic goats. Protein Expr Purif 38: 177-183.

92. Young MW, Meade H, Curling JM, Ziomek CA, Harvey M (1998) Production of recombinant antibodies in the milk of transgenic animals.Res Immunol 149: 609- 610.

93. Pollock DP, Kutzko JP, Birck-Wilson E, Williams JL, Echerlard Y, et al. (1999) Transgenic milk as a method for the production of recombinant antibodies. J Immunol Methods 231: 147-157.

94. Behboodi E, Ayres SL, Memili E, O'Coin M, Chen LH, et al. (2005) Health and reproductive profi les of malaria antigen-producing transgenic goats derived by somatic cell nuclear transfer. Cloning Stem Cells 7: 107-118.

95. Karatzas CN, Zhou FJ, Huang Y, Duguay F, Chretien N, et al. (1999) Production of recombinant spider silk (BioSteel®) in the milk of transgenic animals. Transgenic Res 8: 476-477.

96. Ko JH, Lee CS, Kim KH, Pang MG, Koo JS, et al. (2000) Production of biologically active human granulocyte colony stimulating factor in the milk of transgenic goat. Transgenic Res 9: 215-222.

97. Cerasoli DM, Griffi ths EM, Doctor BP, Saxena A, Fedorko JM, et al. (2005) In vitro and in vivo characterization of recombinant human butyrylcholinesterase (Protexia) as a potential nerve agent bioscavenger. Chem Biol Interact 158: 363-365.

98. Huang YJ, Huang Y, Baldassarre H, Wang B, Lazaris A, et al. (2007) Recombinant human butyrylcholinesterase from milk of transgenic animals to protect against organophosphate poisoning. Proc Natl Acad Sci USA 104: 13603-13608.

14
CHAPTER

FROM "ONE HEALTH" TO "ONE COMMUNICATION": THE CONTRIBUTION OF COMMUNICATION IN VETERINARY MEDICINE TO PUBLIC HEALTH

Micaela Cipolla, Luigi Bonizzi, and Alfonso Zecconi

Department of Veterinary Science and Public Health (DIVET), Università degli Studi di Milano, via Celoria 10, 20133 Milano, Italy

ABSTRACT

Despite the fact that health communication is a discipline developed only recently, its importance in human medicine is well recognized. However, it is less considered in veterinary medicine, even if it has the potential to improve public health because of the role of veterinary medicine in public health. For this reason, an One Health approach is useful for communication as well. This approach leads to a "One Communication" concept, which is the result of the synergy in communicative efforts both in human and in veterinary medicine. Our analysis explores the potential of communication in several veterinary fields: institutions, food safety, companion animal and food-producing animal practice, pharmacology and drugs, wildlife fauna and environment. In almost all the areas of veterinary activity communication can contribute to human health. It takes many forms and use several channels, and this variety of communicative opportunities represent a challenge for veterinarians. For this reason, the communication course should be included in the curricula of Veterinary Medicine Schools. As One Health, One Communication is a strategy for expanding collaborations in health communication and it will enhance public health.

INTRODUCTION

Health Communication is a discipline only recently developed, and it is "The study of how health information is generated and disseminated and how that information affects individuals, community groups, institutions and public policy" [1].

Citation: Micaela Cipolla, Luigi Bonizzi, and Alfonso Zecconi, From "One Health" to "One Communication": The Contribution of Communication in Veterinary Medicine to Public Health, Vet. Sci. 2015, 2(3), 135-149; doi:10.3390/vetsci2030135

The aim of health communication is to inform and influence people's behaviour and attitude in order to improve health [2,3,4]. This is possible because it concerns all aspects of health, including, *i.e.*, research, clinical practice, public health, global health and policy making [5,6]. Different approaches are available to investigate all of the aspects, *i.e.*, health campaigns, risk communication and patient-provider communication.

An effective communication is essential to public health. It can be written and verbal, taking many forms and using various channels such as physicians and other health professionals, family, friends and mass media, Internet, advertisement. For its growing importance, the World Health Organization (WHO) includes health communication in its activities and provides several guides supporting communication strategies development for different situations, such as health emergencies and disease prevention [7,8,9,10,11,12,13]. Moreover, WHO considers communication expertise as essential to outbreak control as well as epidemiological training and laboratory analysis, and demonstrated a significant reduction of cases during an outbreak when applied a proactive communication [14,15]. Many other institutions, such as UNICEF, FAO, CDC, Johns Hopkins University and others agree that communication is a necessary tool for public health [16,17,18,19,20,21,22,23,24,25,26,27,28].

Any advice aiming to enhance health by changing people's behaviour is a communicative act. Health communication allows to identify contexts, channels, messages and factors having the potential to motivate individuals to use correctly health information. Therefore, health communication supports health professionals in their daily work, educates patients and helps policy makers; it has a powerful role in disease prevention and health promotion. It is part of health management, even in settings with limited resources, helping to use information and interacting with the community or other partners.

Due to its pivotal importance, health communication became part of the curriculum in several Medicine and Veterinary Medicine Schools worldwide, but usually health communication refers to human health and it is generally less considered in veterinary medicine. The intended outcome of this article is to describe this new aspect of veterinary medicine—the health communication—and its contribution to public health. With our paper we highlight the role of communication in the main branches of veterinary activity, to help veterinarians to find their role in the "One communication" perspective. Indeed, communication in veterinary medicine has the potential to contribute to public health and should be considered in a One Health perspective.

One Health

The One Health concept links human, animal and environmental health, it is "a worldwide strategy for expanding interdisciplinary collaborations and communications in all aspects of health care for humans, animals and the environment. The synergism achieved will advance health care for the 21st century and beyond by accelerating biomedical research discoveries, enhancing public health efficacy, expeditiously expanding the scientific knowledge base, and improving medical education and clinical care."[29]. This approach considers all global health threats to gain cross-disciplinary collaboration, especially between physicians and veterinarians. The result is a collaborative effort to enhance human and animal health between the health professions.

One Health has its origins in the 1800s, when Rudolf Virchow, the German physician who coined the term "zoonosis", highlighted the linkages between human and veterinary medicine [30]. In the following years, other physicians and veterinarians recognized the importance of good animal health for the public health. One of them, Calvin Schwabe, made important contributions to epidemiology, zoonoses, tropical health and public health. He coined the term "One medicine", emphasizing the close interdependence and similarities between human and veterinary medicine [31]. More recently, the Wildlife Conservation Society promoted a symposium to discuss the movements of diseases among human, domestic animal and wildlife populations. The symposium set twelve priorities—the Manhattan Principles—for an interdisciplinary strategy to combat diseases and maintain the ecosystem integrity. These principles considered, with human and animal health, also environment health [32].

The One Health approach has been endorsed by the main global health organizations, such as WHO, CDC, EFSA, OIE, FAO [33,34,35,36,37]. The collaborative effort between human and veterinary medicine should be applied not only at global level but also at local level, where it could be a new paradigm of health management [38]. This will result in a more effective and sustainable organization of public health, reducing the risk of zoonotic diseases such as rabies, H5N1 avian influenza, West Nile disease, TBC and diseases caused by E. coli STEC, *Staphylococcus aureus*MRSA, Nipah and Hendra viruses, Hantaviruses, Filovirus such as Ebola and Marburg viruses.

VETERINARY MEDICINE AND PUBLIC HEALTH

The purpose of veterinary medicine is to protect public health, through the promotion of animal health and food safety. To fulfil this objective, veterinary medicine has many arenas of activity in public health, including (Figure 1):

- Institutions (health authority, healthcare system)
- Food safety and nutrition
- Clinical practice
  - companion animals
  - food-producing animals
- Pharmacology and drugs
- Wildlife fauna
- Environment

In all these fields, communication has a key role and can contribute to public health by influencing people's behaviour and attitude.

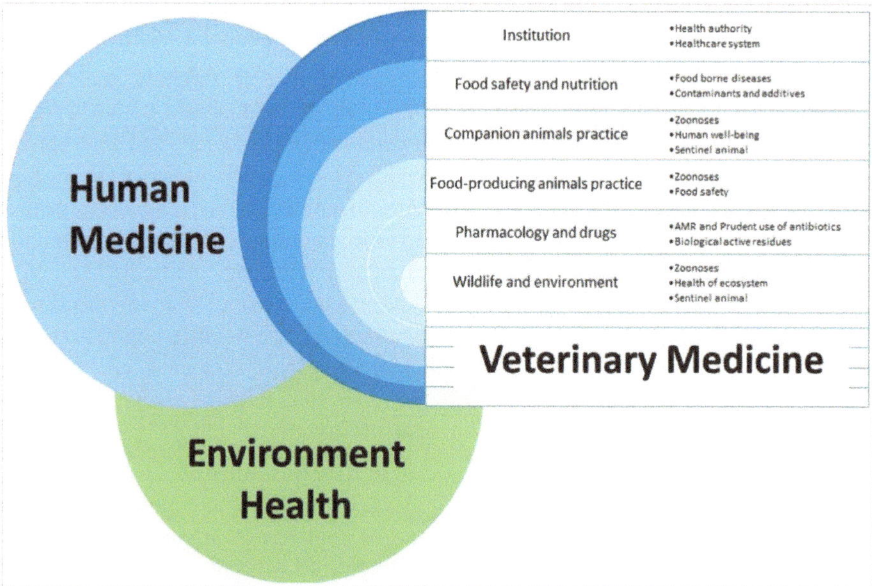

Figure 1: Potential contributes of veterinary medicine to public health in a One Health and One Communication perspective.

Institutions

Health care authorities and systems have the responsibility to manage health system, and communication is part of the management. Therefore, the role of communication is related to the institutional setting. We reported, as example, one European health system. In the Italian health system, communication for human and veterinary medicine is unique at the higher institutional level, because the Ministry of Health (Ministero della Salute) manages both. At lower regional and local institutional level, health authorities work separately on human and animal health, so the communication efforts often are uncoordinated. However, the institutional communication in veterinary medicine gives a high contribution to public health, because of the continuous overlapping between veterinary and human medicine in public health. This institutional activity includes, for example, health campaigns on zoonoses or food safety [39,40].

This organization of veterinary system has both pros and cons. The major benefit of the integration in the Ministry of Health is that the veterinary health system has a peculiar focus on health, and it is much less biased by production aspects, when compared to the systems under the Ministry of Agriculture. However, the focus on health, sometimes, put an excessive pressure on the production system, reducing its efficiency, by applying unnecessary barriers to the production process. At the local level, the system splits into the two components of human and veterinary medicine, and this disconnection gives to the veterinary medicine the opportunity to be more independent and effective in a given area, even if a coordination would be hopeful.

Moreover, the veterinary diseases surveillance networks have a key role in human surveillance and its utility would be increased through a better integration between the two systems, as happens through the joining of health service [41]. Likewise, a coordination also at the communicative level would produce more efficient efforts in enhancing public health. Also at policy and management levels, communication has a key role, as demonstrated by the example of Regional Veterinary Prevention Plan 2012–2014 (Piano Regionale della Prevenzione Veterinaria 2012–2014) of Regione Lombardia [42]. This was a new and powerful tool for public health, supporting veterinary health system at regional level, giving to all the operative units and officers an unique and coherent frame of reference [43]. Indeed, our research group developed a model (scorecard) to assess zoonoses and food safety issues. The scorecard supports daily practice setting priority in prevention and risk management, by assigning different scores to various risk and management aspects of each disease or food safety problem. Once this assignation has been done, the veterinary officers know the priority of each intervention and, also, if there is a lack of information about the specific disease. This model established a completely new approach to risk characterization in Italian public health authorities; it had to be understood and adopted by all the personnel involved in the regional veterinary system and, for this reason, communication was crucial. Both internal and external communication strategies were needed. All the members of the regional healthcare system were the audiences of internal communication: Regione Lombardia, local health authorities (Azienda Sanitaria Locale), regional diagnostic and surveillance laboratory (Istituto Zooprofilattico Sperimentale della Lombardia e dell'Emilia Romagna), research centers. At internal level, the aims of communication were to verify the outcomes of the plan application, to share information and to consolidate cooperation. External communication was addressed to stakeholders, with the aims to involve people, gather information and share results. All the initiatives, planned to inform and involve the target audience, were focused on objectives and results of the prevention plan application. However, the first communication need concerned the plan itself, and the understanding of the new risk characterization praxis. Indeed, the document was very articulated; it had many tables (the scorecards) and schemes for disease control plans, prevention protocols and risk characterization, each one concerning one of the veterinary areas. Indeed, in Italy the veterinary health system has three areas: A for animal health, B for food safety and C for herd management and animal welfare. One of the parameters considered for an effective communication of the plan was its graphic aspect. Due to the high amount and complexity of information delivered, we chose a simple and immediate graphic aspect, assigning a specific colour to each area. Every piece of information addressed to the animal health sector was green, to the food safety sector was red and to the herd management and animal welfare sector was yellow. Everything concerning the past or general topics was blue. This simple color code had a very useful function clarifying the whole document and making it more understandable. Moreover, this code made every local health authority having the same color for the same unit. All the veterinary officers recognized themselves in the color of their area, independently by the district of the local health authority. Therefore, the primary aim of the plan—to make uniform veterinary health system to improve public health—was achieved also with this simple communicative choice, and it was maintained also in the subsequent edition of the plan [44].

Food Safety and Nutrition

Communication on food safety and nutrition frequently pertains to veterinary medicine, being related to food-borne disease, GMO, contaminants, additives and foods of animal origin.

Consumers receive much information about food, but often it is contradictory and conflicting. This includes alerts, recommendation on what is good for health and what could be dangerous, risks and benefits associate in the same food, food components to reduce, nutrients to increase, warning on different diets and eating styles. All this information provide a non-unique frame of reference, which is difficult to manage and to understand by consumers. Sometimes unfounded concerns may overlap reliable messages from health authorities, resulting in more confusion and uncertainty [45]; especially during an alert or an outbreak, this situation may lead to fear and distrust in the product involved. Examples are the recent European food scares on *E. coli* in vegetables, horsemeat scandal, blue mozzarella cheese, BSE and avian influenza.

The health and welfare of food-producing animals during breeding, transportation and slaughtering have consequences for human health and are responsibility of veterinarians. Therefore, due to the pivotal role of veterinary medicine in animal nutrition, animal health, food inspection and food safety, communication in this area is important for public health, contributing to consumers' protection from field to fork.

Communication about food is often risk communication. Accordingly with the Codex Alimentarius Commission (CAC), risk communication is "an interactive exchange of information and opinions concerning risk among risk assessors, risk managers, consumers and other interested parties [46]. Therefore, food risk communication enables informed decision-making to promote health, fosters the understanding of both the real and the perceived food risk, and shares knowledge between government officials, health professionals, academicians, food producers, stakeholders, journalists and public. Misleading messages can have serious consequences not only on public health but also on the entire food supply chain. Thanks to a proper communication, authorities, experts and other stakeholders can communicate more successfully, making the public reacting properly [47].

To meet these needs, many local and international organizations, such as EFSA and FAO, promoted food risk communication [48,49].

Clinical Practice

Companion Animals

Companion animals, due to their close relationship with people, are important in the prevention of zoonoses and in their management. Moreover, pets have a role as sentinel animal and could be used to protect human health. For example, they are useful in cancer prevention and treatment in humans, because often they share the same risk and carcinogen factors, have many of the same types of cancer and are treated almost with the same drugs as humans [50]. Communication on such topics can contribute significantly to public health [51].

However, the focus of veterinary medicine in public health is not limited to zoonoses, because the One Health concept involves all of the aspects of health, including mental health via the human-animal bond phenomenon [52]. This latter aspect gives to the veterinary medicine a further role in public health, through disciplines centred on human-animal bond such as pet therapy. Moreover, the One Health statement amplifies the role of companion animals clinical practice in maintaining and improving human health, because it concerns not only zoonoses but also the owner-pet relationship.

The importance of communication in clinical practice has been widely recognized, even if only recently in veterinary medicine, where effective communication increases client satisfaction and compliance [53,54,55,56,57,58,59,60]. Therefore, this skill has become part of the veterinary education programs in many countries, being as important as other clinical skills [54,61,62,63].

However, in many European countries communication is still poorly considered. This situation may lead to communication errors, failures in meeting client expectations and, eventually, to complaint or malpractice claim as has been observed in human medicine [64]. Recent studies showed that in one of these countries, the large majority of pet owners consider the own pet as family member and this also affected owner responses and attitudes towards the veterinarian [65]. These results confirm the role of communication in improving veterinary practice and promoting clients' comfort, satisfaction and well-being.

Food-Producing Animals

Communication has a key role also in food-producing animals practice, improving management and animal health, as demonstrated for example in dairy farms [66,67,68].

Communication strategies are essential in promoting dairy herd health and are required to support diseases control programs [69,70]. Indeed, how consultant delivers information affects ideas, beliefs and motivation of the farmer, thus his/her behaviour and actions. [71,72,73]. Therefore, the leading role of communication in dairy herds is due to its power in influencing how farmers apply consultants' advice and, thus, in improving animal health and food safety. It is crucial for public health in a "from field to fork" perspective, because farmer's actions and management directly influence the quality of meat, milk and milk products.

All these aspects improve also herd sustainability. An effective communication in food-producing area supports development and improves health and innovation, also in emerging countries.

However, communication in veterinary practice is poorly considered in many countries including Italy. In this country, recent studies showed that dairy farmers are not satisfied with their consultants' communication [74]. This gap in veterinarians' skill represent a problem because an effective farmer-veterinarian communication is essential to improve farm management, herd health, food safety and herd sustainability.

Pharmacology and Drugs

The activity of veterinarians related to pharmacology and drugs is often cross-disciplinary, covering companion and food producing animal practice, food security, and official drugs residue controls. However, the rising importance of prudent use of antibiotics makes this topic suitable to become a specific area under the One Health approach. Indeed, the concern on antimicrobial resistance (AMR) increased in recent years; it is considered a major public health threat, due to misuse of antibiotics in both human and animal therapy. Therefore, it is a cross-disciplinary issue, engaging veterinarians to reduce and monitor antimicrobial usage in livestock [75,76].

Many veterinary organisations promote the responsible and prudent use of antimicrobial agents in animals, such as The World Organisation for Animal Health (OIE) [77]. Moreover, OIE developed standards and guidelines for OIE Member Countries to address the risk of the emergence or spread of resistant bacteria that result from the use of antimicrobial agents in food producing animals [78].

The European Medicines Agency (EMA) implemented the European Surveillance of Veterinary Antimicrobial Consumption (ESVAC) project, to identify possible risk factors that could lead to the development and spread of antimicrobial resistance in animals. The aim was to develop a harmonised approach for the collection and reporting of data on the use of antimicrobial agents in animals from EU Member States. Thus, EMA published reports on sales of veterinary antimicrobial agents in EU/EEA countries [79]. The International Dairy Federation (FIL-IDF) published a Guide to Prudent Use of Antimicrobial Agents in Dairy Production [80] and also the Federation of Veterinarians of Europe (FVE) developed a document on AMR and prudent use of antibiotics in Veterinary Medicine [81]. A specific interest on this topic was shown by U.S. Food and Drug Administration (FDA) and the U.S. Centers for Disease Control and Prevention (CDC) [82,83]. The latter one funded the development of the Antimicrobial Resistance Learning Site (AMRLS), which is a suite of educational materials promoting the prudent use of antimicrobial agents in veterinary practice [84]. Despite the large interest of veterinary sector on AMR, the communication was poorly considered. However, communication in veterinary medicine can promote the prudent use of antimicrobials, being synergic with the initiatives in human medicine. To highlight the problem and to support a rational antimicrobial use, the European Union promoted the European Awareness Day, an health initiative marked annually on 18 November and coordinated by European Center for Diseases Prevention and Control (ECDC). For this event, ECDC provides campaign communication materials for the European national health authorities in order to develop a consistent communication campaign on the prudent use of antibiotics. National campaigns use several communication tools, such as leaflets, poster, videos, websites and social media, that are aimed to both prescribers and the general public. Many communication initiatives take place across Europe, to disseminate messages on risks related to the antibiotic misuse and explaining how to take antibiotics responsibly [85,86,87]. Similar campaigns are promoted also in the United States, Canada and Australia [88,89].

All these programs show the importance of communication in human medicine to contain AMR, but communication in veterinary medicine is equally indispensable to promote a rational use of antibiotics and enhance the collaboration of veterinary organisations with the public health sector to reduce the antimicrobial resistance.

Wildlife Fauna and Environment

The One Health concept considers also the health of ecosystem, being health of humans, animals and environment interrelated. Indeed, both animals and humans live in the same environment, sharing air, water and food. If there is a poor health for the environment, there is a poor health for people and animals. The environmental pollution is a health hazards but it is not the only threat, because the health of plants is indispensable for having food [90]. Through an effective and responsible management of the natural resources, the One Health approach protects human and animal health and ensures a safe food supply [36,37]. Veterinary medicine can contribute to the health of the ecosystem, because agricultural contamination may lead to contamination of foods of animal origin. Moreover, these foods can be used as sentinel for monitoring contamination in the environment. For example, pesticide contamination of honey can be related to the contamination source and could reflect the specific pollution of an environment [91]. The use of animal sentinel for health hazards is very helpful to detect and manage more quickly and efficiently shared health risks [92]. Also when considering toxic risk, as shown by the potentials of "One Toxicology", the protection of domestic and wild animals' health is relevant to protecting humans [93].

In recent years the emerging diseases gained a leading role in epidemics on a global scale, and zoonoses were dominant [94]. These diseases are currently the main and global threat for human health, and are related to both domestic and wildlife fauna. Therefore, the synergy between medicine and veterinary medicine is indispensable for the research, the surveillance, the control and the communication of global health challenges at the animal-human-ecosystem interface [95]. The result of this cooperation is well known in developing countries, where it already resulted in an improved health care for the local populations [96]. Also in this area of veterinary medicine, coordinated communication efforts make an important contribution to public health.

CONCLUSIONS

In almost all the areas of veterinary activity communication can contribute to human health. It takes many forms and employs several channels, and this variety of communication opportunities represent a challenge for veterinarians. For this reason, communication courses should be included in the curricula of Veterinary Medicine Schools, as it happened in some already in North America.

Veterinarians should improve their communication skills because human and animal health are interrelated, as is health communication in human and veterinary sectors. Both of them cover the same issue (zoonoses, food safety *etc.*) and use the same channels. For example, it is not possible to differentiate between food risk communication in human and veterinary areas, having the same target, using the same strategies and considering the same risks.

Despite the fact that health communication is a recent matter, it has a growing importance in human medicine but it is less considered in veterinary medicine. However, because of the role of veterinary medicine in public health, communication in veterinary area also has the potential to improve public health. Therefore, a One Health approach applies to communication as well, leading to the "One Communication" concept, which is the result of the synergy in communicative efforts both in human and in veterinary medicine. As One Health, One Communication is a strategy for expanding collaborations in health communication and it will enhance health care.

AUTHOR CONTRIBUTIONS

Micaela Cipolla conceived and designed the study, wrote the paper; Luigi Bonizzi designed the study, revised the paper; Alfonso Zecconi designed the study, revised the paper.

REFERENCES

1. Harvard School of Public Health. The Field of Health Communication. Available online: http://www.hsph.harvard.edu/health-communication/ (accessed on 17 May 2015).
2. Hornik, R.C. *Public Health Communication—Evidence for Behavior Change*; Routledge-Lawrence Erlbaum Associates: Mahwah, NJ, USA, 2002.
3. CDC. What is Health Communications? Available online: http://www.cdc.gov/healthcommunication/healthbasics/whatishc.html (accessed on 17 May 2015).
4. National Cancer Institute; Public Health Service; National Institutes of Health. *Making Health Communication Programs Work (Pink Book)*; U.S. Department of Health & Human Services: Washington, DC, USA, 2002.
5. Wickremasinghe, D. What makes for good health communication? In *Global Health Communication—Global Health Histories*; WHO: Geneve, Switzerland, 2013.
6. Rajiv, N.; Rimal, M.; Lapinski, K. Why health communication is important in public health. *Bull. WHO* **2009**, *87*, 247–247.
7. WHO. Special theme issue: Public health communication. *Bull. WHO* **2009**, *87*, 565–644.
8. *Afghanistan Report—Health Communication*; WHO: Geneve, Switzerland, 2003; p. 19.
9. Obregón, R.; Chitnis, K.; Morry, C.; Feek, W.; Bates, J.; Galway, M.; Ogden, E. Achieving polio eradication: A review of health communication evidence and lessons learned in India and Pakistan. *Bull. WHO* **2009**, *87*, 624–630.
10. WHO. Create HPV vaccination communication strategies. Available online: http://www.who.int/immunization/hpv/communicate/en/ (accessed on 17 May 2015).
11. WHO. *HPV Vaccine Communication—Special Considerations for A Unique Vaccine*; WHO: Geneve, Switzerland, 2013.

12. Parks, W.; Lloyd, L. *Planning Social Mobilization and Communication for Dengue Fever Prevention and Control*; WHO: Geneve, Switzerland, 2004.
13. *Effective Media Communication During Public Health Emergencies*; WHO: Geneve, Switzerland, 2005.
14. WHO. *World Health Organization Outbreak Communication Planning Guide*; WHO: Geneve, Switzerland, 2008.
15. WHO. *Outbreak Communication Guidelines*; WHO: Geneve, Switzerland, 2005.
16. UNICEF. Communication for development. Available online: http://www.unicef.org/cbsc (accessed on 17 May 2015).
17. Waisbord, S.; Larson, H.J. Why Invest in Communication for Immunization? Evidence and Lessons Learned. A Joint Publication the Health Communication Partnership Based at Johns Hopkins Bloomberg School of Public Health/Center for Communication Programs (Baltimore) and the United Nations Children's Fund (New York). 2005. Available online: http://www.who.int/immunization/hpv/communicate/why_invest_in_communication_for_immunization_unicef_healthcommunicationspartnership_path_usaid.pdf (accessed on 10 July 2015).
18. O'Sullivan, G.A.; Yonkler, J.A.; Morgan, W.; Merritt, A.P. *A Field Guide to Designing a Health Communication Strategy*; Johns Hopkins Bloomberg School of Public Health/Center for Communication Programs: Baltimore, MD, USA, 2003.
19. United Nations Children's Fund Regional Office for South Asia. *Strategic Communication for Behaviour and Social Change in South Asia*; UNICEF: Kathmandu, Nepal, 2005.
20. Wittet, S. *Hepatitis B Vaccine Introduction—Lessons Learned in Advocacy,Communication and Training*; PATH: Seattle, WA, USA, 2001.
21. WHO; UNICEF; FAO. *Communication for Behavioural Impact—A Toolkit for Behavioural and Social Communication in Outbreak Response*; WHO: Geneve, Switzerland, 2012.
22. Feig, C. WHO: Communicating for health. In *Global Health Communication—Global Health Histories*; WHO: Geneve, Switzerland, 2013.
23. Zaman, F.; Underwood, C. *The Gender Guide for Health Communication Programmes*; Johns Hopkins Bloomberg School of Public Health, Center for Communication Programs: Baltimore, MD, USA, 2003.
24. U.S. Department of Health and Human Services Office of Disease Prevention and Health Promotion. *A Quick Guide to Health Literacy: Fact Sheets, Strategies, Resources*; U.S. Department of Health and Human Services, Office of Disease Prevention and Health Promotion: Washington, DC, USA, 2005.
25. Department for International Development. *Radio Broadcasting for Health—A Decision Makers Guide*; Information and Communication for Development, UK Department for International Development: London, UK, 2004.

26. CDC. Gateway to Health Communication & Social Marketing Practice. Available online: http://www.cdc.gov/healthcommunication/about.html (accessed on 17 May 2015).
27. US Department of Health and Human Services. Health Communication, Health Literacy, and E-Health. Available online: http://www.health.gov/communication/Default.asp (accessed on 17 May 2015).
28. FAO; OIE. *Global Animal Health Communication Strategy to Support Prevention and Control of H5N1*; HPAI FAO/OIE International Animal Health Communicators' Roundtable in Support of the FAO/OIE Global Strategy for the Prevention and Control of HPAI: Rome, Italy; Paris, France, 2007.
29. One Health Initiative. About the One Health Initiative. Available online: http://www.onehealthinitiative.com/about.php (accessed on 17 May 2015).
30. CDC. History of One Health. Available online: http://www.cdc.gov/onehealth/people-events.html (accessed on 16 June 2015).
31. Schwabe, C. *Veterinary Medicine and Human Health*; Williams & Wilkins Co.: Baltimore, MD, USA, 1964.
32. The Manhattan Principles. Available online: http://www.cdc.gov/onehealth/pdf/manhattan/twelve_manhattan_principles.pdf (accessed on 16 June 2015).
33. CDC. One Health. Available online: http://www.cdc.gov/onehealth/ (accessed on 17 May 2015).
34. EFSA. *Programming Document 2015-2017*; EFSA: Parma, Italy, 2014.
35. OIE. One Health. Available online: http://www.oie.int/for-the-media/onehealth/oie-involvement/ (accessed on 17 May 2015).
36. FAO. *One Health: Food and Agriculture Organization of the United Nations Strategic Action Plan*; FAO: Rome, Italy, 2011.
37. FAO. FAO workshop leverages country case studies for stronger collaboration on One Health. Available online:http://www.fao.org/ag/againfo/programmes/en/empres/news_041013.html (accessed on 17 May 2015).
38. OIE. One Health at a Glance. Available online: http://www.oie.int/for-the-media/onehealth/ (accessed on 17 May 2015).
39. Ministero della Salute. Influenza Aviaria. Available online: http://www.salute.gov.it/portale/temi/p2_6.jsp?lingua=italiano&id=816&area=Malattie%20infettive&menu=altremalattie (accessed on 17 May 2015).
40. Ministero della Salute. Infezione da Virus West Nile. Available online: http://www.salute.gov.it/portale/temi/p2_6.jsp?lingua=italiano&id=1201&area=Malattie%20infettive&menu=altremalattie (accessed on 17 May 2015).
41. Zinsstag, J.; Schelling, E.; Bonfoh, B.; Fooks, A.R.; Kasymbekov, J.; Toews, D.W.; Tanner, M. Towards a One Health research and application tool box. *Vet. Ita.* **2009**, *45*, 121–133.
42. Bonizzi, L.; Cipolla, M.; Grieco, V.; Grilli, G.; Lanfranchi, P.; Mortarino, M.; Zecconi, A. *Piano regionale della prevenzione veterinaria 2012-2014*; Regione Lombardia: Milano, Italy, 2011.

43. Scali, F.; Bonizzi, L.; Ferrero, F.; Frazzi, P.; Grilli, G.; Lanfranchi, P.; Mortarino, M.; Sala, V.; Taloni, D.; Zecconi, A. Risk prioritization as a tool to guide veterinary public health activities at regional level. *Vet.Ita.* **2014**. in press.

44. Alfonso Zecconi, U.O.V.R. *Piano regionale integrato della sanità pubblica veterinaria 2015-2018*; Regione Lombardia DG Sanità: Milano, Italy, 2014.

45. EFSA. Risk Communication. Available online: http://www.efsa.europa.eu/en/efsawhat/riskcommunication.htm(accessed on 17 May 2015).

46. FAO; WHO. *Codex Alimentarius Commission Report of the Twenty-Second Session*; FAO: Rome, Italy, 1997.

47. EFSA. Risk communication: Making it clear, timely and relevant. Available online: http://www.efsa.europa.eu/en/press/news/120711e.htm (accessed on 17 May 2015).

48. FAO. *The Application of Risk Communication to Food Standards and Safety Matters*; FAO: Rome, Italy, 1998.

49. EFSA. *When Food is Cooking Up a Storm—Proven Recipes for Risk Communications*; EFSA: Parma, Italy, 2012.

50. Thamm, D.; Dow, S. How companion animals contribute to the fight against cancer in humans. *Vet. Ita.* **2009**, *45*, 111–120.

51. Ministero della Salute. *Rabbia—conoscere per prevenire*; Istituto Zooprofilattico Sperimentale delle Venezie: Legnaro, Italy, 2010.

52. One Health Initiative. Mission Statement. Available online: http://www.onehealthinitiative.com/mission.php(accessed on 17 May 2015).

53. Grant, C.H.; Cissna, K.N.; Rosenfeld, L.B. Patients' perceptions of physicians communication and outcomes of the accrual to trial process. *Health Commun.* **2000**, *12*, 23–39.

54. Shaw, J.R.; Adams, C.L.; Bonnett, B.N. What can veterinarians learn from studies of physician-patient communication about veterinarian-client-patient communication? *J. Am. Vet. Med. Assoc.* **2004**, *224*, 676–684.

55. Kurtz, S.M. *Teaching and Learning Communication Skills in Medicine*, 2nd ed.; Radcliffe Publishing: Oxford, UK, 2005.

56. Kanji, N.; Coe, J.B.; Adams, C.L.; Shaw, J.R. Effect of veterinarian-client-patient interactions on client adherence to dentistry and surgery recommendations in companion-animal practice. *J. Am. Vet. Med. Assoc.* **2012**, *240*, 427–436.

57. Chadderdon, L.M.; King, L.J.; Lloyd, J.W. The skills, knowledge, aptitudes, and attitudes of successful veterinarians: A summary of presentations to the NCVEI subgroup (Brook Lodge, Augusta, Michigan, December 4–6, 2000). *J. Vet. Med. Educ.* **2001**, *28*, 28–30.

58. Coe, J.B.; Adams, C.L.; Bonnett, B.N. A focus group study of veterinarians' and pet owners' perceptions of veterinarian-client communication in companion animal practice. *J. Am. Vet. Med. Assoc.* **2008**, *233*, 1072–1080.

59. Shaw, J.R.; Bonnett, B.N.; Roter, D.L.; Adams, C.L.; Larson, S. Gender differences in veterinarian-client-patient communication in companion animal practice. *J. Am. Vet. Med. Assoc.* **2012**, *241*, 81–88.

60. Shaw, J.R.; Adams, C.L.; Bonnett, B.N.; Larson, S.; Roter, D.L. Veterinarian satisfaction with companion animal visits. *J. Am. Vet. Med. Assoc.* **2012**, *240*, 832–841.

61. Adams, C.L.; Kurtz, S.M. Building on existing models from human medical education to develop a communication curriculum in veterinary medicine. *J. Vet. Med. Educ.* **2006**, *33*, 28–37.

62. Latham, C.E.; Morris, A. Effects of formal training in communication skills on the ability of veterinary students to communicate with clients. *Vet. Rec.* **2007**, *160*, 181–186.

63. Martin, F.; Ruby, K.L.; Deking, T.M.; Taunton, A.E. Factors associated with client, staff, and student satisfaction regarding small animal euthanasia procedures at a veterinary teaching hospital. *J. Am. Vet. Med. Assoc.* **2004**,*224*, 1774–1779.

64. Beckman, H.B.; Markakis, K.M.; Suchman, A.L.; Frankel, R.M. The doctor-patient relationship and malpractice. Lessons from plaintiff depositions. *Arch. Intern. Med.* **1994**, *154*, 1365–1370.

65. Cipolla, M.; Bonizzi, L.; Zecconi, A. Attitude toward companion animals and breaking bad news: The role of caretakers' attitude and other factors on client-veterinarian communication. *Soc. Anim.* **2015**. submitted.

66. Kleen, J.L.; Atkinson, O.; Noordhuizen, J.P. Communication in production animal medicine: Modelling a complex interaction with the example of dairy herd health medicine. *Ir. Vet. J.* **2011**, *64*, 8.

67. Jansen, J.; Steuten, C.D.; Renes, R.J.; Aarts, N.; Lam, T.J. Debunking the myth of the hard-to-reach farmer: Effective communication on udder health. *J. Dairy Sci.* **2010**, *93*, 1296–1306.

68. Jansen, J.; Lam, T.J. The role of communication in improving udder health. *Vet. Clin. North Am. Food Anim. Pract.* **2012**, *28*, 363–379.

69. Jansen, J.; Renes, R.J.; Lam, T.J. Evaluation of two communication strategies to improve udder health management. *J. Dairy Sci.* **2010**, *93*, 604–612.

70. Lievaart, J.J.; Noordhuizen, J.P.T.M.; Buckley, D.; Van Winden, S.C.L. The marketing of herd health and production management services on dutch dairy farms: Perceptions of dairy farmers and their veterinary surgeons. *Ir. Vet. J.* **2008**, *61*, 668–676.

71. Jansen, J.; van den Borne, B.H.P.; Renes, R.J.; van Schaik, G.; Lam, T.J.G.M.; Leeuwis, C. Explaining mastitis incidence in dutch dairy farming: The influence of farmers' attitudes and behaviour. *Prev. Vet. Med.* **2009**, *92*, 210–223.

72. Valeeva, N.I.; Lam, T.J.G.M.; Hogeveen, H. Motivation of dairy farmers to improve mastitis management. *J. Dairy Sci.* **2007**, *90*, 4466–4477.

73. Kristensen, E.; Jakobsen, E.B. Challenging the myth of the irrational dairy farmer; understanding decision-making related to herd health. *N. Z. Vet. J.* **2011**, *59*, 1–7.

74. Cipolla, M.; Zecconi, A. Short communication: Study on veterinarian communication skills preferred and perceived by dairy farmers. *Res. Vet. Sci.* **2015**, *99*, 60–62.

75. WHO. Antimicrobial Resistance. Available online: http://www.euro.who.int/en/health-topics/disease-prevention/antimicrobial-resistance (accessed on 17 May 2015).

76. WHO Regional Office for Europe. Tackling antibiotic resistance from a food safety perspective in europe. WHO Regional Office for Europe: Copenhagen, 2011.

77. OIE. Antimicrobial agents and antimicrobial resistance. Available online: http://www.oie.int/our-scientific-expertise/veterinary-products/antimicrobials/ (accessed on 17 May 2015).

78. OIE. Antimicrobial Resistance (AMR). Available online: http://www.oie.int/en/for-the-media/amr/ (accessed on 17 May 2015).

79. EMA. European surveillance of veterinary antimicrobial consumption (ESVAC). Available online: http://www.ema.europa.eu/ema/index.jsp?curl=pages/regulation/document_listing/document_listing_000302.jsp (accessed on 17 May 2015).

80. International Dairy Federation. *Guide to Prudent Use of Antimicrobial Agents in Dairy Production*; International Dairy Federation: Brussels, Belgium, 2013.

81. Federation of Veterinarians of Europe. *Antibiotic Resistance & Prudent Use of Antibiotics in Veterinary Medicine*; FVE: Brussels, Belgium, 2012.

82. FDA. Antimicrobial Resistance. Available online: http://www.fda.gov/AnimalVeterinary/SafetyHealth/AntimicrobialResistance/default.htm (accessed on 17 May 2015).

83. CDC. Antibiotic use in food-producing animals. Available online: http://www.cdc.gov/narms/animals.html(accessed on 17 May 2015).

84. College of Veterinary Medicine, Michigan State University; College of Veterinary Medicine, University of Minnesota. Antimicrobial resistance learning site. Available online: http://amrls.cvm.msu.edu/ (accessed on 17 May 2015).

85. ECDC. European antibiotics awareness day. Available online: http://ecdc.europa.eu/en/eaad/Pages/Home.aspx(accessed on 17 May 2015).

86. ECDC. Antimicrobial resistance. Available online: http://www.ecdc.europa.eu/en/healthtopics/antimicrobial_resistance/Pages/index.aspx (accessed on 17 May 2015).

87. AIFA. Campagne di comunicazione. Available online: http://www.agenziafarmaco.gov.it/it/content/campagne-di-comunicazione-0 (accessed on 17 May 2015).

88. CDC. Get smart about antibiotics week. Available online: http://www.cdc.gov/getsmart/campaign-materials/week/index.html (accessed on 17 May 2015).

89. NPS MedicineWise. Join the fight against antibiotic resistance. Available

online: http://www.nps.org.au/about-us/what-we-do/campaigns-events/antibiotic-resistance-fighter (accessed on 17 May 2015).

90. Fletcher, J.; Franz, D.; LeClerc, E. Healthy plants: Necessary for a balanced One Health concept. *Vet. Ita.* **2009**,*45*, 79–95.

91. Panseri, S.; Catalano, A.; Giorgi, A.; Arioli, F.; Procopio, A.; Britti, D.; Chiesa, L. Occurrence of pesticide residues in italian honey from different areas in relation to its potential contamination sources. *Food Control***2014**, *38*, 150–156.

92. Rabinowitz, P.; Scotch, M.; Conti, L. Human and animal sentinels for shared health risks. *Vet. Ita.* **2009**, *45*, 23–24.

93. Beasley, V. One Toxicology, ecosystem health and One Health. *Vet. Ita.* **2009**, *45*, 97–110.

94. Gibbs, E.P.; Anderson, T.C. One World—One Health' and the global challenge of epidemic diseases of viral aetiology. *Vet. Ita.* **2009**, *45*, 35–44.

95. FAO; OIE; WHO; UN System Influenza Coordination; UNICEF; The World Bank. *Contributing to One World, One Health—A Strategic Framework for Reducing Risks of Infectious Diseases at the Animal–Human–Ecosystems Interface*; FAO: Rome, Italy, 2008.

96. FAO. *FAO's Support to the One Health Regional Approach—Towards Integrated and Effective Animal Health—Food Safety Surveillance Capacity Development in Eastern Africa*; FAO: Rome, Italy, 2013.

15
CHAPTER

A REVIEW ON THE PUBLIC HEALTH IMPORTANCE OF BOVINE SALMONELLOSIS

Jelalu Kemal

College of Veterinary Medicine, Haramaya University, Ethiopia

ABSTRACT

Salmonellosis is an infectious disease of human and animal caused by organisms of the two species of Salmonella (S. enterica and S. bongori). A Salmonella pathogen are highly adaptive and potentially pathogenic to human and other domestic animals; young, pregnant and lactating animals are the most susceptible and are capable of producing a serious of infections having foodborne zoonosis importance. Enteric disease is the commonest clinical manifestation, but a wide range of clinical signs, which include acute septicaemia, abortion, arthritis and respiratory disease, may be seen.Worldwide there are 16 million annual cases of typhoid fever, 1.3 billion cases of gastroenteritis and 3 million deaths. Poultry, egg, meat, dairy products and fruits and vegetables serve as vehicles of transmission. Most human salmonellosis cases are foodborne, but each year infections are also acquired through direct or indirect animal contact in homes, veterinary clinics, zoological gardens, farm environments or other public, professional or private settings. Salmonella passes through M-cells overlying Peyer's patches, through dendritic cells or through the epithelial lining in the lower part of small intestine or proximal colon to arrive in the sub epithelial location which is also transported to extra intestinal sites such as the liver, spleen and mesenteric lymph nodes. Salmonella pathogens are common in cattle and potentially infect human that come in contact with cattle. Bovine salmonellosis is caused by S. typhimurium and dublin. The disease in cattle is characterized by septicemia, acute or chronic entritis or abortion. Salmonella entrica sub species entrica develop a resistance to multi antibiotics in which results in increasing failure of treatment and severity of infection. Basic hygiene practices and the implementation of scientific based management strategies can efficiently

---

Citation: Kemal J (2014) A Review on the Public Health Importance of Bovine Salmonellosis. J Veterinar Sci Technol 5: 175. doi:10.4172/2157-7579.1000175

mitigate the risks associated with animal contacts. However, the general public is frequently unaware of the specific disease risks involved and high-risk behaviors are common. The disease can be also controlled by vaccination of cattle.

INTRODUCTION

The genus Salmonella was named after Daniel E. Salmon who first reported the isolation of Salmonella from a pig in 1885 and named the organism Bacterium choleraesuis (currently known as Salmonella enterica serovar Choleraesuis) [1,2]. Salmonella causes gastroenteritis and typhoid fever and is one of the major foodborne pathogens of significant public health concern [3]. Salmonella is considered as one of the most wide spread foodborne zoonosis in industrialized as well as developing countries even though the incidences seems to vary [4]. Salmonellosis is a disease caused by many serotypes of Salmonella and characterized clinically by one or more of the three major syndromes; septicemia, acute and chronic enteritis [5].

Salmonellae are common in cattle. They are often concern due to disease of cattle and the potential to infect human that come in contact with cattle or consume dairy product or bovine meat product. Meat processing and packaging at the whole sale or retail level contribute to higher levels of contamination in minced beef product compared to beef carcass. The presences of even small number of Salmonella in carcass meat and edible offal may lead to heavy contamination of minced meat. When meat is cut in to pieces more microorganisms are added and increased surface area of exposed tissue from the contaminated equipment. Raw meat particularly, minced meat has a very high total count of microorganisms of which Salmonella are likely to present large number [6].

Bovine salmonelosis usually manifest clinically as a syndrome of septicemia, acute or chronic enteritis and abortion [7]. There are few serotypes that are associated with cattle and of this Salmonella enterica subspecies enterica serotype Dublin (S. dublin) and Salmonella enterica subspecies enterica serotype Typhimurium (S. typhimurium) is the most common [8]. The presence of S. typhimurium in cattle and the cross contamination of beef carcass tissue is one of the most common cause of Salmonella infection in developed countries [9].

In addition to causing infection many Salmonella isolates particularly S. typhimurium definitive type (DT) 104 have developed resistance to multiple antibiotics. Many isolate of this phage type are resistance to ampicillin, chloramphinicol, streptomycin, sulfonamides and tetracycline (ACSUT) with increasing number of isolate showing resistance to trimethoprim and fluoroquinolones [10,11].

The resistance organism may act as donor of resistant determinant to another facultative pathogen of the human commensal flora of intestinal tract which may later be associated with disease and, in turn, supply the resistances gene to other pathogen [12].

There are more than 2500 different Salmonella serotypes and all are considered potentially pathogenic to human [13]. In human Salmonella is one of the most common causes of bacterial gastroenteritis. Death from Salmonella food poisoning estimated 1,000 deaths each year in USA [14]. The economic loss associated in human salmonellosis is due to investigation, treatment and prevention of illness [15]. Therefore, the objective of this review paper is to show the effect of eating of raw or undercooked meat, drinking of unpasteurized milk from the perspective of public health and to forward recommendation based on conclusion.

GENERAL OVERVIEW OF BOVINE SALMONELLOSIS

Classification

The current nomenclature of the genus Salmonella adopted worldwide through different publications is the one used by CDC is based on the recommendations from the WHO collaborating centre and it adequately addresses the concern and requirements of clinical and public health microbiologists (Table 1) [16]. Scientifically Salmonella classification is described under:

- Domain: Bacteria
- Phylum: Protobacteria
- Class: Gamma Protobacteria
- Order: Enterobacteriales
- Family: Enterobacteriaceae
- Genus: Salmonella, and

Species: Salmonella enterica and Salmonella bongori [17]. The species Salmonella enterica being divided into six subspecies (I–VI); S. enterica subsp. enterica (I), S. enterica subsp. salamae (II), S. enteric subsp. arizonae (IIIa), S. enterica subsp. diarizonae (IIIb), S. enterica subsp. houtenae (IV) and S. enterica subsp. indica (VI) [18] on the basis of biochemical characteristics (biotype), differences observed in multilocus enzyme electrophoresis (MLEE), phylogenetic analysis using 16S rRNA or other sequences, or analyses using other molecular techniques such as amplified-fragment length polymorphism (AFLP). Members of Salmonella enterica subspecies I account for 99% of all human infections [19].

Etiology and characteristics

Strains of genus Salmonella obey the definition of the family Enterobacteriaceae, they are straight rod usually motile with peritrichous flagella (except S. pullorum and S. gallinarum), facultative anaerobe, ferment glucose usually with production of gas (except S. typhi and S. dublin), but failed to ferment lactose, sucrose, salicin and urea, reduce nitrate to nitrite and most are phototropic [20,21]. Salmonella multiply optimally at a temperature of 35°C to 37°C, pH about 6.5-7.5 and water activity between 0.94-0.84. They are chemo-organotrophic organisms [22]. They are also able to multiply in the environment with low level or no oxygen [23]. The bacteria are sensitive to heat and will not survive a temperature above 70°C; so it is sensitive to pasteurization, but resist to drying even for years. Especially in dried feces, dust and other dry materials such as feed and certain food [24].

Salmonella strains are serologically classified using Kauffmann- White scheme, and at the present the genus contains more than 2500 serotypes [13,25,26]. However, a report from the Centre for Infectious Disease Research and Policy (CIDRAP) classifies members of the Salmonella species into more than 2541 serotypes (serovars) according to their somatic lipopolysaccharide (O), flagellar (H) antigens and at times capsular (Vi) antigen and most strains show diphasic variation of the flagellar antigns [27,28]. Recently, Dignostic Services of Monitoba (DSM) suggested the number of Salmonella serotypes that causes disease in human now approaches 3000 and new serotypes are identified continuously [29] (Table 2).

Epidemiology

The epidemiology of Salmonella is complex which often makes control of disease difficult. Epidemiological pattern of prevalence of infection and incidences of disease differ greatly between geographical area depending on climate, population density, land use farming practice, food harvesting and processing technologies and consumer habits. In addition, the biology of serovar differs so widely that Salmonella infection or Salmonella contamination are inevitably complex [24].

Geographical distribution: S. entritidis is the most prevalent species followed by S. typhimurium which are a worldwide distribution. Change in the relative frequency of serotypes can be observed over a short period of time. Some times within one or two years only limited number of serotypes is isolated from man or animals in a single region or country and the predominance of one or other can vary over a time. Some serotypes like S. entritidis and S. typhimurium are found worldwide in contrast to S. weltevreden which seems to be confined to Asia [30]. Sibhat et al. [31] found the serovars Newport, Anatum and Eastbourne to be the most prevalent in Ethiopia.

Occurrences: The rate of infection in domestic animal has been estimated from 1-3%. In 1980, 16274 strains of 183 serotypes of Salmonella were isolated in USA from samples of meat obtained from slaughter house. In other examination of animals positive culture was obtained from 4.59% of 141, 827 bovine fecal samples. Epidemiological surveillance of animals including bird is of the most important since source of large majority of non-typhoidal salmonellosis cases are of food animal origin. There is scarce of data from developing countries in this regard [30].

Morbidity and mortality: In a case control study of S. typhimurium DT 104 infection in cattle in Great Britain, Evans and Davies [32] reported an overall case fatality rate of 44%. In the herd with outbreak of S. typhimurium DT 104 the case fatality rate was 51.2% in calves, 37.4% in adult cattle and 26.2% in fattening cattle [32]. In dairy sucker and mixed herd the case fatality rate was found 44% where in calf rearing unit and dealer herd was found 50%-100% [33]. However modern antibiotic therapy may have reduced this rate. In an outbreak of S. dublin in calf rearing unit 29 (13.5%) of 214 calves died [34]. Mortality was significantly higher in group reared calves (19.25%) than in calves in single pens (9.2%). Mortality and morbidity is usually highest in calves under 12 week of age. In all species case fatality rate often reach 100% if treatment is not provided [24].

Economic importance: Salmonellosis is a significant cause of economic loss in farm animals because of the cost of clinical disease, which include death, diagnosis and treatment of clinical cases, diagnostic laboratory cost, the cost of cleaning and disinfection and cost of control and prevention. In addition when the disease is diagnosed in the herd, it can create a considerable apprehension in the producer because of difficulty on identifying infected animals. An estimation of economic impact of an outbreak of S. dublin infection in calf rearing unit indicate that the cost of disease represented a substantial proportion of gross margin of rearing calves [24]. Estimated annual costs for salmonellosis have ranged from billions of dollars in United States to hundreds to millions of dollars in Canada and millions of pounds in United Kingdom. Analysis of five Salmonella outbreak due to manufactured food in North America gave direct cost with range from $36,400-$62 million, there have been few studies in to the cost and benefit of preventing Salmonella infection, but it has been suggested that for every £1 spent on investigation and curtailment of the outbreak there is a saving of £5 [35].

Source of infection and transmission : Most Salmonella infection in farm animals are likely to acquire from animals of the same species, especially in the case of the host adapted serovars. In adult cattle there are important differences in the behavior of S. dublin and S. typhimurium. Those animals which recover from clinical S. dublin infection may become persistent excreters, shedding up to 106 organisms per gram of feaces daily. Other herd may harbor infection and excrete the organisms only when stressed particularly at parturition. Aerosol transmission has long been suggested as a means by which Salmonella may be transmitted and experimental infection of calves by aerosol has been reported recently. In addition pasture contamination results when flooding occurs and there are many reports of clinical case in adult cattle arising from grazing recently flooded pasture [35] (Figure 1).

Pathogenesis

The outcome of infection with Salmonella depends essentially on three factors: the infective dose, predisposing factor influencing the host and the level of immunity [7]. In cattle the common route of infection is ingestion of the bacteria through contaminated feed and water. It may disseminate to the rest body part of the host via the lymph fluid or blood and usually also lead to faecal excretion of bacteria. Salmonellae are normally inhibited by the high concentrations of volatile fatty acids and the normal pH below 7 in the rumen [36]. These bacteria have developed mechanisms to survive and cope with the host inhibiting factors, but the normal inhibition of Salmonella is primarily disrupted in the rumen and small intestine when (i) starvation or reduced feed intake occur [37], (ii) the feeding strategy leads to an increased pH in the abomasum, and (iii) antibiotic treatment kills the normal competing microflora of the intestine [38]. The bacteria adhere to and invade intestinal cells in the mucosa mainly associated with the Peyer's patches in the terminal jejunum and ileum through the columnar enterocytes and specialized microfold enterocytes (M cells). Once the bacteria have crossed the intestinal epithelium they enter macrophages in the underlying lymphoid tissue from where they are drained to the local lymph nodes, which are important barriers for further dissemination. If this barrier is overcome, the bacteria reach the reticuloendothelial tissue containing organs while surviving and replicating inside the macrophages [39].

The virulence of Salmonella is related to their ability to invade host cell and resist both digestion by phagocytes and destruction by complement system [40].The specific O antigen is important for the virulence strain of Salmonella (specific antigen) by decreasing the susceptibility of phagocytosis and ability to activate the alternative complement pathway [41]. Three toxins namely endotoxin, enterotoxin and cytotoxin play an important role in the pathogenesis of Salmonella. The endotoxin produce fever, the enterotoxin produce mucosal damage in the cell culture and cytotoxin inhibit protein synthesis [42] (Figure 2).

In human the bacteria travel to the stomach and pass to the intestine, where they invade the cells, causing diarrhoea to their infected host body. Salmonella Pathogenicity Island (SPI1) function is required for the initial stages of salmonellosis, i.e. the entry of Salmonella into nonphagocytic cells by triggering invasion and the penetration of the gastrointestinal epithelium. Furthermore, SPI1 function is required for the onset of diarrheal symptoms during localized gastrointestinal infections. The function of SPI2 is required for later stages of the infection, i.e. systemic spread and the colonization of host organs. The role of SPI2 for survival and replication in host phagocytes appears to be essential for this phase of pathogenesis [43] (Figures 2 and 3).

Post mortem findings: There may be no gross lesion in animals that have died peracutely but extensive submucosal and subserosal petechial heamorrhage are usually evident [24]. In adult cattle, a typical case reveals acute muco/necrotic enteritis, especially of the ileum and large intestine. The wall is thickened and covered with yellow-grey necrotic material overlying a red, granular surface. The mesenteric lymph nodes and spleen may be enlarged. In calves, the small intestine typically shows a diffuse mucoid or mucohaemorrhagic enteritis and the mesenteric lymph nodes are oedematous, congested and greatly enlarged [44].

Pathological findings : In adult cattle acute heamorrhagic entritis with necrotic change usually most pronounced in the mucosa of large intestine is commonly found at postmortem examination and similar change may be seen in the small intestine. The mesenteric lymph node are in variably swollen, edematous and in many case heamorrhagic. The liver may show degenerative change and the wall of gall bladder may be thickened. In calves, the clinical sign are those of septicemia which resemble those described for adult cattle i.e. congestion and heamorrhagic areas in the intestine, enlarged lymph node and congested spleen. Petechial heamorrhages may be seen in the cortex of the kidney and epicardium [35].

The chronic form is manifested by discrete areas of necrosis of the wall of the cecum and colon. The wall is thickened and covered with yellow gray necrotic material overlying a red granular mucosal surfaces. Salmoneaella are present in the heart, blood, spleen, liver, bile, mesenteric lymph node and intestinal contents in both septicemic and acute forms. In the chronic form the bacteria may be isolated from the intestinal lesions and less commonly from other viscera [24].

Clinical Sign

Adult cattle generally contract either acute or subacute enteric salmonellosis and pregnant animal may abort during the early stage of acute enteric disease. Severely affected animals show fever, depression, inappetence and drop in milk yield. These sign are followed by diarrhea which is fowl smelling, the faces being mucoid and usually containing a clot of blood and shred of necrotic intestinal mucosa. Sign of colonic congestion of mucus membrane and dehydration may be evident. The acute disease last for about a week. S. dublin in particular but also other serovars may cause abortion in cows at any stage of pregnancy (Table 3). Abortion may either precede the onset of dysentery or follow it within two or four weeks. Alternatively abortion may occur in cows that show no sign of illness, septicemia and/or placentitis being the case of death of fetus. Retention of the placenta occurs in approximately 70% of cases that abort but subsequent fertility is not usually affected [7].

In calves clinical disease is most common 2-6 week of age. Clinical sign vary but typically the enteric form of diseases predominate which is characterized by pyrexia, dullness and anorexia, followed by diarrhea that may contain fibrin and mucus. The feaces may become blood stained and "stringy" due to the presences of necrotic intestinal mucosa. Calves rapidly become weak and dehydrated unless treated. Infected calves usually die 5 7 days after the onset of disease. At this stage the organisms has become systemic as a result of reduced innate immunity and may be isolated from variety of tissue including blood. Calves that recover from infection do not typically remain carrier. Salmonellosis is very variable and in some animals particularly in very young animals rapid multiplication occur both in intestine and systemically associated with poor absorption of specific immunoglobulin G from colostrums or with calves receiving in sufficient or no colostrums [45].

DISEASE IN HUMAN

Distribution

Worldwide there are 16 million annual cases of typhoid fever, 1.3 billion cases of gastroenteritis and 3 million deaths due to Salmonella. In the US annually there are 2-4 million cases with a death rate of 500-1,000 and an economic loss of about 3 billion dollars. A recent CDC report indicates that the incidence of S. typhimurium decreased significantly (42% decline) from 1996–1998 to 2005; however, the incidence of other serotypes are on the rise such as S. enteritidis and S. heidelberg, each of which increased by 25% and S. enterica serovar Javiana increased by 82% [46].

Physiology

The Salmonella, in the family Enterobacteriaceae, are facultatively anaerobic, gram negative and rod-shaped bacteria. Given the close relationship with E. coli and the many years devoted to its study, the overall metabolism of Salmonella is well understood. The cells are typically 0.7-1.5 μm by 2-5 μm. They grow at 7-48°C with an optimum growth at 37°C (mesophile) and at pH 4.05-9.5 with an optimal growth at pH 6.5-7.5

(neutrophile). Salmonella grows optimally at a water activity of 0.995 and are chemo-organotrophs. They have both fermentative and oxidative metabolism. The primary route for metabolism of carbohydrates is the Embden-Meyerhof pathway (glycolysis). They ferment glucose to formate (with the production of gas) and to ethanol, acetate, or lactate [19].

Transmission to human

Human salmonellosis is generally foodborne and is contracted through consumption of contaminated food of animal origin such as meat, milk, poultry and eggs. Dairy products including cheese and ice cream were also implicated in the outbreak. However, fruits and vegetables such as lettuce, tomatoes, cilantro, alfalfa-sprouts and almonds have also been implicated in recent out-break [35].

Acute gastroenteritis is usually acquired from consumption of food which may be directly or indirectly contaminated with Salmonella. A wide variety of animal species have been shown to be capable of harboring the organisms and in the developed world turkey, chicken, swine and cattle are found to be infected carriers in the studies conducted in the abattoirs. These carriers may readily shed Salmonella during transportation to the abattoir and contaminate abattoir workers or equipment during slaughter. The progressive trend forwards mass processing and distribution of food products has been an important factor in the increase incidences of Salmonella foodborne diseases. Person to person spread has been demonstrated on many occasions and may take place in young children and group living under poor socioeconomic condition where effective sanitation is lacking. Person to person spread also may occur in hospitals, nursing homes, mental institution in which large number of outbreak has occurred. Amplification of infection in these institutions may occur from contaminated food or asymptomatic carrier's babies being at special risk [35]. Direct or indirect contact with animals colonized with Salmonella is another source of infection, including contact during visits to petting zoos and farms [47].

Fecal oral route and vehicle born infection may result from ingestion of food or water that have been contaminated with human or animal feaces or from direct exposure to animals or their waste. A lower infectious dose of organism is usually required in the elderly, the immunocompromised, antibiotic users and those with achlorhydria or regular use of antacid and related medication. The commonly recognized vehicle of transmission includes inadequate cooked or raw meat, unpasteurized milk or milk product, contaminated and inadequately treated drinking water. www.dol.gov.

Contamination of milk may occur by a variety of route. Animal may occasionally, excrete the organisms in milk during the febrile stage of the disease or more likely infected feaces, from either a clinically infected cow or healthy carrier may contaminate the milk during the milking process. Milk also may be contaminated from use of polluted water from dirty equipment or from dairy workers. Indirect contamination also has been described when cattle have become contaminated with Salmonella. Contamination of food also may occur directly from Salmonella infected food handlers or indirectly from sewage polluted water [48].

Clinical Sign in Human

The incubation period depends on the number of bacteria ingested and varies from 5-72 hours. Affected individual's experience sudden nausea, vomiting and watery fowl smelling diarrhea which is in most case last only a few hours. If the colon is affected, the stool may also contain blood and or mucus. Fever up to 39°C is not uncommon. Convalescences within 1-2 days but the illness may last for 5-7 days [49].

More severe symptom may occur in people who are at high risk like those extreme age groups (the young because their immune system are immature and the elderly because the immune system are declining), person with decreased gastric acidity (because gastric acid is the first line of defense for the ingested Salmonella), person with altered gastric intestinal bacteria (including those taking broad spectrum antibiotics, purgatives or who have had bowl surgery) and person taking opiate drug in which the bowl movement is decreased. In these highest risk groups of people Salmonella may invade beyond the gastrointestinal tract (GIT) to cause severe systematic illness.

Salmonella gastroenteritis is usually a self-limiting illness and fatality is uncommon. Biopsy and endoscopic examination have demonstrated the colon to be a major site of infection. The change in the colon ranges from edema of lamina propria with a focal or diffuse inflammatory infiltrate to a more intensive inflammation with disruption of the surface epithelium and multi-focal micro abscesses. In more severe cases, vascular congestion, infiltration of the lamina proporia with polymorphonuclear leucocytes and abscess formation has been recorded [35].

PUBLIC HEALTH ASPECT OF BOVINE SALMONELLOSIS

Salmonellosis is an important global public health problem causing substantial morbidity and thus also has a significant economic impact. Although most infections cause mild to moderate self-limited disease, serious infections leading to deaths do occur [50]. In spite of the improvement in hygiene, food processing, education of food handlers and information to the consumers, foodborne diseases still dominate as the most important public health problem in most countries [51].

A salmonellosis incidence is defined as the identification of Salmonella from animals or group of animal's product or surrounding which can be specifically related to identifiable animals or from animals feed. On the human side, a registered medical practitioner in the US required under the Public Health (Control of Disease) act to notify the local authority, if the patient is suffering from or suspected of having foodborne disease [35].

Studies provide increasing evidence of adverse human health consequences due to the occurrence of resistant microorganisms. Use of antimicrobial agents in human and animal affects the intestinal tract placing those concerned at increased risk of certain infection. This is defined as the proportion of Salmonella that would not have occurred if the Salmonella were not resistant. In addition antimicrobial agent used in animal can result in increased transmission of resistant microorganisms between animal and therefore would results in case of transmission of such microorganisms to human through food. Increased frequency of treatment failure and increase severity of infection may be manifested by prolonged duration of illness. www.who.int.mediacenter.

Salmonella dublin is largely but not entirely specific to cattle with average 10 human case reported in each year in Ireland. Apart from its pathogenicity two other characteristics of S. dublin make it particularly important for Ireland from a public health viewpoints. First, it is very prevalent on Irish farms and secondly in evolutionary terms, it is only one step away from S. enteritidis, a common Salmonella serotype in poultry and the main case of clinical salmonellosis in humans. In genetic terms, difference between the serovars S. dublin and S. enteritidis are no greater than those found within each serotypes. This indicates that, S. dublin and S. enteritidis share a common ancestor. One branch evolved in to a poultry adapted serotype capable of causing disease in human, the other in to host specific cattle pathogen. If S. dublin has been confirmed in breeding herd there is a significant risk of persistent infection in carrier cows for as long as animal which were present at the time of the outbreak remain in the herd [53].

DIAGNOSIS OF SALMONELLOSIS

The clinical sign and finding at postmortem examination are not unique to salmonellosis although a tentative diagnosis may be made. They should confirm either in diseased animal or at necropsy by isolation of organisms in their feces and determination of viable counts. Fecal samples rather than swabs should be taken and these should obviously be obtained before administration of antibiotics. It may be also possible to isolate organism from oral secretion and by blood culture although these are less reliable than feces culture and must be taken with care to avoid contamination. Animal that died of salmonellosis usually have large number of Salmonella distributed throughout their tissue and sample of spleen, liver, hepatic, mediastinal and bronchial lymph nodes may yield count in excretion of 106 organisms/gram. Similar concentration may be present in the wall and content of the ileum, cecum, colon and associated lymph nodes. Sample should be taken from internal organs in order to distinguish animal that have died of enteritis without septicemia [53].

CULTURE METHODS

The traditional Salmonella culture method involves pre-enrichment, selective enrichment, isolation of pure culture, biochemical screening and serological confirmation, which requires 5-7 days to complete. The USDA and FDA recommended method involves a 6-24 h preenrichment step in a nonselective broth such as lactose broth, tryptic soy broth, nutrient broth, skim milk, or buffered peptone water with a recommended incubation temperature of 37°C. The selective enrichment step requires additional 24 hours incubation in Rappaport- Vassiliadis (RV) broth, selenite cystine (SC) broth, or Muller Kauffmann tetrathionate broth. The inoculation temperature of 41.5°C ± 1°C for RV broth and 37°C ± 1°C for SC and MKTT broth is used. Bacterial cells are isolated from selective agar plates such as Hektoen enteric agar (HEA), xylose lysine deoxy-cholate (XLD), and/or brilliant green agar (BGA). Biochemical testing is done using triple sugar iron agar and lysine iron agar, which requires an additional 4–24 hours [54,55].

Rapid detection methods

Detection of antibodies to Salmonella by enzyme immunoassay (EIA): The detection of antibodies to Salmonella by EIA offers a sensitive and cost-effective method for mass screening of animal flocks/herds for indications of a past/present Salmonella infection. The limitation of the method is that the immune response of the individual animal is not elicited before 1-2 weeks after infection takes place. A number of commercial kits are available for testing poultry, cattle and pigs. An obvious advantage of this method is that it can be automated and no incubation is required to increase the numbers of bacterial cells [56].

The EIA is a well-established technique for assaying antigens. Antibodies labeled with an enzyme are bound to Salmonella antigens, and the level of antigen present is determined by enzymatic conversion of a substrate, usually resulting in a color change which can be read visually or by a spectrophotometer. The EIAs rely on the standard cultural procedures for pre-enrichment and selective enrichment to provide enough Salmonella cells for detection. EIA technology that enables detection at an earlier stage of resuscitation and/or culture can provide even more rapid results. Serological test, such as ELISA, serum agglutination and complement fixation can be used for the retrospective diagnosis of salmonellosis or the detection of carriers [55].

Nucleic acid-based assays: Real-time quantitative polymerase chain reaction using PCR (Q-PCR), reverse transcriptase PCR (RTPCR), and nucleic acid sequence-based amplification (NASBA) have been used for detection of Salmonella from various food matrices. Salmonella enterica was detected at 1 cfu ml−1 after a culture enrichment of 8-12 h in the TaqMan-based Q-PCR using invA gene as target. NASBA method has been used for detection of viable Salmonella cells and it has been demonstrated to be more sensitive than RT-PCR, and moreover, it requires fewer amplification cycles than the conventional PCR methods [46].

Differential diagnosis

The differential diagnosis of Salmonella enterocolitis in humans include viral gastroenteritis and bacterial enteric infections including those caused by Shigella, Enterotoxigenic E-coli, Campylobacter species, Vibrio species and Yersinia enterocoliticia. The disorder must also be differentiated from toxin-mediated foodborne illness including those caused by Staphylococcus aureus, Bacillus cereus and Clostridium perfringens. Compared to the patient with toxin mediated disorder person with salmonellosis usually have less prominent vomiting and are the more likely have prolonged diarrhea and fever. The shorter incubation period of toxin mediated foodborne illness can be important to distinguish them from salmonellosis. A recent history of ingestion of raw milk, undercooked meat and contact with farm animals 48 hours before the onset of illness suggests the diagnosis of salmonellosis [49].

Treatment

Treatment of non-typhoidal Salmonella infection is different from typhoidal infection. In treatment of non-typhoidal Salmonella infection antibiotics should not be used routinely, as used in typhoid. Antibiotic should be only used if required as most infection with non-typhoidal Salmonella is self-limiting type and duration of diarrhea and fever are not much affected by use of antibiotics. Additionally antibiotic therapy can increase relapse of infection and also prolong the duration of gastrointestinal carrier states. The main treatment should be aimed at correcting dehydration that may arise due to prolonged diarrhea by fluid and electrolyte replacement. www.webcan.gogleuserconten.com.

Although Salmonellae are usually sensitive in vitro to many antibiotics, their use for treatment of uncomplicated gastroenteritis until recently has been generally contraindicated by their lack of favorable effect on the course of the disease and by prolongation of Salmonella shedding. Following the introduction of fluoroquinolones a number of clinicians have advocated their use for treatment of only on enteric fever but also of Salmonella gastroenteritis because of their efficacy in reducing the duration of illness and of Salmonella shedding. In case of patient with bacteremia and other complication antimicrobials are used. Likewise the treatment of enteric fever necessitates the use of antimicrobial drugs with chloramphinicol, ampicillin, amoxicillin, trimethoprimsulfamethoxazole and newer fluoroquinoazoles being drug of choice against sensitive Salmonella. Proper management of fluid and electrolyte balance is impotant in all patients with Salmonella gastroenteritis but is crucial in young children and elder individuals [35].

In animal treatment supportive treatment with intravenous fluid is necessary for patients that have anorexia, depression, significant dehydration. Individual patient may be treated aggressively following acid base and electrolyte assessment. Oral fluid and electrolyte may be somewhat helpful and much cheaper than IV fluid for cattle demand to be mildly or moderately dehydrated. The effectiveness of oral fluid may be somewhat compromised by malabsorption and maldigestion in salmonellosis patient but still should be considered useful. Cattle that are willing to drink can have specific electrolyte (NaCl, KCl) added to drinking water to help correcting electrolyte [57].

The implementation of broad prophylactic strategies that are efficacious for all Salmonellae may be required in order to overcome the diversity of Salmonella serovars present on farms, and the potential for different serovars to possess different virulence factors [58]. Early treatment is essential for septicemic salmonellosis but there is controversy regarding the use of antimicrobial agent for intestinal salmonellosis. Oral antibiotic may alter the intestinal micro flora and interfere with competitive antagonism and prolong shading of the organism. There is also a concern that antibiotic resistance strain of Salmonella selected by oral antibiotic may subsequently infect human. Antibiotic such as ampicillin or cephalosporin lead to lyses of bacteria with release of endotoxin. NSAID may be used to reduce the effect of endotoxemia [5].

PREVENTION AND CONTROL

Prevention and control in animals

Condition that contribute to an increasing incidence of epidemic salmonellosis include large herd size, more intensive and crowded husbandry and the trend of free-stall barn with loose housing, which contribute to the feacal contamination of the entire premise. When salmonellosis has been confirmed in a herd, the following control measure should be considered; isolate obviously affected animals to one group if possible, treat severely affected animals, affected animals institute measure to minimize public health concern like (no raw milk should be consumed) physically clean the environment and disinfect the premise following resolution of the outbreak or crises period. A mastitis survey should be conducted that include bulk tank surveillance. Prevention is best accompanied by maintaining a cross herd and culturing new feed additives and components before using the entire ration [57].

It is generally agreed that supportive therapy and good nursing are important. These include oral or parentral re-hydration, correction of electrolyte balance and stabilization of acid base equilibrium [7].

Salmonella vaccinology: Calves vaccinated at 1-3 weeks of age with a modified aromatic dependant S. dublin bacteria have detectable anti-lipoplisaccharide immunoglobins after immunization. Safe live oral vaccine against S. typhimurium and S. dublin has been constructed and shown to control protection against experimental infection with virulent wide type strain of the organisms. A virulent S. choleraesuis vaccine is efficacies experimentally against salmonellosis due to S. dublin in calves to protect young calves. The best program is to vaccinate the cow during pregnancy which will give passive protection to calves for 6 weeks [24].

Generally, both live and attenuated vaccines produced from rough strain in bacteria commercially. There is some evidence that inactivated bacterins can induce a lower level of protection [59]. The veterinarian research institute produced vaccine against bovine salmonellosis in activated bacteria prepared from isolate of S. dublin, S. typhomurium and S. bovismorbificans and a live attenuated vaccine containing a virulent rough mutant of S. dublin [7].

Prevention and control in human

There is no vaccine to prevent salmonellosis in human whereas, vaccine against Salmonella typhi has been developed, especially in children, but is only 60% effective. A person given this vaccine would still have a strong chance of developing salmonellosis. It is not expected that there will be a single vaccine that is effective against all the different forms of Salmonella soon. Ongoing research is investigating what can be done to produce a useful human vaccine for Salmonella [59]. People should not eat raw or uncooked meat, they should not drink raw milk or unpasteurized dairy product, cross contamination of food should be avoided. Uncooked meat should be kept separate from cooked food ready to eat. Hands, cutting boards or knifes and other utensils should be washed thoroughly after handling uncooked food. Hands should be washed before handling any food and in between handling different food items. People should have to wash their hands after contact with animal's feces [46].

Pasteurization of milk and treating municipals water supply for reducing risk of Salmonella infection, improvement in farm animal hygiene in slaughter process in food harvesting and in packaging operation have helped to prevent salmonellosis [55]. A periodic surveillance of the level of Salmonella contamination in different food product and environment is necessary to control spread of the pathogen. Reducing Salmonella prevalence requires comprehensive control strategy in animal and animal foodstuff with restriction in the infected flock until they have been cleaned from infection. In addition mandatory testing before slaughter should be conducted like the one implemented in Sweden [60]. Ensuring safe food production requires knowledge on the nature and origin of animal, animal feed, the health status of animals at the farm, the use of veterinary medicinal data regarding antimortem and postmortem findings and the risk association with post harvests production strategies [61].

CONCLUSION AND RECOMMENDATION

Salmonella is a leading cause of foodborne disease in human and consumption of both meat and milk has been implicated in salmonellosis outbreaks of people. Having animals and raw products it is not possible to be free from zoonotic agent; however the occurrences can be minimized by applying high standard of hygiene in all steps of the food production. Infected animals can present with a great variety of clinical symptoms, and risk factors for transmission to humans clearly differ by animal species, age groups, animal purpose and geographic region. In addition, strains of Salmonella resistant to multiple antibiotics have been isolated from dairy cow during salmonellosis outbreak on dairy operation. The same strains have also been isolated from ill people. A high degree of interaction between medical and veterinarian surveillance is needed. Finally, implementing basic and applied research to the agent that cause foodborne salmonellosis will be a crucial point for new approaches to prevent and control the disease

Based on the above facts the following recommendations are forwarded:

- Strict hygiene of the slaughter house and lairage
- People should not drink unpasteurized milk or milk products and should not eat raw meat.
- Establishment of HACCP
- Education of food handlers
- Vaccination of cattle
- Maintenance of cold chains
- Setting import standards
- Sanitary examination of the product

- Collaboration between government agencies, professional organizations and special interest groups.
- New legislations or public awareness campaigns have leads to dramatic decreases in Salmonella incidence.

REFERENCES

1. Rao PV (2004) Essential of Microbiology. Satish Kumar Jain for CBS publishers and Distributors, New Delhi. India. 146-148.
2. FDA/CFSAN (2008) Food Safety A to Z Reference Guide Salmonnella.
3. Fluit AC (2005) Towards more virulent and antibiotic-resistant Salmonella? FEMS Immunol Med Microbiol 43: 1-11.
4. BayleyegnM, Dainal A, Woubit S (2003) Source of Salmonella serotypes isolated from animals, slauther house personnel and retail meat product in Ethiopia 1997-2002. Ethio.J.Health.Dev.17: 63-70.
5. Davison, S. 2005. Salmonellosis. In: Merck veterinary manual 10th edition. Edited by Cynthia, M. kahn. Merik and Co.J (inc. White House Station, N.J U.S.A).
6. EjetaG, Molla B, Alemayehu D, Muckle A (2004) Salmonella serotypes isolated from mincied meat beef, mutton and pork in Addis Ababa, Ethiopia Reve.med. Vet 155: 547-551.
7. Venter BJ, Myburgh JG, Van der Walt ML (1994) Bovine Salmonellosis. In: Infectious diseases of Livestock with Special Reference to South Africa. Eds. Coetzer, J.W., Thomson, G.R. and Tustin, R.C. Oxford University Press, Cape Town, Pp: 1104-1112.
8. McEvoy JM, Doherty AM, Sheridan JJ, Blair IS, McDowell DA (2003) The prevalence of Salmonella spp. in bovine faecal, rumen and carcass samples at a commercial abattoir. J ApplMicrobiol 94: 693-700.
9. Gomez TM1, Motarjemi Y, Miyagawa S, Käferstein FK, Stöhr K (1997) Foodborne salmonellosis. World Health Stat Q 50: 81-89.
10. Threlfall EJ, Ward LR, Rowe B (1997) Increasing incidence of resistance to trimethoprim and ciprofloxacin in epidemic Salmonella typhimurium DT104 in England and Wales. Euro Surveill 2: 81-84.
11. Piddock LJ (2002) Fluoroquinolone resistance in Salmonella serovars isolated from humans and food animals. FEMS Microbiol Rev 26: 3-16.
12. SalyersAA (1995) Antibiotic resistance transfer in the mammalian intestinal tract: Implication for human health, food safety and Biotechnology New York.
13. Popoff MY, Bockemühl J, Gheesling LL (2003) Supplement 2001 (no. 45) to the Kauffmann-White scheme. Res Microbiol 154: 173-174.
14. Mead PS, Slutsker L, Dietz V, McCaig LF, Bresee JS, et al. (1999) Food-related illness and death in the United States. Emerg Infect Dis 5: 607-625.
15. Wray C, Wray A(2000) Salmonella in domestic animals, Veterinary Microbiology 81: 281-282.

16. Deb M, Kapoor L (2005) Salmonella nomenclature seen in the literature. Indian J Med Microbiol 23: 204-205.

17. Hafez, H.M. 2005. Government regulation and control of some important poultry diseases. World's Poult. Sci. J. 61: 574-575.

18. Brenner FW, Villar RG, Angulo FJ, Tauxe R, Swaminathan B (2000) Salmonella nomenclature. J ClinMicrobiol 38: 2465-2467.

19. Craig DE, James MS(2006)The genus Salmonella In: The Prokaryotes 3rd Edition. 6: 123-158.

20. Lund, Barbara, Baird-Parker, Anthony C, Gould et al.(2000) The Microbiology safety and quality of food (II). Gaithersburg, Malaysia. Food Microbiology 12: 3-8.

21. Johnson TJ, Wannemuehler YM, Johnson SJ, Logue CM, White DG, et al. (2007) Plasmid replicon typing of commensal and pathogenic Escherichia coli isolates. Appl Environ Microbiol 73: 1976-1983.

22. Food Research International (FRI) (2010) Salmonella in Foods. Evaluation, Strategies and Challenges 43:1557-1558.

23. European Commission(2000)An opinion of the scientific committee on veterinary measure relating to public health on foodborne zoonoses. Health and consumer protection directorate general, Directorate B, Scientific health opinions, Unit B3-Managements of Scientific committees II 24-27.

24. Radostitis OM, Gay CC, Hinchliff KW, Constable PD (2007) Veterinary Medicine: A text book of the disease of cattle, horses, sheep, pigs, and goats. 10th ed. Elsevier Ltd. 325-326.

25. Popoff MY, Bockemühl J, Brenner FW, Gheesling LL (2001) Supplement 2000 (no. 44) to the Kauffmann-White scheme. Res Microbiol 152: 907-909.

26. Tindall BJ, Grimont PA, Garrity GM, Euzéby JP (2005) Nomenclature and taxonomy of the genus Salmonella. Int J SystEvolMicrobiol 55: 521-524.

27. Centre for Infectious Disease Research and Policy (CIDRAP) (2006) Academic Health Centre, University of Minnesota.

28. Scott S (2010)The most probable number method and its use in Enumeration, Qualification and validation. J of Validation Technology 16: 35-38.

29. Diagnostic Services of Manitoba (DSM) (2009) Salmonella Nomenclature and the Reporting of Results on Salmonella Species: Memorandum.

30. Acha PN, Szyfres B (2001) Zoonosis and communicable disease common to man and animals 3rd ed. 233-245.

31. SibhatB, Molla B, Zerihun A, Muckle A, Cole L, et al. (2011) Salmonella Serovars and Antimicrobial Resistance Profiles in Beef Cattle, Slaughterhouse Personnel and Slaughterhouse Environment in Ethiopia. Zoonoses public health 58: 102-109.

32. Evans S, Davies R (1996) Case control study of multiple-resistant Salmonella typhimurium DT104 infection of cattle in Great Britain. Vet Rec 139: 557-558.

33. Richardson A (1975) Salmonellosis in cattle. Vet Rec 96: 329-331.

34. Peters AR (1985) An estimation of the economic impact of an outbreak of Salmonella dublin in a calf rearing unit. Vet Rec 117: 667-668.

35. Wray C (1994)Mamalian salmonellosis In: Hand book of zoonosis 2nd Edition. Edited by BeranGW, New York, C.R.C, press: 291-300.

36. Mattila T, Frost AJ, O'Boyle D (1988) The growth of Salmonella in rumen fluid from cattle at slaughter. Epidemiol Infect 101: 337-345.

37. Morisse JP, Cotte JP (1994) Evaluation of some risks factors in bovine salmonellosis. Vet Res 25: 185-191.

38. Bäumler AJ, Tsolis RM, HeffronF(2000) Virulence Mechanisms of Salmonella and their Genetic Basis. In: Wray, C., Wray, A. (Eds.), Salmonella in Domestic Animals. CABI Publishing, New York, pp. 57-72.

39. Scherer CA, Miller SI (2001) Molecular Pathogenesis of Salmonellae. In: Groisman, E.A. (Ed). Principles of Bacterial Pathogenesis. Academic Press, New York, pp. 265-333.

40. Quinn J, MarkeyBK (2003) Concise Review of Veterinary Microbiology: Blackwell publishing.

41. Mekaloson JJ (1990) Microbiology 4th edition. Lippincotcompany New York.

42. Koo FC, Peterson JW, Houston CW, Molina NC (1984) Pathogenesis of experimental salmonellosis: inhibition of protein synthesis by cytotoxin. Infect Immun 43: 93-100.

43. Hansen-Wester I, Hensel M (2001) Salmonella pathogenicity islands encoding type III secretion systems. Microbes Infect 3: 549-559.

44. Wray C, Davies RH (2000) Salmonella Infections in Cattle. Veterinary Laboratories Agency (Weybridge), New Haw, Addlestone, Surrey KT15 3NB, UK.

45. Barrow PA, Jones MA, Thomson N (2010) Pathogenesis of bacterial infection in animals 4th edition. Edited by Gyles, C.L., Songer, G. Theon, C.O: Blackwell publishing 233.

46. ArunK Bhunia (2008) Mechanisms and Pathogenesis In: Foodborne Microbial Pathogens: pp. 201-215.

47. Friedman CR, Torigian C, Shillam PJ, Hoffman RE, Heltzel D, et al. (1998) An outbreak of salmonellosis among children attending a reptile exhibit at a zoo. J Pediatr 132: 802-807.

48. Jones BD (2005) Salmonella invasion gene regulation: a story of environmental awareness. J Microbiol 43 Spec No: 110-117.

49. Krauss HM, Albert W, Appel M, Henery B, Lesenberg D, et al. (2003) Zoonosis infectious disease from animals to humans. 3rd edition. American Society, for Microbiology: 234-236.

50. de Jong B, Ekdahl K (2006) The comparative burden of salmonellosis in the European Union member states, associated and candidate countries. BMC Public Health 6: 4.
51. Domínguez C, Gómez I, Zumalacárregui J (2002) Prevalence of Salmonella and Campylobacter in retail chicken meat in Spain. Int J Food Microbiol 72: 165-168.
52. Mee JF, Moyes T, Gleeson D, Brien B (2002)A questionnaire survey of fertility management on dairy farms in the Republic of Ireland. Irish Veterinary Journal, 55: 122-128.
53. Jones PJ, Weston PR, SwailT (2007) Salmonellosis In: Bovine medicine, diseases and husbandry of cattle. Edited by Andrew, A.H. 2nd Edition: Blackwell publishing 215-230.
54. International Organization for Standardization (ISO) (2002) Microbiology of Food and Animal Feeding Stuff-Horizontal Method for the Detection of Salmonella. 4th ed. ISO 6579.
55. Hans PR, Dean OC, Morris P(2006) Salmonella infection In: Foodborne Infections and Intoxications 3rd Edition. Food Science and Technology International Series: 57-136.
56. Zamora BM, Hartung M (2002) Chemiluminescent immunoassay as a microtiter system for the detection of Salmonella antibodies in the meat juice of slaughter pigs. J Vet Med B Infect Dis Vet Public Health 49: 338-345.
57. Rebhun CW (1995) Disease of Dairy cattle: 1st Edition. Awa Verly Company.
58. Mohler VL, Izzo MM, House JK (2009) Salmonella in calves. Vet Clin North Am Food AnimPract 25: 37-54, vi.
59. Danielle AB (2006) Deadly Diseases and Epidemics: Salmonella. David Heymann; Communicable Diseases Section. World Health Organization, Geneva, Switzerland. CHELSEA HOUSE PUBLISHERS pp. 8-74.
60. Boqvist S, Vågsholm I (2005) Risk factors for hazard of release from Salmonella-control restriction on Swedish cattle farms from 1993 to 2002. Prev Vet Med 71: 35-44.
61. SnijdersJMA, Kanapen FV (2002) Prevention of human disease and integrated quality control system. Livestock production Science 76: 203-206.
62. GrimontPAD, Weill FX (2007)Antgenic formulae of the Salmonella serovars 9th edition. Paris: WHO.
63. CoetzerJA, Thomson GR, Tustin RC (1994) Disease of livestock (2): Oxford University Press.

INDEX

T

U

V

W